EMERGENCY MEDICINE

EMERGENCY MEDICINE

Second Edition

Arjun Mehta MBBS (AIIMS) FRCP (London)
Consultant Physician
Royal Victoria Hospital
Edinburgh, UK

Catherine Culley MBBS MRCGP
Registrar in Dermatology
Princess Royal Hospital, Haywards Heath
Brighton, UK

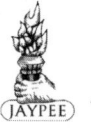

The Health Sciences Publisher
New Delhi | London | Philadelphia | Panama

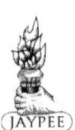

Jaypee Brothers Medical Publishers (P) Ltd.

Headquarters
Jaypee Brothers Medical Publishers (P) Ltd.
4838/24, Ansari Road, Daryaganj
New Delhi 110 002, India
Phone: +91-11-43574357
Fax: +91-11-43574314
E-mail: jaypee@jaypeebrothers.com

Overseas Offices

J.P. Medical Ltd.
83, Victoria Street, London
SW1H 0HW (UK)
Phone: +44-20 3170 8910
Fax: +44(0) 20 3008 6180
E-mail: info@jpmedpub.com

Jaypee-Highlights Medical Publishers Inc.
City of Knowledge, Bld. 237, Clayton
Panama City, Panama
Phone: +1 507-301-0496
Fax: +1 507-301-0499
E-mail: cservice@jphmedical.com

Jaypee Medical Inc.
The Bourse
111, South Independence Mall East
Suite 835, Philadelphia, PA 19106, USA
Phone: +1 267-519-9789
E-mail: jpmed.us@gmail.com

Jaypee Brothers Medical Publishers (P) Ltd.
17/1-B, Babar Road, Block-B, Shaymali
Mohammadpur, Dhaka-1207
Bangladesh
Mobile: +08801912003485
E-mail: jaypeedhaka@gmail.com

Jaypee Brothers Medical Publishers (P) Ltd.
Bhotahity, Kathmandu, Nepal
Phone: +977-9741283608
E-mail: kathmandu@jaypeebrothers.com

Website: www.jaypeebrothers.com
Website: www.jaypeedigital.com

© 2016, Jaypee Brothers Medical Publishers

The views and opinions expressed in this book are solely those of the original contributor(s)/author(s) and do not necessarily represent those of editor(s) of the book.

All rights reserved. No part of this publication may be reproduced, stored or transmitted in any form or by any means, electronic, mechanical, photocopying, recording or otherwise, without the prior permission in writing of the publishers.

All brand names and product names used in this book are trade names, service marks, trademarks or registered trademarks of their respective owners. The publisher is not associated with any product or vendor mentioned in this book.

Medical knowledge and practice change constantly. This book is designed to provide accurate, authoritative information about the subject matter in question. However, readers are advised to check the most current information available on procedures included and check information from the manufacturer of each product to be administered, to verify the recommended dose, formula, method and duration of administration, adverse effects and contraindications. It is the responsibility of the practitioner to take all appropriate safety precautions. Neither the publisher nor the author(s)/editor(s) assume any liability for any injury and/or damage to persons or property arising from or related to use of material in this book.

This book is sold on the understanding that the publisher is not engaged in providing professional medical services. If such advice or services are required, the services of a competent medical professional should be sought.

Every effort has been made where necessary to contact holders of copyright to obtain permission to reproduce copyright material. If any have been inadvertently overlooked, the publisher will be pleased to make the necessary arrangements at the first opportunity.

Inquiries for bulk sales may be solicited at: jaypee@jaypeebrothers.com

Emergency Medicine

First Edition: 2005

Second Edition: **2016**

ISBN: 978-93-5250-017-8

Printed at Sanat Printers

Dedicated to
*The memory of my Mother and Father
whose love, sacrifice and
dedication helped me in life.*

Foreword

In *Emergency Medicine*, Dr Arjun Mehta, has set out to produce a clear, concise and comprehensive text of acute medicine. Medical students and junior doctors alike will appreciate its brief, informative style and easy portability. Dr Mehta has accumulated experience of acute care over many years of clinical practice, and the text of the book summarizes the essential elements of care of the commonly encountered medical emergencies.

Andrew Elder FRCP (Edin)
Consultant Physician
Western General Hospital
Edinburgh, UK

Preface to the Second Edition

There are many books on clinical medicine and emergency medicine, but being very big, they are either in the library or in the office but never at the bedside where it is needed most. The second edition of *Emergency Medicine* has been extensively revised and updated to include essential information about diagnosis, differential diagnosis and management of acute medical problems. It also includes a chapter on emergency dermatology. It is helpful for final year medical students and practicing junior and senior doctors who are likely to encounter these medical problems.

Arjun Mehta
Catherine Culley

Preface to the First Edition

There are many books on clinical medicine and emergency medicine, but being too big to put in the coat pocket, they are either in the library or in the office and never at the beside where it is most needed. The book has been written with this ideal in mind. It is pocket size and is readily available at the bedside at times of emergency. The aim of the book is to give confidence in differential diagnosis and management of acute medical problems, and is intended to complement the standard textbooks in clinical medicine. It is useful for medical students, and practicing doctors, who are likely to encounter these clinical problems.

Arjun Mehta

Acknowledgments

I would like to thank Gautam for his constant encouragement and Andy Elder for reading the book and helpful suggestions. I express my thanks Catherine Culley for writing the dermatology chapter for the book. Finally, I would like to thank my wife Satya for her love and patience.

Arjun Mehta

Contents

1. **Introduction** — 1
   Factors for Prevention of Cardiac Arrest *1*
   Unexplained Hypotension *1*
   - **Septic Shock** *2*; Diagnosis *2*; Treatment *2*
   - **Acute Anaphylaxis** *3*; Causes *3*; Treatment *3*
   - **Disseminated Intravascular Coagulation** *3*
     Causes *4*; Investigation *4*; Management *4*
   - **Antibiotics** *5*

2. **Resuscitation** — 10
   - **Adult Basic Life Support (BLS)** *10*
   - **Advanced Life Support (ALS)** *11*
   - **Syncope** *14*; Vertigo (Merry Go Round),
     not Vertigo (Rocking Like a Boat) *17*;
     Benign Positional Paroxysmal Vertigo (BPPV) *17*
   - **Red Flags** *19*

3. **Neurological Emergencies** — 20
   - **Acute Stroke** *20*; Exclusion Criteria for
     Thrombolysis *22*; Stroke Mimics *27*
     Investigations and Differential Diagnosis
     of Stroke *28*; Where is the Stroke? *29*
   - **Thrombosis of Cerebral Veins and Sinuses** *40*;
     Pathogenesis *40*; Risk Factors *41*; Clinical Signs *42*
     Diagnosis *42*; Treatment *42*
   - **Anterior Spinal Artery Thrombosis** *43*
   - **Coma** *43*; History *43*; Causes *43*; Assessment
     Usually GCS <8 *44*; Document GCS *45*
   - **Hypothermia** *47*; Causes *47*; Examination *48*
     Investigations *48*; Complications *49*
     Management *50*
   - **Meningitis** *51*; History *51*; Examination *52*
     Investigations *52*
   - **Viral Encephalitis** *55*; Treatment *56*
   - **Acute Wernicke's Encephalopathy** *56*; History *56*
   - **Subarachnoid Hemorrhage (SAH)** *57*
     Management *59*; Grading of Subarachnoid
     Hemorrhage (SAH) *60*; Priorities *60*
     Investigations *60*; Prevention and Treatment *61*
     Neurological Deterioration or Complications *61*
     Screening *62*
   - **Epilepsy (Status Epilepticus)** *62*; First Epileptic
     Seizure *62*; Status Epilepticus *64*; Syncope *65*
   - **Headache** *68*; Migraine (*6–18%*) *68*; Chronic
     Tension Headache *70*; Coital Headache *70*; Benign
     Intracranial Hypertension *70*; Temporal Arteritis
     (Giant-cell Arteritis) *71*

xiv *Emergency Medicine*

- **Malaria** 72; Clinical Features 72; Severe Malaria 72
  Investigations 72; Treatment 72
- **Spinal Cord Compression** 73; History 73; Causes 73
  Anterior Spinal Artery Thrombosis 73
- **Spastic Paraparesis** 74
- **Brown-Sequard Syndrome (Hemisection of Spinal Cord)** 75
- **Acute Inflammatory Polyneuritis, Guillain-Barré Syndrome (GBS)** 75; History 75; Examination 75
  Case History 76
- **Myasthenia Gravis (MG)** 77; Differential Diagnosis 78
- **Delirium** 79; Delirium Tremens 82
  Management 82
- **Cerebellopontine Angle Syndrome** 83
- **Horner's Syndrome** 83
- **Ptosis** 84
- **Vertigo** 84
- **Benign Paroxysmal Positional Vertigo (BPPV)** 85
- **Ménière's Disease** 85
- **Peripheral Neuropathy** 86
- **Median Nerve Palsy (Carpal Tunnel Syndrome)** 88
- **Ulnar Nerve Palsy** 90; Differential Diagnosis
  Syringomyelia 91
- **Radial Nerve Palsy** 91
- **Foot Drop (Common Peroneal Nerve Palsy)** 92
  Cervical Myelopathy 92
- **Absent Ankle Jerks and Extensor Plantars** 93
- **Cauda Equina Syndrome** 94
- **Spinal Stenosis** 95
- **Multiple Sclerosis (MS)** 95; Optic Neuritis 95
  Cervical Cord 95; Brainstem and Cerebellum 96
  Paroxysmal Symptoms 96
- **Motor Neurone Disease (MND)** 98
- **Syringomyelia** 99
- **Sub-acute Combine Degeneration (SACD)** 100
- **Friedreich's Ataxia (Hereditary Spinocerebellar Degeneration)** 101
- **Taboparesis** 101
- **Tuberous Sclerosis/Adenoma Sebaceum** 102
- **Neurofibromatosis Type *1* (NF*1*, Von Recklinghausen's Disease)** 102
- **Lateral Medullary Syndrome (Wallenberg's Syndrome)** 104
- **Gait Disturbances** 105
- **Parkinson's Disease** 107
- **Differential Diagnosis** 110; Essential Tremor (ET) 110; Parkinsonism Plus 111
- **Multisystem Atrophy (MSA)** 111
  Lewy Body Dementia (LBD) 112
- **Dementia (De-Ment) Apart Brain** 115; Alzheimer's Disease AB (Bet- Amyloid) is the Cause 116; Vascular Dementia 117; Frontotemporal Dementia 118

Contents **xv**

4. Metabolic, Renal and Endocrine — 119

- **Acute Kidney Injury** *119*; Nephrotoxic Drugs *119*
- **Adult Polycystic Kidney Disease** *124*
- **Nephrotic Syndrome** *125*
- **Chronic Renal Failure (Chronic Kidney Disease)** *126*
  Renovascular Disease *127*; Renal Artery Stenosis
  Presentation *127*; Anemia *129*; Rhabdomyolysis *132*
- **Hyperkalemia** *133*
- **Diabetic Ketoacidosis and Hyperglycemic Hyperosmolar Syndrome (HHS)** *135*; Ketosis Prone Type 2 Diabetes Mellitus *135*; Hyperosmolar Hyperglycemic Syndrome (HHS) *140*
- **Diabetic Foot** *141*; Antibiotics *141*
- **Diabetic Neuropathic Pain** *142*
- **Surgery and Diabetes** *142*; Noninsulin Dependent Diabetes Mellitus (NIDDM) *144*
- **Hypokalemia** *144*
- **Hypoglycemia, Diabetic Management and New Drugs in Type 2 Diabetes Mellitus** *146*
  Diabetic Management *148*; Newer Agents in Type 2 Diabetes Mellitus *150*
- **Hyponatremia** *151*
- **Syndrome of Inappropriate Antidiuretic Hormone Secretion (SIADH)** *153*
- **Primary Adrenal Failure (Addison's Disease) and Secondary Adrenal Failure** *154*; Adrenal Crisis *157*
- **Hypocalcemia** *157*
- **Hypercalcemia** *158*
- **Hyperthyroidism or Thyrotoxicosis** *160*; Thyroid Acropachy *162*; Subclinical Hyperthyroidism *164*
- **Thyrotoxic Crisis** *164*
- **Goiter** *165*; Toxic Multinodular Goiter *165*; Solitary Nodule *166*; Sick Euthyroid Syndrome (SES) *168*
- **Amiodarone Effect** *168*
- **Hypothyroidism** *169*
- **Subclinical Hypothyroidism** *170*
- **Pheochromocytomas and Paraganglioma** *171*
- **Pituitary Apoplexy (Infarction)** *172*
- **Cushing Syndrome** *173*; Cushing Disease *173*
- **Polycystic Ovarian Syndrome (PCOS)** *175*
- **Acromegaly** *175*
- **Hypopituitarism** *176*
- **Acid-base Balance** *177*; Respiratory Acidosis *179*

5. Musculoskeletal — 181

- **Acute Arthritis** *181*; Gout (Supersaturation of Serum for Urate) *181*; Pseudogout *185*; Septic Arthritis *186*; Reactive Arthritis *188*
  Osteoarthritis *188*; Rheumatoid Arthritis (RA) *189*
- **Polymyalgia Rheumatica, Temporal Arteritis, Vasculitis** *196*; Churg-Strauss (Allergic Granulomatosis) *198*; Microscopic Angiitis (Necrotizing Small Vessel Vasculitis) *199*

6. Cardiovascular — 200

- **Acute Chest Pain: Acute Coronary Syndrome (ACS)** *200*; Troponins *203* Thrombolytics *207*
- **Stable Angina** *210*
- **Unstable Angina** *210*
- **Implantable Cardioverter Defibrillator and Pacing** *213*
- **Pericarditis** *215*
- **Right Ventricular Infarction/↑ JVP Clear Lungs, Breathlessness** *215*; Tachyarrhythmia *217*
- **Atrial Fibrillation and Paroxysmal Atrial Fibrillation** *218*; Atrial Fibrillation Ablation Therapy *218*
- **Atrial Flutter** *224*
- **Supraventricular Tachycardia** *224*
- **Broad Complex Tachycardia** *227*; Diagnosis *228*
- **Sudden Cardiac Death** *229*; Hypertrophic Cardiomyopathy *230*; Arrhythmogenic Right Ventricular Cardiomyopathy (ARVC) *231*; Brugada Syndrome *231*; Long QT Syndrome (A Disease of the Young, Unusual After 40) *231*; Torsades-De-Pointes Tachycardia *232*; Bradycardia and Pacemaker *233*; First Degree Heart Block *233* Second Degree Heart Block *234*; Third Degree Atrioventricular Block *234*; Transvenous Temporary Pacing *234*; Risk of Pacemaker *235*; Suspected Malfunction of Permanent Pacemaker *235*
- **Heart Failure (Mild/Moderate) in Acute Coronary Syndrome** *235*; Severe Heart Failure *237*; Digoxin Toxicity *238*
- **Hypertensive Emergencies and Resistant Hypertension** *238*; Resistant Hypertension *241*
- **Acute Aortic Dissection** *242*
- **Infective Endocarditis** *244*; High Risk Patients *244* Moderate Risk Patients *245*
- **Aortic Stenosis** *247*
- **Aortic Regurgitation** *250*
- **Mitral Regurgitation** *251*
- **Mixed Mitral Valve Disease** *252*
- **Mitral Stenosis** *253*; Prosthetic Mitral and Aortic Valves *254*; Dextrocardia *255*
- **Dilated Cardiomyopathy** *255*
- **Hypertrophic Cardiomyopathy** *256*; Pulmonary Embolism, Deep Vein Thrombosis *257*
- **Pulmonary Hypertension** *264*
- **General Surgery and Cardiac Patient** *266*

7. Gastrointestinal — 268

Abdominal Pain *268*
- **Acute Upper Gastrointestinal Hemorrhage** *269* Heyde's Syndrome *274*

Contents **xvii**

- **Variceal Bleeding** *275*; Preventive Strategies in Cirrhosis or Management of Portal Hypertension *277*
- **Lower Gastrointestinal Bleeding** *278*
  History *278*; Examination *278*
- **Acute or Chronic Liver Failure** *279*
  Fulminant Liver Failure *279*; Subfulminant *279*
- **Signs of Chronic Liver Disease** *281*
- **Hepatorenal Syndrome** *283*
- **Viral Hepatitis (HBV, HCV)** *284*; Hepatitis A and E *284*

8. **Nonalcoholic Fatty Liver Disease and Nonalcoholic Steatohepatitis**   **291**
   - **Alcoholic Hepatitis** *293*; Alcohol Withdrawal Syndrome (DT) *295*

9. **Primary Biliary Cirrhosis**   **296**
   - **Hemochromatosis** *297*
   - **Wilson's Disease** *297*

10. **Autoimmune Hepatitis**   **299**
    - **Budd-Chiari Syndrome (Hepatic Vein Obstruction)** *300*; Cholestatic Hepatitis *300*
    - **Indications for Liver Transplant** *301*
      Fulminant Hepatic Failure *301*
    - **Ascites** *305*
    - **Acute Pancreatitis and Ascending Cholangitis** *308*
    - **Acute Diarrhea** *313*; *Clostridium Difficile* Colitis *314*; Complicated *Clostridium Difficile* Colitis *315*; Campylobacter Enteritis *317* Nontyphoid Salmonellas *317*
    - **Known Inflammatory Bowel Disease or Sigmoidoscopy Suggests Ulcerative Colitis** *317*
      Acute Severe Colitis *319*
    - **Microscopic Colitis** *320*
    - **Toxic Megacolon** *321*
    - **Crohn's Disease** *321*; Extra Intestinal Manifestation of Crohn's Disease *322*

11. **Blood**   **326**
    - **Sickle Cell Crisis** *326*; Hand-foot Syndrome *326* Acute Pain in Limbs and Back *326*; Acute Chest Syndrome *327*; Anemia *327*; Prevention of Complications in HbSS and HbS/Beta-Thalassemia *328*
    - **Chronic Myeloid Leukemia** *328*
    - **Chronic Lymphatic Leukemia (CLL)** *329*
    - **Polycythemia Rubra Vera (PRV)** *330*
      Anemia *332*

12. **Pulmonary**   **334**
    Respiratory failure *335*
    - **Acute Asthma** *335*

xviii *Emergency Medicine*

- **Allergic Bronchopulmonary Aspergillosis** *341*
- **Community-acquired Pneumonia (CAP)** *342*
  Community-acquired (CA) Methicillin-resistant *Staphylococcus aureus* (MRSA) *345*; Methicillin-resistant *Staphylococcus aureus* (MRSA) Panton–valentine LeukocidIn (PVL) *345*; Hospital-acquired (HA) Methicillin-resistant *Staphylococcus aureus* (MRSA) *345*
- **Aspiration Pneumonia** *347*; Indications for Bronchoscopy *347*
- **Pleural Effusion and Empyema** *348*
- **Mesothelioma** *351*
- **Acute Exacerbation of Chronic Obstructive Pulmonary Disease (COPD), Long-term Oxygen Therapy (LTOT) and Noninvasive Ventilation (NIV)** *351*; Definition *351*; Pneumothorax *359* Secondary Pneumothorax *359*; Primary Pneumothorax *359*; Tension Pneumothorax *360*

13. Bronchiectasis — 364
- **Antibiotics** *365*; *Pneumocystis Pneumonia* *366*

14. Carcinoma of Bronchus — 368
- **Idiopathic Pulmonary Fibrosis (IPF) or Usual Interstitial Pneumonia (UIP)** *369*

15. Obstructive Sleep Apnea Syndrome — 370
- **Mechanism** *370*
- **Percutaneous Needle Stick Injury** *371*
- **Malaria** *373*
- **Human Immunodeficiency Virus** *376*

16. Toxicology — 379
- **Calcium Channel Blockers Overdose** *379*
- **Tricyclic Overdose** *380*
- **Opioid (Heroin) Overdose** *380*
- **Cocaine** *380*
- **Ecstasy (MDMA)** *382*; Clinical Features *382*
- **Aspirin** *383*; Clinical Features *383*
- **Paracetamol** *384*
- **Carbon Monoxide Poisoning** *385*

Index — *387*

1

Introduction

- Need for consideration of deep vein thrombosis (DVT) prophylaxis in every admitted patient in the hospital.
- Hand washing and hand hygiene is crucial in every patient.
- Consider the need for coagulation screen and blood grouping before undertaking any invasive procedure.

FACTORS FOR PREVENTION OF CARDIAC ARREST

Consider and avoid hypoxia, hypovolemia, hyperkalemia, hypokalemia, hypocalcemia. For regular monitoring with pulse oximetry, blood pressure (BP) monitoring and electrocardiography (ECG).

Respiratory rate (RR) >35/min or <6/min, BP <90 mm Hg are at risk of cardiac arrest.

UNEXPLAINED HYPOTENSION

Machine derived BP is not accurate at extremes of BP or in fast tachycardia or in atrial fibrillation (AF).

Consider
- Sepsis (Septic shock)
- Myocardial infarction (MI) without any pain (early ECG changes though)
- Occult blood loss
- Poisoning
- Pulmonary embolus (PE)
- Anaphylaxis
- Addison's disease
- Cardiac tamponade
- Autonomic dysfunctions.

Emergency Medicine

Septic Shock

Septic shock is, as a result of severe infection and sepsis and can cause multiple organ dysfunction and death. It is common in children, immune compromised individuals and elderly.

DIAGNOSIS

- Systemic inflammatory response syndrome (SIRS) is present.
- Any two of the following (tachypnea RR >20/min, white blood cells <4000 or >12000 cells/mm^3, heart rate >90 beats/min, temperature >38.5°C (101.3°F) or <35°C (95°F).
- There must be sepsis with evidence of infection like positive blood culture or sign of pneumonia on chest X-ray or other radiological or laboratory evidence of infection.
- Signs of organ dysfunction such as renal failure, liver dysfunction or change in mental status or elevated serum lactate.
- Finally refractory hypotension.

TREATMENT

- Begin resuscitation immediately if hypotension, or hypotension and serum lactate 4 or more. Goals—urine output >0.5 mL/kg/hr, mean arterial pressure >65 mm Hg.
- Intravenous (IV) fluids—Crystalloids (normal saline or Hartmann's solution) 1 L or colloids (gelofusine) 300–500 mL over 30 minutes as fluid challenge, consider pack cells if hematocrit <30%.
- Early antibiotics—Appropriate cultures before broad-spectrum antibiotics, at least 2 blood cultures (one percutaneous and other from vascular access) and imaging studies promptly to confirm or sample the source of infection and source control (abscess drainage or tissue debridement).
- Use hospital guideline in *Pseudomonas* infections or neutropenic patient.
- Vasopressors—Norepinephrine or dopamines are initial vasopressors administered centrally. Use dobutamine infusion maximum 25 µg/kg/min in patients with MI.

- Hydrocortisone 300 mg/day IV if hypotension responds poorly to fluids challenges.
- Blood transfusion if hemoglobin <7.0 g/dL, platelet transfusion if platelets <5000 (asymptomatic), <5000–30,000 (significant bleeding risk), <50,000 (invasive procedure or surgery).
- Use IV insulin to control hyperglycemia, keeping BM 8.3 mmol/L (150 mg/dL).
- Use bicarbonate if pH <7.15.
- Use H_2RA (H_2 receptor antagonist), TEDS (stockings) or LMWH (low molecular weight heparin) or both (TEDS + LMWH) in view of high risk of DVT.

Acute Anaphylaxis

Acute allergic response to a substance to which the individual has been exposed previously results in mast cell degranulation and histamine release. Anaphylactic shock is twice as common in women and 1/3 suffer from atopy.

CAUSES

Nuts, fish, nonsteroidal anti-inflammatory drugs (NSAIDs), antibiotics, anesthetics and stings.

Present as bronchospasm and/or cardiovascular collapse.

TREATMENT

- Airway, breathing and circulation (ABC)
- Maintain airway and O_2 by high flow O_2 mask and reservoir bag, intubate if stridor.
- Give adrenaline 500 μg (0.5 mL 1.1000) intramuscular (IM) and repeat in 5–10 min if no better.
- Secure IV access and give IV fluids (Hartmann's solution or normal saline or gelofusine).
- Monitor O_2 saturation and BP.
- Hydrocortisone 200 mg IV.
- Antihistamine chlorpheniramine 10–20 mg IV slowly
- Salbutamol 5 mg, nebulizer if wheeze present.

Disseminated Intravascular Coagulation

It is a systemic disorder in which hemorrhage (main problem 90%) and thrombosis can occur at the same time.

It involves generation of intravascular fibrin and consumption of clotting factors and platelets. It can be acute or chronic. History—Bleeding—Extensive superficial bruising and oozing from venipuncture, IM injection sites, around indwelling catheters and tubes. Bleeding from mucosa, mouth, nose, gastrointestinal (GI), lungs, renal tract.

CAUSES

- Sepsis—bacterial, viral, fungal, parasitic, malaria.
- Major trauma, burns, surgery.
- Toxins—venom.
- Obstetric—placental abruption, eclampsia, and amniotic fluid embolism.
- Cancer—metastatic carcinoma of stomach, colon, pancreas, breast, lung, mucin secreting adenocarcinoma, leukemia.
- Severe pancreatitis.
- Liver disease—acute liver failure.
- Others—heat stroke, prosthetic devices, purpura fulminants, recreational drugs, severe transfusion reaction, transplant rejection, giant hemangioma and large vessel aneurysm (aortic).

INVESTIGATION

- Low platelet count
- PT (prothrombin time) and activated PTT (partial thromboplastic time) both increased
- FDP (fibrinogen degradation product) and/or D-dimer present or increased
- AT3 (antithrombin 3) level reduced
- Fibrinogen reduced
- Thrombin time prolonged
- Blood film—red cell fragmentation/microangiopathic hemolytic anemia.

MANAGEMENT

- Treat aggressively.
- Broad-spectrum antibiotics for sepsis.
- When established DIC diagnosed by laboratory then give FFP (fresh frozen plasma) (15 mL/kg or 1L = 4 units = 1 adult dose) to keep PT (prothrombin time) and PTT (partial thromboplastin time) <1.5 times upper limit of control value.

- Give cryoprecipitate to keep fibrinogen >1 g/L (1–1.5 pack/10 kg = 10 units = 1 adult dose)
- Give platelets (4–8 units) to keep platelets >50,000.
- Give blood to keep hematocrit >0.30
- Sepsis related DIC activated protein C can be used as 96 hrs infusion, provided platelet count > 30,000 × 10^9/L. Apart from acting as anticoagulant, it also has anti-inflammatory and anti-apoptotic properties.
- If patient continues to bleed after 6 hr of treatment of underlying cause and supportive measures then with hematological advice consider AT3 and heparin 20–30,000 U/24 hr.
- Used when thrombosis is main problem.
- If hypotension or shock, consider an adrenal infarction (Waterhouse-Friderichsen syndrome) and give hydrocortisone 100 mg 6 hrly.

Antibiotics

- Amoxycillin 500 mg tds oral or IV, 1.0 g tds in pneumonia if CURB >2
- Cefuroxime 1.5 g tds IV
- Ciprofloxacin 750 mg bd IV
- Clarithromycin 500 mg bd oral or IV
- Co-amoxiclav 1.2 g tds IV
- Flucloxacillin 1.0 g qid IV
- Gentamycin 5 mg/kg IV
- Penicillin G 1.2 g tds IV
- Vancomycin 1.0 g bd IV
- Tazocin 4.5 g tds IV
- Doxycycline 200 mg stat and 100 mg oral daily
- Levofloxacin 500 mg IV bd

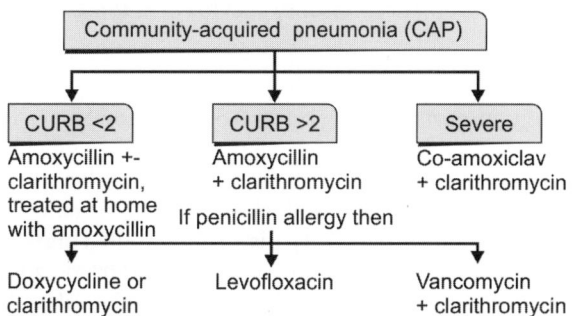

- CURB-65 Score
  - C (confusion) AMT <8/10,
  - U (urea >7 mmol/L),
  - R (respiratory rate 30 or >30),
  - B (blood pressure systolic <90 mm Hg or diastolic 60 or <60 mm Hg),
  - Age 65 or >65.

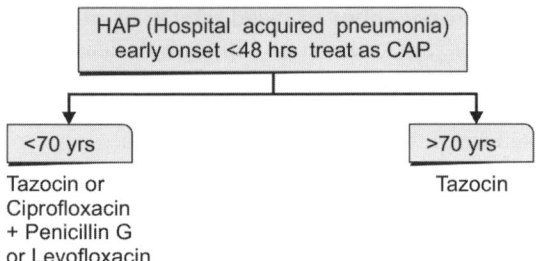

If Penicillin allergy Vancomycin + Clarithromycin or Levofloxacin or Ciprofloxacin + Metronidazole if aspiration

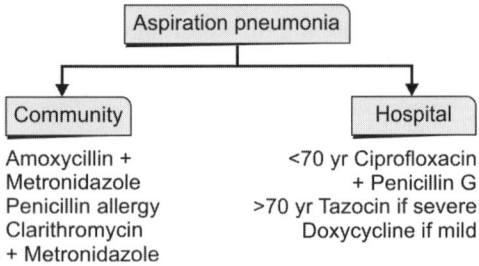

Chronic Obstructive Pulmonary Disease (COPD)

Amoxycillin 500 mg tds. If penicillin allergy or recent failure of amoxycillin—Doxycycline 200 mg stat and then 100 mg/day and if severe then ciprofloxacin to cover *Pseudomonas*.

Urinary Tract Infection (UTI)

- Trimethoprim 200 mg bd for 3 days in females.
- In males, trimethoprim failure, catheter associated, immune suppressed, hospital acquired, pyelonephritis, renal failure, recent urological surgery, co-amoxiclav 625 mg oral tds or IV 1.2 g tds + gentamycin 5 mg/kg for 2 doses. If penicillin allergy, ciprofloxacin 500 mg bd oral or IV 400 mg bd + stat dose of gentamycin for 7 days.

- Gentamycin 80 mg IV or IM stat with in 30 minutes before catheter manipulation.

Nonlocalized Sepsis

- *<70 yrs*: Penicillin G 1.2 g qid + flucloxacillin 1 g qid + ciprofloxacin 750 mg bid.
- *>70 yrs*: Penicillin G + Flucloxacillin + Gentamycin or Tazocin 4.5 g IV + Gentamycin 5 mg/kg. If penicillin allergy then cefuroxime 1.5 g tid or vancomycin + ciprofloxacin + metronidazole or teicoplanin 400 mg IV 12 hrly 3 doses and then OD.

Biliary Sepsis or Spontaneous Bacterial Peritonitis (SBP)

- Tazocin IV 4.5 g tds or ciprofloxacin + metronidazole or gentamycin + metronidazole.
- Prophylaxis for SBP—Norfloxacin 400 mg daily life long.

Diverticulitis

- *<70 yrs*: Cefuroxime 1.5 g tid + Metronidazole.
- *>70 yrs*: Gentamycin + Metronidazole if creatinin >260 then ciprofloxacin 375 mg bid + metronidazole.

Acute Surgical Abdomen (Peritonitis)

Cefuroxime 1.5 g tid + Metronidazole or Gentamycin + Metronidazole or Tazocin 4.5 g tds.

Neutropenic Sepsis

If neutrophils <1 × 10 × 9/L, tazocin 4.5 g tid + gentamycin 4–6 mg/kg/day, if non-IgE penicillin allergy then Ceftazidime 2 g tid + gentamycin. If IgE penicillin allergy then ciprofloxacin IV 400 mg bd + gentamycin. Also consider granulocyte colony stimulating factor (GCSF). Add Teicoplanin IV 400 mg 12 hrly for 3 doses then od if central line infected.

Meningitis

Ceftriaxone IV 2 g/d for 7–10 days, add amoxycillin IV 2 g 4 hrly if over 55, immune suppressed or alcoholic. If penicillin allergy then vancomycin 1 g bd + IV chloramphenicol 25 mg/kg qds for 7–14 days. Add dexamethasone

10 mg qds IV for 4 days with IST dose of antibiotic unless septic shock or immune compromised or neurosurgery.

Septic Arthritis

Flucloxacillin 1 g qid + penicillin G 1.2 g 4 hrly 2 weeks. If penicillin allergy then teicoplanin IV 400 mg bd for 3 doses then od.

Septic Arthritis in Prosthetic Joint

Vancomycin 1 g bd + Rifampicin 600 mg od.

Discitis

Flucloxacillin 2 g qid + Penicillin G 1.2 g qid for 6 weeks.

Prostatitis

Ciprofloxacin 500 mg bd or Trimethoprim 200 mg bd for 28 days.

Endocarditis

Indolent presentation—Penicillin G 1.2 g 4 hrly + Gentamycin 1 mg/kg tds maximum (80 mg), if penicillin allergy vancomycin 1 g bd + gentamycin 1 mg/kg tds.

Acute onset, intravenous drug users (IVDU), methicillin-resistant *Staphylococcus aureus* (MRSA), prosthetic valve—Vancomycin 1 g bd IV + Gentamycin + Rifampicin oral 600 mg bd.

Cellulitis

- Mild—Flucloxacillin 500 mg qid
- Severe—Penicilin G 1.2 g qds + Flucloxacillin 1 g qds or if penicillin allergy or MRSA colonized then Teicoplanin 400 mg bd IV for 3 doses and then od or if non-IGE mediated penicillin allergy ceftriaxone 1.2 g od.

Diabetic Foot

- If no systemic toxicity and no comorbidities then treat as mild cellulitis.
- Otherwise teicoplanin IV 400 mg bd for 3 doses and then od + tazocin IV 4.5 g tds OR if penicillin allergy

then teicoplanin + metronidazol IV 500 mg tds + gentamycin.

Orbital Cellulitis

Co-amoxiclav 1.2 g IV tds or if penicillin allergy clarithromycin 500 mg IV bd + metronidazole 500 mg IV tds.

Human or Animal Bites

Co-amoxiclav 625 mg tds oral or if penicillin allergy then doxycycline 100 mg bd + metronidazole 400 mg tds.

2

Resuscitation

Adult Basic Life Support (BLS)

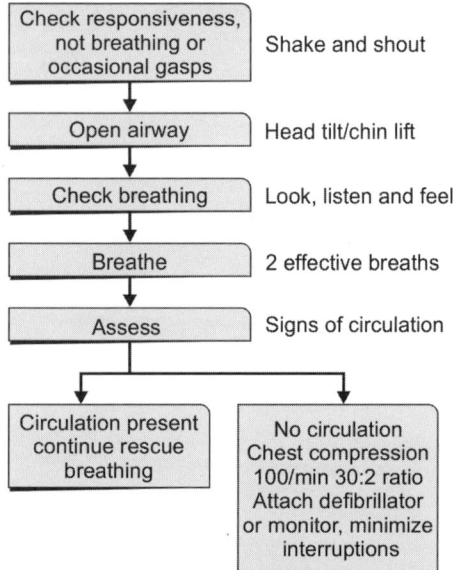

- Shake the shoulder and ask loudly are you alright?
- If responds by answering or moving, leave in a safe place and get help.
- If no response, open the airway by head tilt and chin lift, if neck injury is underlying then just jaw thrust.
- Keeping airway open, look at the chest, listen at the mouth and feel the air on your cheek as signs of breathing for 10 seconds, if breathing, turn to recovery position, monitor for continued breathing and get help.
- If not breathing, send someone for help or if you are on your own then leave the victim momentarily to telephone for help.
- Return and commence rescue breathing.

- Remove visible obstructions from the mouth.
- Give two effective rescue breaths and check the carotid pulse and signs of circulation, movements, swallowing, and breathing for maximum 10 secs.
- If there are definite signs of circulation continue rescue breathing 100 breaths/min checking for circulation every minute.
- If the victim starts to breathe on his own but remains unconscious, put in recovery position and continue monitoring.
- If no sign of circulation, start chest compression 100/min.
- Combine compression and rescue breathing 30:2 ratio.
- Continue till victim shows signs of life or apply advanced life support technique.

Advanced Life Support (ALS)

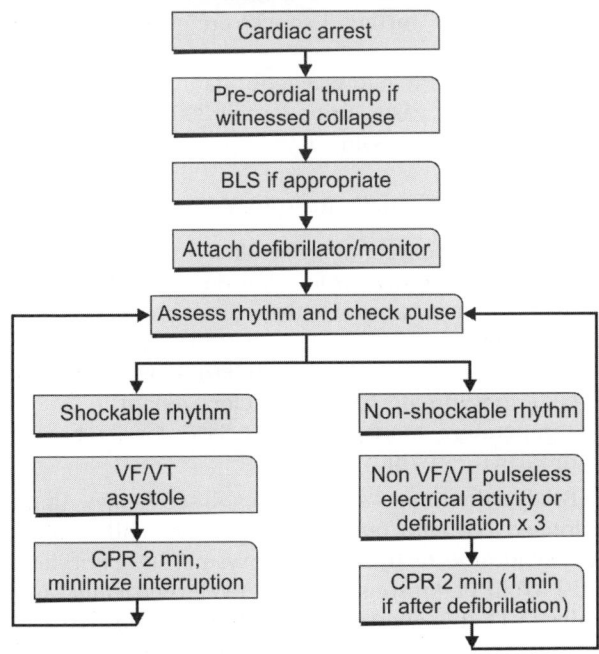

During CPR

- Ensure high quality CPR (chest compression 100–120/min 5–6 cm depth, pressure released fully between chest compressions and interruptions minimized). Plan actions before interrupting CPR. Give adrenalin

every 3–5 min. Adrenalin increases aortic relaxation (diastolic) and augments coronary and cerebral blood flow. Correct reversible causes hypoxia, hypovolemia, hypo/hyperkalemia, metabolic disorders, hypothermia, tension pneumothorax, tamponade, and thromboembolic/mechanical obstruction.
- Attempt and verify IV access, O_2 and airways. Check electrodes' position and contact. Consider amiodarone, Atropine/pacing. BLS is commenced in unmonitored situations while monitor/defibrillator is obtained and attached.
- In VF/pulse less VT, defibrillation is given as soon as possible. 1st shock 150 J ensuring good contact with chest wall, use of gel pads and appropriate paddle position, 2nd shock 200 J and 3rd 360 J.
- Three shocks should be administered within 45 sec. A pulse check is performed if after defibrillation ECG rhythm or morphologic changes.
- If VF persists, further 3 shocks are given in the same sequence.
- A 1 minute CPR follows 3 defibrillation shocks.
- In refractory cases, amiodarone 300 mg in prefilled syringes of 10 mL saline IV.

Immediate Treatment Postcardiac Arrest

- Controlled reoxygenation 94–98%.
- Controlled arterial carbon dioxide, aim for normal as hypocapnia is harmful to the injured brain.
- Blood glucose control between 4–10 mmol/L
- Control seizures with benzodiazepines, phenytoin, sodium valproate, propofol or clonazepam.
- Temperature management 32–34°C for 24 hrs and rewarm 0.25°C/hr.

Bradyarrhythmia—sinus pauses >3 sec, Stokes-Adams, prolonged P-R with bundle branch block (BBB), brady-tachy syndrome, tachycardia, paroxysmal atrial fibrillation (PAF), Wolff-Parkinsons-White (WPW), ventricular tachycardia (VT) in hypertrophic cardiomyopathy (HOCM), aortic stenosis (AS), prolonged QT interval, drugs, atrial myxoma, PE, PH (pulmonary hypertension), drugs, electrolytes calcium (Ca), magnesium (Mg), potassium (K) and prosthetic valve thrombosis.

Syncope—Transient loss of consciousness (TLOC) or postural tone. Return of consciousness is prompt and brief in syncope while it is prolonged and slow after the seizure.

Resuscitation 13

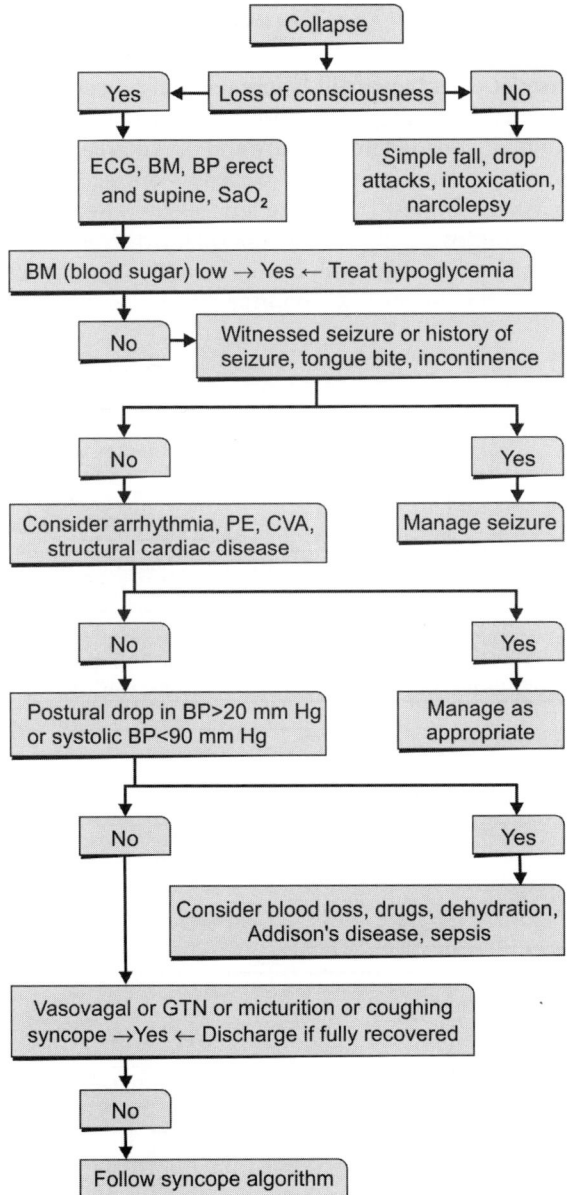

Presyncope symptoms—Light headedness, dizziness, feeling of warmth, nausea, sweating, visual blurring. Three-fourth blood volume in venous bed.

Consider also loose carpet, poor vision, osteoarthritis (OA) knees as a cause for falls.

Syncope

History of what happened before (circumstances, posture, prodromal symptoms), during (appearance, color, movement, tongue bite or injury and duration) and during recovering period (confusion, weakness during one side). Also ask the witness (by phone if necessary). Red flags are syncope during exertion, new or unexplained breathlessness, heart failure, age < 40, family history of sudden cardiac death, heart murmur or any ECG abnormality.

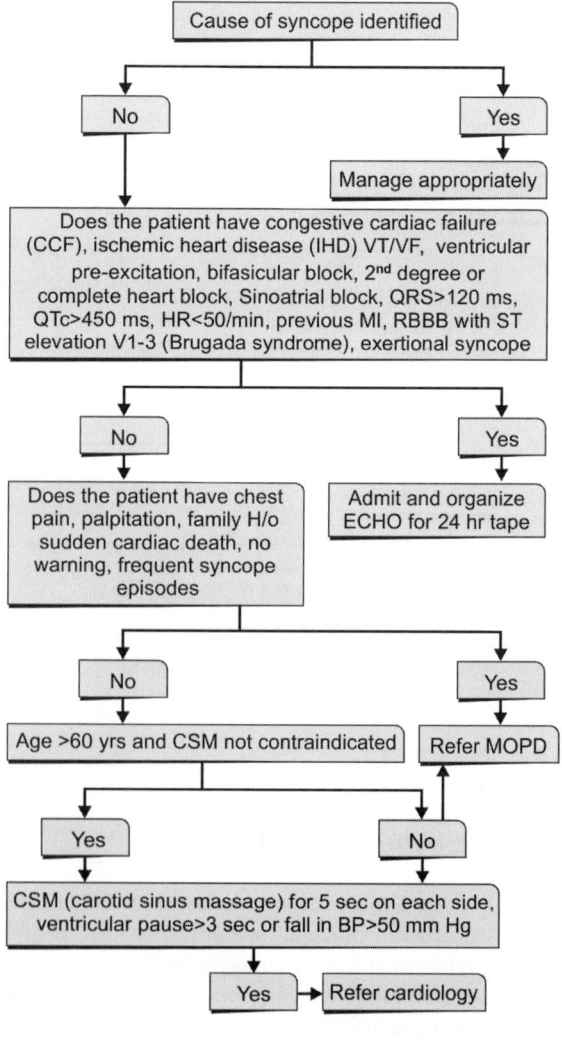

transient loss of conscious (TLOC) neurogenic, orthostatic hypotension and cardiac. Syncope is transient, self-limited with loss of consciousness leading to collapse and recovery is spontaneous and complete.

Syncopy—50% neurogenic, reduced sympathetic outflow causing bradycardia and activation of vagal efferents causing vasodilatation (vasovagal, situational, carotid hypersensitivity), diagnosed by tilt table test, drop in BP 30 mm Hg or sinus pauses >3 sec. In this, the patient cannot remember falling and hitting the head.

Vasovagal syncope—After sudden unexpected sights, sound, smell or pain, fear, emotional distress, instrumentation, prolonged standing or prolonged sitting in crowded hot places or during or after meal. Prodromal symptoms of light headedness or ringing in the ears or visual disturbances or sweating, pallor, nausea or vomiting are often common.

Cardiac—20% usually have facial injury, sinus node disease or atrioventricular (AV) conduction system disease or structural cardiac disease. Prolonged ECG recording 24 hrs or 7 days or ECHO and rarely implantable loop recorder (ILR) is required.

Cardiac arrhythmia (bradycardia <40, sinus pauses >3s, heart blocks), tachycardia (SVT, VT, PAF). Structural (MI, aortic stenosis, HOCM (hypertrophic cardiomyopathy), PE, PH (pulmonary hypertension), drugs, and low calcium, potassium or magnesium.

Orthostatic hypotension—Volume depletion, brief duration, pallor prior to and during and cold to touch are common symptoms.

Causes—Autonomic neuropathy, Parkinson's disease, drugs and Addison's diseases.

Postural orthostatic tachycardia syndrome (POTS)— Palpitation, sweating, headache, giddiness but no vertigo and near syncope on standing from lying without hypotension with in 10 minutes of standing. Diagnosed by tilt table test with increase in heart rate >120 or >30 of base line within 10 minutes of 70 O up tilt.

Cause—Failure of peripheral resistance to increase on standing. Age 12–50 M: F 1:5.

Offending drugs—Alpha blockers, β blockers, ACE, calcium antagonists, diuretics, nitrates, ethanol, opiates, phenothiazines, sildenafil and tricyclic antidepressants.

1. Primary (partial dysautonomic) post-viral, pregnancy, surgery, immunization, hyperadrenergic, secondary—diabetes, sarcoidosis, amyloidosis, alcoholism and paraneoplastic.
   Treatment—exercise lower legs, hydration and increase salt, fludrocortisone, labetalol, SSRI (Fluoxetine or venlafaxine) and pyridostigmine in paraneoplastic syndrome.
   Nonsyncope—seizure (bitten tongue, head turning to one side, no memory of abnormal behavior before, during or after TLOC, confusion after syncope, prolonged jerking of limbs and unusual posturing), TIA's, hypoglycemia, intoxication, migraine, vertebrobasilar insufficiency. If persistent TLOC consider psychogenic. Acute illnesses—infections, ACS, bleeding, PE, dissection.
   Carotid sinus syncope with head rotation.
2. *Situational syncope*—if after urination, defecation, cough, swallowing or eating and ECG is normal.
   Orthostatic syncope—orthostatic hypotension with syncope occurs soon after standing or after prolonged standing in crowded hot places or recent change or introduction of antihypertensive drugs or anti-Parkinson's drugs. This occurs frequently in autonomic neuropathy.
   Vertebral basilar insufficiency—episodes occur on extension of the neck, neck pain, nausea and vertigo.
   Nonsyncopal—metabolic, epilepsy, falls, drop attacks, intoxicants, psychogenic, TIA and falls.

Fits

Any warning of lip smacking or fiddling with clothes or stereotype movements suggests complex partial seizures. Prolonged tonic-clonic movements, coinciding with LOC (loss of consciousness), tongue bite lateral side, blue face, 5 minutes or more with aura and prolonged confusion post-LOC, family history, incontinence, injury, headache, and pins and needles. Usually waking up in hospital or ambulance. Return of consciousness is prompt and brief in syncope while it is prolonged and slow after seizure.

Jerking limb and incontinence do not prove epilepsy.

Faints

- Tonic-clonic movements shorter duration <15 sec, after LOC, may have tongue bite but no incontinence. Usually waking up at the home.
- Beware syncope masquerading either epilepsy or mechanical fall when person denies loss of consciousness because of retrograde amnesia.
- *Tilt table*—single event in high-risk setting (pilots, commercial vehicle driver) or recurrent event. Specificity 90%, sensitivity 20–74% and reproducibility 90%.
- *Treatment*—avoid climbing ladders, swimming alone, operating heavy machinery.
- Treat the cause, if postural hypotension, avoid offending drugs, thromboembolic deterrent stockings (TEDS), fludrocortisone or midodrine.

VERTIGO (MERRY GO ROUND), NOT VERTIGO (ROCKING LIKE A BOAT)

Vestibular organ detects head motion, so abnormal activity in vestibular nerves is interpreted by brain as self-motion. Vertigo with facial numbness or weakness (stroke) and with auditory distortion is Mennier's disease.

Vestibular ocular reflex (VOR)—to stabilize the eyes during fast head movements (when walking or running). This is tested by head thrust test—patient is asked to fixate on visual target high acceleration low amplitude head movements will activate the VOR. Normally, eye does not deviate from target, but VOR + (positive) when eye produce saccade movements to refixate the target. Side towards which produces saccade movements of the eyes is the side of lesion.

BENIGN POSITIONAL PAROXYSMAL VERTIGO (BPPV)

Cause—calcium carbonate crystals in semicircular canals. Vertigo with nystagmus on change in position of head (bending down, looking upward or turning over in bed) lasts few seconds and confirmed by Halpike test and treated by Epley maneuver.

Dix-Hallpike test patient is sitting upright with legs extended and patients head is then rotated 45 degrees. Clinician helps the patient to lie down quickly with head held in 20 degrees extension by placing the pillow under the upper back or supporting the head of the edge of the bed. Eyes are observed for 45 seconds for rotatory nystagmus.

Treatment is by Eply maneuver (relocation maneuver of free floating crystals in the semicircular canals in to utricle). Like Dix-Hallpike patients sits with extended legs and head rotated 45 degrees to the affected side. Patients lie down quickly with head held 30 degrees extended and affected ear facing the ground for 1–2 minutes. Head is turned 90 degrees so that unaffected ear faces the ground for 1 minute. Keeping head position fixed patient rolls on to their shoulder and can sit up after 1 minute.

Eyes are constantly being observed for nystagmus. Usually there is 90% success rate but rarely vestibular sedatives can be used for only 2–3 months.

Vestibular Neuronitis

Subacute onset, spinning vertigo, persists for days and weeks and aggravated by head motion and associated with nausea, vomiting, sweating, pallor, veers towards affected side. Head impulse test positive when head is turned towards affected side.

Cerebellar stroke—abrupt onset of vertigo (within seconds) with occipital headache, gait and limb ataxia, hemiparesis and facial numbness. Head impulse test normal. Urgent CT or MRI scans.

Migrainous—spontaneous positional vertigo lasting hours at the same time of migraine with headache, photophobia, nausea and phonophobia. A diagnosis of exclusion, so acute imaging at 1st presentation.

Bilateral Vestibular Failure (BVF)

The most common cause of BVF is aminoglycosides toxicity and 90% of these will not develop.

Deafness, so vestibular functions are much more sensitive to aminoglycosides. Initially, they present with spontaneous episodic vertigo before developing BVF. Patients have gait disturbance and disabling head movement induced oscillopsia. The diagnosis is made by head impulse test and confirmed by caloric testing. The symptoms improve slowly with vestibular rehabilitation.

Red Flags

- Glycemic control in ACS (acute coronary syndrome) if BM >11 mmol/L with insulin infusion sliding scale with target blood glucose 5–8 mmol/L.
- Back pain, bilateral sciatica, saddle sensory loss and bladder dysfunctions, consider cauda equina lesion and needs urgent MRI.
- Headache with occipital pain, consider posterior fossa lesion. Young obese patient presenting with headache consider idiopathic intracranial hypertension (ICH).
- LQTS (long QT syndrome) QT >450 ms in men and >460 ms in women. It has propensity for ventricular dysrhythmia and sudden cardiac death. Avoid antipsychotics, exercise, and swimming and consider beta-blockers.
- Heart failure with BBB or QRS duration >120–149 ms and on optimal therapy, consider CRT-P (resynchronization therapy with biventricular pacing).
- Young person with abdominal pain, low sodium and hypertension, consider acute intermittent porphyria.
- In females over 40 with abdominal pain, bloating and early satiety, consider ovarian cancer and CT abdomen.
- In AKI (acute kidney injury) look out for metformin and omeprazole as they can cause acute interstitial nephritis.

3

Neurological Emergencies

Acute Stroke

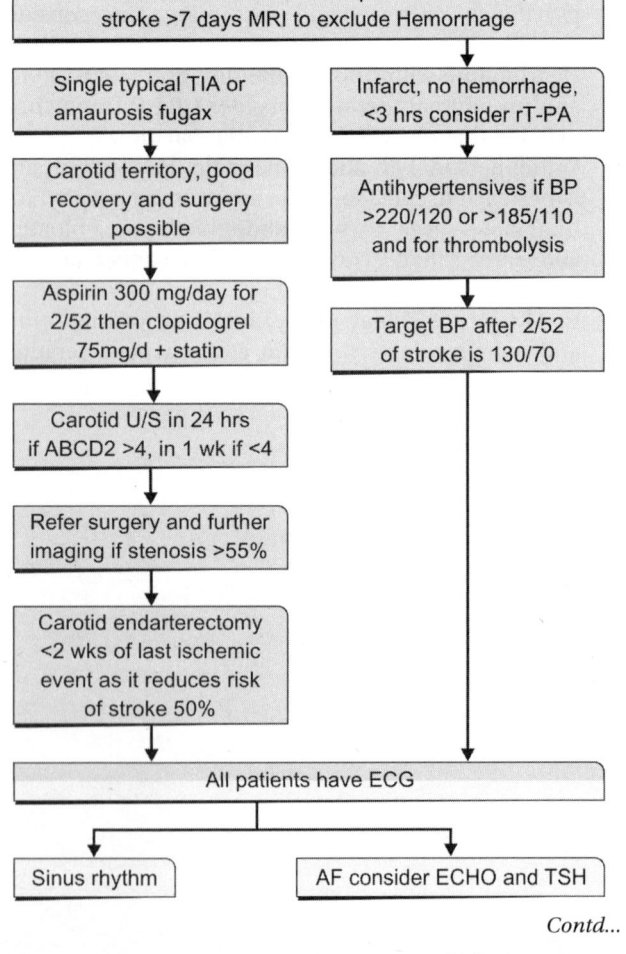

Contd...

Contd...

> Aspirin 300 mg/d for 2/52 then clopidogrel 75 mg/d. Aspirin 75 mg/d +Dipyridamole MR 200 mg bd If clopidogrel intolerant

> Clopidogrel or aspirin as in SR, Warfarin in 2/52 in ischemic stroke if no contraindication. Contraindicated in recurrent falls, binge drinking, poor compliance, then aspirin 300 mg stat and 75 mg/d.

↓

> All for simvastatin 40 mg/day or pravastatin (if on digoxin or warfarin) after 2 days, and ACE inhibitors after 2 wks.

Risk of stroke after TIA is 3.1% in 2 days and 5.2% in 1 wk. 40% of these strokes occur within 24 hrs.

If raised homocystein >10 µmol/L in a young patient with ischemic stroke then for vitamin B_6 4.7 mg/day, B_{12} 2.4 µg/day and folic acid 400 µg/day.

Comparison of anterior and posterior circulation stroke

	Anterior circulation (carotid territory)	Posterior circulation (vertebrobasilar)
Fast	Highly sensitive	Moderate
CT head	Moderate sensitivity	Poor sensitivity
MRI	Excellent sensitivity	Very good sensitivity
Isolated hemianopia	+	++
Quadrantanopia	–	+
Pupil abnormalities	+ (Horner's syndrome)	+++ (may be bilateral)
Diplopia	–	+++
Unilateral sensory motor	+++	++
Bilateral sensory motor	–	+++
Unsteady/ataxia	+	++
Vertigo	–	+++
Dysarthria	++	++
Dysphasia	+++	+ (thalamic infarct)
Coma	+ (unusual unless mass effect)	+++ (thalamic or brainstem infarct)

IV tPA with in 4.5 hr (used up to 24 hrs in basilar occlusion)

Crossed syndrome (ipsilateral cranial nerve dysfunction and contralateral sensory or motor tract dysfunction), motor or sensory deficits in any combination of arms or legs and sometimes involving all four limbs, homonymous hemianopia, ataxia, vertigo, imbalance and dysphagia or dysarthria are the main symptoms of posterior circulation stroke.

Causes of post-circulation stroke—occlusion or embolism from atherosclerotic vertibrobasilar artery or from the heart and dissection of extracranial vertebral artery (in young people presenting as dizziness or vertigo, headache and neck pain without any history of trauma) are the main causes. Treatment is the same as for anterior stroke except MRI is needed for assessing TIA. Cerebral angiography is essential to diagnose basilar artery occlusion.

FAST (Face numbness or weakness one side, Arm numbness or weakness one side, Speech slurred or difficulty in speaking or understanding, time to summon emergency ambulance).

Alteplase if stroke <3 hrs over 80 yrs, and <4.5 hrs in under 80 yrs and after 24 hrs of alteplase, aspirin 300 mg/day.

Benefit from thrombolysis 1:3 in 3 hrs and 1:6 in 3–4.5 hrs. Benefit from thrombolysis is in reducing long-term disability and not in improved survival.

EXCLUSION CRITERIA FOR THROMBOLYSIS

Exclusion because of Clinical Features

- Stroke >4.5 hrs since the onset of symptoms, prior stroke with diabetes, seizures or headache at the onset. Recent (21 days) severe bleed or major surgery. Improving symptoms before starting thrombolysis is not exclusion. Prior stroke or head trauma in the last (3 months) or any history of intracranial hemorrhage (ICH) or SAH, brain tumor, bleeding disorders, intracranial AVM. Severe liver disease, heparin with in last 48 hrs with APTT > 1.2, or warfarin with INR > 1.4.

Exclusion on Examination
- Coma GCS <8, severe stroke NIHSS >25, systolic BP>185 or diastolic >110, hemorrhagic retinopathy in diabetes, blood glucose <2.8 or >22 and platelets <100.

Exclusion in Radiology
- CT signs of large infarct >1/3 of middle cerebral artery (MCA) or entire anterior cerebral artery (ACA) or posterior cerebral artery (PCA) territory.
- Cerebral hemorrhage on CT (Amyloid angiopathic (AA) hemorrhage has irregular border or indistinct, inhomogeneous density, at the border of gray and white matter and multiple or lobar hemorrhages). AA in old people while SVD (small vessel disease) in young and old. Recurrent hemorrhage at the same site—AVM and at different site AA.
- Loss of gray-white interface.
- Loss of sulci (sulcal effacement).
- Parenchyma acute hypodensity and mass effect.
- Factors that predict favorable outcome with alteplase—younger age, good prestroke function, less severe stroke, normal blood glucose and renal functions and absence of early infarct signs or hyperdense cerebral artery an CT.

National Institute of Health Stroke Scale (NIHSS)
- 1a—Level of cosciousness (LOC)
  0—alert
  1—not alert but arousable with minor stimulation
  2—not alert needs strong or painful stimulation to make movements
  3—responds with reflex motor or unresponsive
- 1b—LOC questions ask month and his/her age
  0—answers both correctly
  1—one question correctly
  2—neither question correct.
- 1c—Commands open and close the eyes, grip and release the hand
  0—performs both task correct
  1—one task correct
  2—neither task correct.
- 2—Best gaze, only horizontal eye movements will be tested
  0—normal

    1—partial gaze palsy
    2—total gaze paresis.
- 3—Vision by confrontation method
    0—no visual loss
    1—partial hemianopia
    2—complete hemianopia
    3—bilateral hemianopia.
- 4—Facial palsy ask to show teeth, raise eyebrows or close eyes
    0—normal symmetrical
    1—minor paralysis (flattened nasolabial fold, asymmetry on smiling)
    2—partial paralysis (total paralysis of lower face)
    3—complete paralysis upper and lower face.
- 5—Motor arm
    0—no drift (limb holds 90 degrees (45 degrees when lying) full 10 secs
    1—drifts before 10 sec but does not hit the bed
    2—some effort against gravity
    3—no effort against gravity
    4—no movement.
    5a—left arm and 5b right arm.
- 6—Motor leg
    0—no drift leg holds 30 degrees 5 sec
    1—drift leg falls before the end of 5 sec but does hit the bed
    2—some effort against gravity
    3—No effort against gravity
    4—no movement
    6a—left leg and 6b right leg
- 7—Limb ataxia finger-nose and heel-shin test for unilateral cerebellar lesion
    0—absent
    1—present in one limb
    2—present in two limbs.
- 8—Sensory
    0—no sensory loss
    1—mild to moderate sensory loss (pin prick is less sharp)
    2—severe to total sensory loss.
- 9—Best language
    0—no aphasia
    1—mild to moderate aphasia
    2—severe aphasia
    3—mute or global aphasia no usable speech.

- 10—Dysarthria clarity of articulation of speech
  0—normal
  1—mild to moderate dysarthria (slurs some words)
  2—severe dysarthria (extremely slurred).
- 11—Inattention
  0—no abnormality
  1—visual, tactile, auditory or personal in attention
  2—profound hemi in attention.

History

- Sudden or rapid onset of focal neurological deficit, differentiated from TIAs by the persistence of symptoms for >24 hr (differential diagnosis seizure, encephalopathy, migraine; patients are alert in ischemic stroke while drowsy and stuporous in encephalopathy).

  About 80% strokes are ischemic and 20% hemorrhagic caused by thromboembolism (20% carotid artery stenosis, 25% cardioembolic AF and 25% lacunar small vessel disease) and 15% by cerebral hemorrhage and 5% subarachnoid hemorrhage).

  The presence of headache, vomiting and coma at onset are more common in hemorrhagic stroke. Stroke is responsible for 12% of all deaths and is the most common cause of physical disability in adults. 25% of men and 20% of women who live beyond 80 can expect to suffer. 25% of strokes occur in working life. Consider stroke mimics (tumor, MS, postictal, hemiplegic migraine) in cases discovered waking from sleep, so MRI needs to be considered.
- If the patient has dysphasia then as much information as possible should be obtained from friends, relatives, ambulance crew and bystanders.
- Previous episodes of stroke, TIA or amaurosis fugax. After a TIA, the risk of stroke is 5.2% within 7 days. The ABCD2 score helps to identify high-risk patients.
  A—age 60 or > = 1,
  B—BP systolic >140 mm Hg and or diastolic 90 or > mm Hg =1 each,
  C—clinical features unilateral weakness = 2, speech disturbance without clinical weakness = 1
  D—duration of symptoms in minutes 60 minutes or > = 2,
  10–59 minutes = 1,
  <10 minutes = 0.

Diabetes-1
High risk (score >5) 8.1% 2-day risk 7-day risk 11.7%
of stroke,
Moderate (4–5) 4.1% 2-day risk 7-day risk 5.9%
Low (<4) 2-day risk 1%. 7-day risk 1.2%

Score of 4 or crescendo TIA's (>2 TIA's/wk) should be admitted and investigated while a score of less than 4 can be investigated as outpatients. With score of 4 and diabetes, risk of stroke within 7 days is 5% so should be rapidly investigated.

Anterior circulation TIA—sensory or motor weakness, dysphasia or inattention.

Posterior circulation TIA—dysarthria, imbalance, diplopia or visual field defect.

- Risk factors—age, hypertension (each diastolic rise of 7.5 mm Hg doubles the risk), atrial fibrillation (AF), ischemic heart disease (IHD), hyperlipidemia, diabetes mellitus, obesity (BMI >30), smoking.

  In young people, raised homocysteine, sickle cell disease, migraine with aura, carotid and vertebral artery dissection, PFO (patent foramen ovale), PAF (paroxysmal atrial fibrillation), oral contraceptive pill containing estrogen, lupus anticoagulant, vasculitis and cerebral autosomal-dominant arteriopathy with subcortical infarcts and leukoencephalopathy (CADASIL) disease.

  Risk of stroke in AF (AF 1% of population, stroke risk 5%/yr) is high in valvular AF or large left atrium >5.5 cm or score >1 in CHADS2 (moderate with 1 and low with 0).

C = CCF = 1,
H = hypertension = 1,
A = age = >75 = 1,
D = diabetes = 1,
S = stroke or TIA = 2.

Annual stroke risk— Score 0—2%, 1—3%, 2—4%, 3—6%, 4—8.5%, 5—12.5% and 6-18%.

All patients with AF (>2 CHADS2 score) or moderate (score 1) risk of stroke should receive warfarin or dabigatran (thrombin inhibitor) or rivaroxaban (factor X inhibitor).

Low risk (score 0) <65 yrs should receive aspirin. PAF <75 yrs alone carries a low risk

AF over 75 yrs should be treated with warfarin unless contraindicated, then aspirin or clopidogrel.

Risk of intracranial embolism in patients with A-V valve disease (MR, MS, TR, AS, AR) is 4% off warfarin, 2% on aspirin and 1% on warfarin.

Cardioversion—warfarin 3–4 wks before and after for AF >48 hrs for electrical or pharmacological cardioversion.

Cardiac ablation for AF, warfarin 3 wks before, heparin during the procedure and warfarin for 3 months after the ablation.

Risk Factors for Stroke <55 yrs

These are carotid and vertebral artery dissection, oral contraceptive pill containing estrogen, lupus anticoagulant, antiphospholipids syndrome and vasculitis.

Helicobacter pylori, *Chlamydia* infections, infective endocarditis, raised CRP, metabolic syndrome, factor V leiden, lipoprotein a, ↑ fibrinogen, ↑ homocysteine and PFO (patent foramen ovale with atrial septum aneurysm). Other risk factors are sickle cell disease, migraine with aura.

PFO is present in 20% of adult population but it is with atrial septum aneurysm shall undergo bubble study to confirm paradoxical embolism.

Cerebral venous thrombosis is responsible for 1% of strokes, occurs in hypercoagulation states such as dehydration, polycythemia, thrombocythemia, oral contraceptive pill, protein C, S, or AT3 (antithrombin 3) deficiency or vessel occlusion by tumor or abscess.

Postpartum stroke—cerebral venous thrombosis, antiphospholipid syndrome, systemic lupus erythematosus (SLE) should be considered,

Migraine with aura in people who smoke or use oral contraceptive.

STROKE MIMICS

- History of trauma or alcohol abuse (consider extradural or subdural hematoma).
- Progressive onset over days (? subdural hematoma or tumor).
- Fever (? brain abscess, meningitis, encephalitis, endocarditis, and cerebral lupus).

- Neck stiffness (? meningitis, subarachnoid hemorrhage).
- Todd's paresis (reversible neurological deficits after the seizure due to depression of postepileptogenic cortical area lasting less than 48 hrs) and cerebral vasculitis.
- Vertigo, benign paroxysmal positional vertigo (BPPV) dizziness when lying in bed on turning and transient global amnesia (TGA) with antigrade and retrograde amnesia, repetitive, asking the same question, lasts1hr or more with recurrence rate <5% and are considered to be due to venous congestion in the hippocampal area of the brain related to Valsalva like activity. So, in TGA, ask for sexual activity in the history.

INVESTIGATIONS AND DIFFERENTIAL DIAGNOSIS OF STROKE

- Urgent BM to exclude hypoglycemia.
- Full blood count (FBC), ESR, C reactive protein (CRP), U and E, coagulation studies, glucose, TSH, calcium and Lactate in MELAS.
- Thrombophilia screen, including for protein C, S, AT3 and leiden factor V deficiency in cerebral venous thrombosis or unexplained stroke or TIA in young person.
- LFT, cholesterol, ECG, CXR and ECHO for mural or atrial appendage thrombosis and PFO.
- Doppler ultrasound of carotid arteries in all anterior circulation (anterior and middle cerebral artery) TIA's and selected patients with stroke.
- CT/MRI scan should be requested in all patients with stroke or TIA's (>1 hr) and can be done over the next 24 hrs if not for thrombolysis otherwise ASAP. Patent foramen ovale (PFO) should be considered in all cryptogenic strokes whether over or less than 55.
- MRI may not identify acute hemorrhage correctly with in 1st few hrs. Diffusion weighted imaging (DWI) can identify ischemia and stroke with in few minutes. DWI is useful up to two wks.
- The presence of bilateral acute infarcts is suggestive of cardioembolism where as one acute infarct with several old infarct is suggestive thromboembolism.
- If a patient presents one wk after a stroke and it is extremely important to know whether it was infarct or hemorrhage then MRI T2 images should be used.

- MRI contraindicated in patients with pace makers, claustrophobic and very ill patient.
- About 50% of infarcts never become visible on CT. After 7 days 20% infarcts become invisible.

Urgent CT

- If thrombolysis is being considered (stroke presenting within 3–4.5 hrs).
- Depressed level of consciousness or coma GCS <13.
- Patient on anticoagulants, who develop headache or focal neurological signs.
- Unexplained progressive or fluctuating symptoms.
- History of severe headache at onset, or presence of fever, neck stiffness and papilledema, likelihood of nonstroke diagnosis, i.e. subdural hematoma, subarachnoid hemorrhage, meningitis, encephalitis, brain abscess and evidence of head injury.
- MRI should be considered in patients with brain stem or cerebellar symptoms and when CT is normal in stroke presenting after 1 wk to exclude hemorrhage.
- ECG—Prolongation of QT interval, ST depression or elevation, paroxysmal SVT, AF may precede or follow stroke.
- ECHO should be considered for cardioembolic stroke.
- *Urine*: Testing urine may reveal diabetes, vasculitis or infective endocarditis. A drug screen (amphetamine, cocaine, ecstasy) should be considered in a young patient with a stroke and no obvious cause.
- Genetic testing is undertaken in MELAS syndrome (mitochondrial encephalopathy, lactic acidosis and stroke like episode) or cerebral autosomal dominant arteriopathy with subcortical infarcts and leukoencephalopathy (CADASIL).

WHERE IS THE STROKE?

Total Anterior Circulation Infarct (TACI)

- *Large cortical stroke in middle cerebral artery, or middle and anterior cerebral artery territories*: Anterior cerebral artery infarction may be asymptomatic or may cause weakness primarily in the leg.
  Middle cerebral artery stroke may cause hemiparesis (worse in the arm if cortical infarction or affecting

arm face and leg equally if subcortical), hemi sensory loss, hemianopia (involvement of optic radiation), dysphasia (if in the dominant hemisphere), inattention (sensory and visual) and neglect. The 1st branch of internal carotid is the ophthalmic artery and emboli from carotid stenosis can cause amaurosis fugax (a curtain descending from above leading to complete transient loss of vision).

New higher cerebral dysfunction (dysphasia, dyscalculia, visuospatial disorder),

homonymous visual field defect, and

Ipsilateral motor and/or sensory deficit involving 2 out of 3 of face, arm, or leg.

- *Partial anterior circulation infarct (PACI)*: Cortical stroke in middle or anterior cerebral artery territories.
  - 2 out of 3 components of TACI,
  - New higher cerebral dysfunction alone (dysphasia, sensory inattention and conscious levels).
- *Lacunar infarct (LACI)*: Many lacunar strokes are asymptomatic. Commonly when affecting posterior limb of internal capsule, presents as pure motor stroke, pure sensory stroke, clumsy hand with dysarthria (slight weakness and clumsiness of hand with slurred speech) or ataxic hemi paresis (ataxia and mild hemiparesis on the same side).

  Sub cortical stroke due to small vessel disease:
  - Pure motor stroke,
  - Pure sensory stroke,
  - Sensorimotor stroke,
  - Ataxic hemi paresis,
  - Dysarthria and clumsy hand.
  - Evidence of higher cortical involvement or disturbance of consciousness excludes lacunar syndrome.
- *Posterior circulation syndrome (PCS)*: Posterior cerebral artery infarction results in hemianopia. Posterior circulation supplies the brainstem and cerebellum and infarction can result in hemiparesis or hemi sensory loss (from involvement of descending or ascending tracts), ataxia or involvement of cranial nerve nuclei (vertigo, eye movement abnormalities, facial palsy, tongue weakness, dysphagia). Basilar ischemia may result in bilateral weakness or sensory loss or bilateral loss of vision.

- Ipsilateral cranial nerve palsy with contralateral motor/sensory deficit
- Bilateral motor and/or sensory deficit
- Disorder of conjugate eye movement or brainstem dysfunction
- Cerebellar ataxia
- Isolated homonymous visual field defect.

Management of Acute Stroke

- The ABC standard acute initial assessment is to ensure that patient is maintaining adequate airway, breathing and has an adequate circulation.
    - Check blood glucose (maintain 4–11 mmol/L) to exclude hypo or hyperglycemia in an unconscious patient.
    - Glucose infusions are avoided as large load of carbohydrate causes surge of insulin; with influx of glucose, water and phosphorus in the cell results in hypophosphatemia with resultant exhaustion and possibility of vital organ failure. So for rehydration normal saline or Hartmann's solution should be used.
    - Blood glucose of 11 mmol/L or higher insulin treatment is needed as hyperglycemia worsens outcome.
- Nurse the patient in recovery position if impairment of consciousness.
- O_2 only if SpO_2 <95%, high flow (humidified) with reservoir bag if needed to keep SpO_2 >95%.
    - Normal cerebral blood flow 50–60 mL/100 mg/hr.
    - Irreversible tissue damage at 10–15 mL/100 mg/hr.
    - Between these is potentially salvageable tissue.
- Intravenous access.
- Check swallowing prior to allowing free fluids. If there are doubts about the swallowing then the patient should be kept nil by mouth and given IV fluids (usually 2 L/24 hr). Use normal saline or Hartmann's solution in the first 24 hrs and dextrose should be avoided as high blood glucose levels may worsen the prognosis. Avoid plasma volume contraction and raised hematocrit.

Patients with swallowing difficulty should be assessed by speech and language therapist.

Hyperglycemia is a risk factor and insulin sliding scale should be used if blood glucose is >11 mmol/L

- Venous thromboembolism—If high risk, use LMWH after 2 days (previous DVT, thrombophilia).

  Heparin is indicated in AF (after 2 wks).

  For prosthetic valves stop anticoagulant for 7 days and for aspirin 300 mg/day for 7 days.
- Stroke with dissection and acute venous stroke (cerebral venous sinus thrombosis) are treated LMWH followed by warfarin 3–6/12.
  - Ischemic stroke with symptomatic DVT or PE are treated with either anticoagulant or inferior vena cava filter.
  - Tight carotid stenosis prior to surgery and crescendo TIAs are treated with LMWH and warfarin.
  - If high INR give FFP and vitamin K.
  - If BM >11 then IV insulin on sliding scale.
  - Hemorrhagic stroke with symptomatic DVT, full dose of LMWH for 5–10 days and then prophylactic dose for 3/12.
  - If BP >180 mm Hg then antihypertensive IV Labetalol 10–20 mg over 1–2 min or nicardipine infusion 5 mg/hr or nitro paste or oral antihypertensive.
  - Routine H2RA or PPI.
  - In intracranial artery stenosis give aspirin + clopidogrel
  - EEG in lobar hemorrhage to detect subclinical seizures, anticonvulsive for 30 days and if seizure then for long term.
  - Consider IV mannitol if coning or sudden deterioration in cerebellar or ventricular hemorrhage.
- Urinary catheterization should be avoided in the acute phase unless there is urinary retention. Catheterize if high risk of pressure sore or urinary out put needs to be monitored.
- Aspirin 300 mg/d for 2/52 and then clopidogrel 75 mg/day, once cerebral hemorrhage has been excluded by CT scan. If intolerant of clopidogrel then aspirin 75 mg/d.

  Aspirin 300 mg (oral, nasogastric tube, rectal or IV) should be given preferably with in 48 hrs.

  In patients treated with thrombolysis, aspirin should be delayed for 24 hrs.

  Effective treatment for stroke:

	rTPA	Stroke unit	Aspirin
NNT (number needed to treat)	10	20	100
Proportion Eligible	10%	100%	70–80%

NNT for secondary prevention
Aspirin—100, Aspirin + Dipyradimol—53,
Clopidogrel—62
Warfarin—11, carotid endartectomy—26.
Decompressive surgery should be done within 48 hrs for malignant infarction of MCA.

Thrombolysis: On arrival in the A and E, FAST test +, duration of stroke <3 hrs if over 80 yrs and <4.5 hrs if <80 yrs of age, assess briefly GCS, contraindications to thrombolysis, NIHSS and order CT and blood test.

While waiting for CT complete the exclusion and inclusion criteria, take bloods for FBC, U and E, coagulation screen and ECG.

Accompany the patient to the CT scan and talk to relatives about consent for thrombolysis. Inform the stroke unit of imminent admission and thrombolysis.

Discuss the CT with radiologist to exclude hemorrhage and other conditions and examine the patient again to ensure patient is not improving rapidly before starting thrombolysis treatment.

- Thrombolysis with IV r-tPA (tissue plasminogen activator), Alteplase 0.9 mg/kg (max 90 mg) 10% bolus and rest over 1 hr increases survival free of disability for a few selected patients who can be assessed and treated within 3 hrs of onset of symptoms.

Risk of death 2–3%, 6% will have hemorrhage and 33% will improve.

Number needed to treat (NNT) 1:7 to improve disability, 1:18 to prevent death for anterior and postcirculation stroke

Fixed or progressive, no recent surgery, alert or somnolent, INR <1.4, platelet >100,000, BP <185/110, <80 yrs, no notable infarction or swelling on CT (sulcal effacement, frontoparietal attenuation, dense MCA).

>80, (no increase in ICH but increased mortality × 3 in 3/12). >ICH if BM >8.4 and 25% if BM >11.1

Contraindication for use of r-tPA in acute ischemic stroke
General: Severe bleeding within past 6/12, known bleeding diathesis, warfarin use INR >1.4, history of intracranial hemorrhage, recent (<10 days) cardiopulmonary resuscitation, bacterial endocarditis or pericarditis, acute pancreatitis, peptic ulcer (<3/12) disease, recent puncture of noncompressible vessel,

neoplasm with bleeding risk, major surgery or trauma (<3/12), recent obstetric delivery and severe liver disease.

Specific: Intracranial hemorrhage, onset of symptoms > 4.5 hrs, unclear time of onset, age <18 yrs, mild stroke NIHSS <5 or rapid improvement, severe stroke NIHSS >25 or imaging contraindications, seizure at the onset of stroke, symptoms indicating SAH, platelet count <100 × 10^6/L, heparin with in last 48 hrs with raised prothrombin time (PTT), previous stroke within 3/12, previous stroke and concomitant diabetes, BP systolic >185 or diastolic >110.

Outcome
The earlier the better <90 min better, established benefit <3 hrs over 80 yrs and <4.30 hrs <80 yrs of age.

Caution is advised in severe stroke or if CT demonstrates sulcal effacement, mass effect or edema or any evidence of intracranial hemorrhage.

There is 5% risk of fatal intracranial hemorrhage with thrombolysis.

Streptokinase is not used because of high ICH rate.

After r-tPA, vital sign observed every 15 min for 2 hrs, then every 30 min for 6 hrs and every 1 hr for 16 hrs.

Arterial punctures avoided for 24 hrs and antiplatelets and anticoagulants withheld for 24 hrs.

If suspicion of hemorrhage on r-tPA, stop r-tPA, give 6–8 U cryoprecipitate and 6U of platelets and FFP and notify neurosurgeon.

Oro-lingual angio edema often in patients on ACE and can be managed with antihistamines and IV hydrocortisone.

Intra-arterial r-tPA is not used because of increased risk of ICH.

Anticoagulants are only used in venous sinus thrombosis and arterial dissection.

High BP is associated with increased risk of hemorrhagic transformation.

- Avoid and treat hypotension or drastic reduction in BP. Hypotension after stroke is usually due to MI, aortic dissection or GI bleed. Antihypertensive medication may be continued if the patient is able to swallow. Do not actively lower BP in the 1st wk after stroke.

New antihypertensive medication can be initiated after 2 wk with ACE + diuretics (indapamide or thiazides) or calcium channel blockers), unless there is hypertensive encephalopathy (diastolic BP >120 mm Hg with papilledema retinal exudates and hemorrhages), aortic dissection, acute renal failure or intracerebral hemorrhage. Treatment may be considered if sustained rise in BP >180/120 in cerebral infarction and >180/105 in cerebral hemorrhage. If indicated use IV labetolol or IV nicardipine or modified release nifedipine 10 mg orally.

- Patients with ischemic stroke and AF or thrombophilia disorder should be considered for anticoagulation after 2 wks, if AF symptomatic then chemical or electrical cardioversion should be considered. Low dose heparin can be used for DVT prophylaxis in high risk patients after 2 days.
- If febrile at presentation consider brain abscess, meningitis or endocarditis. Pyrexia increases infarct size so if febrile after 12 hrs (rectal temp 37.5°C) of presentation then consider UTI, aspiration pneumonia.
- Patients with ischemic stroke or transient ischemic attack (TIA) with in last 6/12 and ipsilateral internal carotid artery stenosis >70% should be considered for early carotid arterectomy, <3-6 wks after the TIA's or stroke in patients who are clinically stable provided surgical risk of stroke is <6%. Over 70 yrs endartectomy better than carotid artery stenting while under 70 yrs both procedures are equal. Patients not fit for surgery, dissection, radiation induced stenosis or stenosis after surgery, carotid artery stenosis (CAS) stenting should be considered. Vertebral artery stenosis, symptomatic in spite of best medical therapy should be considered for stenting and angioplasty.

If SAH or ICH or subdural hematoma—stop aspirin, warfarin and give vitamin K +FFP.

- Start the patient on simvastatin 40 mg/day or atorvastatin irrespective of cholesterol level after 2 days.

Reduction in low density cholesterol (LDL) with various statins in mg/day

Statin	5 mg	10 mg	20 mg	40 mg	80 mg
Fluvastatin			21%	27%	33%
Pravastatin		20%	24%	29%	
Simvastatin		27%	32%	37%	42%
Atorvastatin		37%	43%	49%	55%
Rosuvatatin	38%	43%	48%	53%	

Aim to achieve 40% reduction in LDL cholesterol in secondary prevention

Consider pravastatin if the patient is on digoxin or warfarin. Risk of rhabdomyolysis increases if diltiazem or amiodarone or verapamil, antifungal, HIV drugs or grapefruit juice are used. There is increased risk of myopathy with 80 mg of simvastatin. Control of 4 risk factors—Blood pressure (BP) <120/89, LDL cholesterol <70 mg/dL, Triglyceride <150 mg/dL and HDL cholesterol >50 mg/dL enables risk reduction of 70–80%.

- If the patient is unable to swallow by 24 hrs after the stroke; nasogastric tube feeding should be considered and if swallowing not recovered by 2 wks, feeding via PEG should be considered.

  Loss of consciousness is rarely due to TIA. Transient global amnesia (TGA) is not due to TIA. Isolated vertigo is rarely due to TIA. TIA and AF consider anticoagulation if unable to take warfarin then aspirin 300 mg/day. Risk of stroke greatest in 1st 72 hrs after the TIA If >1 TIA, admit, investigate and consider heparin. Goal for HbA1c <7% in diabetics.

- TIA or strokes after anterior septal MI, consider ventricular thrombus diagnosed by ECHO, treated by warfarin for 3–12 months and aspirin 75–150 mg for ischemic heart disease (IHD). Patients with TIA or stroke and dilated cardiomyopathy may benefit from warfarin or aspirin. Patients with rheumatic heart disease (RHD) with mitral valve disease with or without AF need warfarin. If recurrent embolism in spite of warfarin add aspirin. For mitral valve prolapse, aortic valve disease with out AF aspirin is the best therapy for TIA or stroke. With prosthetic valves warfarin or warfarin plus aspirin in recurrent TIA or stroke.

Pregnancy with stroke: In pregnancy (last trimester) and 6 wks after birth there is high incidence of thrombo embolic disease (particularly 2 days before and 1 day after birth). 25–45% of patients with pregnancy associated stroke have pre-eclampsia or eclampsia. Investigations in pregnancy include MRI, MRA, ANCA, thrombophilia screen, antiphospholipid antibody and ECHO. If evolving deficit rather than sudden onset then consider migraine with aura. Peripartum or pastpartum angiopathy with thunderclap headache, seizures and neurological deficits are not due to eclampsia as their BP is normal without proteinuria but is due to migraine and use of sympathomimetic or vasoactive drugs. Reversible posterior leukoencephalopathy presenting as altered behavior, alertness, seizures, visual loss is treated with IV magnesium sulfate, lowering BP and rapid delivery of the baby.

Risk factors: Pre-eclampsia, cesarean section, known coagulopathy (presence of anticardiolipin, anti-phospholipid antibody, lupus anticoagulant), presence of medical conditions, hypertension, diabetes mellitus, sickle cell disease, thrombophilia, smoking, alcohol, use of cocaine, age >35, multiple gestation, greater parity and migraine headaches. In pregnancy with confusion, headache, seizure, TIA, variable neurology, anaemia and thrombocytopenia consider TTP and plasma exchange may be lifesaving. In prosthetic heart valve or cerebral venous thrombosis or dissection, LMWH till 13 wks then warfarin till middle of 3rd trimester and then UFH or LMWH till delivery or LMWH all through pregnancy. If low risk then LMWH till 13 wks then aspirin. Aspirin is safe in pregnancy and while breast feeding. Heparin safer after 24 hrs of delivery. Warfarin started 2–3 days if postpartum. Warfarin and heparin are safe in breast feeding. No thrombolytics in pregnancy and 4 wks after.

- TIA or ischemic stroke after bioprosthetic valve treat with warfarin. TIA or ischemic stroke after MI or LV thrombus warfarin for 3/12 to 1 yr along with concurrent aspirin for IHD.
- Stop smoking, alcohol no more than 1 drink/day for non pregnant women and 2 drinks/day for men, BMI 18.5–24.9, waste < 35 cm in females and <40 cm in men. Homocysteine >10 micromoles/L give B_6 1.7 mg/day + B_{12} 2.4 micro gm/day + Folate 400 µg/day.
- *PFO*: Aspirin and warfarin for high risk patients and if recurrent TIAs the closure of PFO.
- AF or paroxysmal AF treat with warfarin or direct oral anticoagulants unless recurrent falls risk then aspirin 300 mg/day. If antiphospholipid antibody present then treat with aspirin, but if venous or arterial occlusive disease, miscarriage or livido reticuolaris present then treat with warfarin.

- *Prognosis*: Risk of recurrent stroke is 8-12% in 7 days and 18% in 1 month after TIA's or minor stroke; hence assessment of patients with TIA'S must be rapid and comprehensive.
- After stroke 10% mortality in 1st month (half due immobility related causes and ¼ direct neurological sequele). Of those who survive 50% remain disabled at 6 months and 30% are functionally dependent at 1 yr. Any patient after stroke suspected of shoulder subluxation should be considered for electrical stimulation of supraspinatus and deltoid muscles. For neuropathic pain treat with amitriptyline or pregabalin or gabapentin or amitriptyline + pregabaline.
- *Driving*: After TIA or stroke group 1 (social driving)—Stop driving for 4/52 and assess.

  For group 2 (heavy goods) stop for 12/12. If visual or cognitive impairment inform DVLA.

  Any epileptic seizures stop driving for 12/12 except seizure with in 24 hrs of stroke.

Basilar Artery Thrombosis

Often sub acute 6-24 hrs in onset, presents with vertigo, headaches, vomiting, dysarthria, motor weakness, visual disturbance, ataxia or altered consciousness.

Signs: Eye movement abnormalities, facial palsy, lower cranial nerve palsies, crossed signs, extensor plantar, stupor or coma.

CT: Hyperdense basilar artery.

MRI diagnostic.

Treatment: Thrombolysis is best if unavailable consider heparin.

Carotid Arterial Dissection

Tear in intima with intramural hematoma and possible stenosis. It should be excluded in all young patients with stroke.

People with Marfan syndrome, Ehlers-Danlos syndrome or autosomal dominant polycystic kidney disease can have carotid dissection without injury.

Suggestive features: Neck injury (rapid deceleration, hyperextension and rotation of the neck) or manipulation.

Pulsatile tinnitus, Hornor's syndrome, lowers cranial nerve palsies and ischemic stroke.

Treated with anticoagulation and stenting of carotid artery.

Potentially Treatable Causes of Stroke

Urgent neurosurgical assessment is required for subarachnoid hemorrhage, large cerebellar hematoma and hydrocephalous. All cerebellar hemorrhages should have neurosurgical opinion because of risk of obstructive hydrocephalus.

Embolism from heart: This accounts for 15–20% of ischemic strokes.

Dysphasia or hemianopia without any other neurological deficit. Recent anterior MI, AF, LBBB, LV hypertrophy with strain pattern. Single cortical or subcortical branch territory infarct on CT or MRI. Fever at presentation (? Endocarditis). Preceding systemic illness (? Endocarditis, myxoma). Pan systolic or mid systolic murmur, signs of heart failure. Replacement heart valve (mechanical) in the mitral valve position.

Chronic Subdural Hematoma (SDH) (Fig. 3.1)

It is due to tearing of the veins linking cerebral cortex and dural sinuses causing blood to accumulate in between

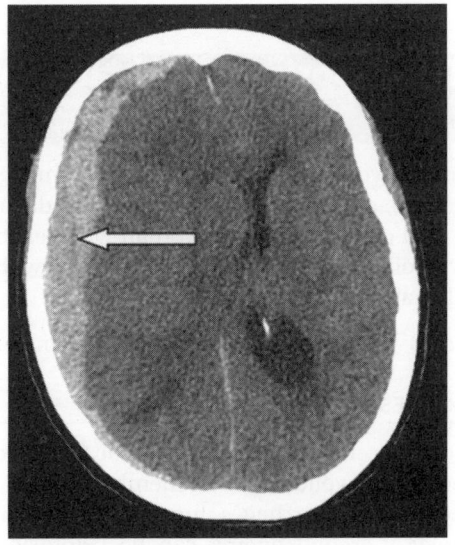

Fig. 3.1 Subdural hematoma

dura and arachnoid maters. Brain atrophy or dementia stretches these fragile veins such that they are prone to tearing with trivial fall or head injury (often forgotten). Anticoagulation increases the risk.

There may be a long delay between fall or head injury and onset of symptoms (15–49 days) and initial CT head may sometimes be normal after the fall or head injury. Subdural hematoma (SDH) usually presents with confusion, headache, reduced consciousness, seizure, wandering, behavior or personality change, delirium, gait disturbances and focal transient neurological deficits. There should be high index of suspicion in patients on anticoagulants, these patients often present within a wk with symptoms of raised intracranial pressure headache, nausea, vomiting, reduced consciousness, hemiparesis and ataxia.

Investigation: CT head shows crescent shape clot around the cerebral hemisphere. Initially it is hyper dense but in chronic stage it can be iso dense or hypo dense and at that stage presence of mid line shift or effacement of sulci points toward subdural hematoma (SDH).

Management: Rapid reversal of anticoagulants and stoppage of antiplatelet therapy. Evacuation of the clot by neurosurgery. Small asymptomatic SDH can be managed conservatively with follow-up repeat CT scanning.

Thrombosis of Cerebral Veins and Sinuses

Often affects young adults (70–80% in women of child bearing age), a teenager with recent headaches after starting oral contraceptives, a woman with seizures after delivery in obstetric ward or a comatose man with dilated pupil, all may have sinus thrombosis.

Incidence: 3–4 cases/million, more common in females.

PATHOGENESIS

Occlusion of cerebral veins causes localized edema of brain, enlarged swollen veins, ischemic neuronal damage and petechial hemorrhages merging to become large hematomas. Cerebral edema can be cytotoxic (caused by ischemia causing intracellular swelling) or vasogenic (caused by disruption of blood brain barrier and leakage of blood plasma in interstitial space). Vasogenic edema is reversible, if underlying condition is treated successfully.

Intracranial hypertension develops without ventricular dilatation as a result of occlusion of sinuses. Normally cerebrospinal fluid (CSF) is transported from ventricles through subarachnoid spaces from the base and surface of the brain to arachnoid villi, where it is absorbed and drains into superior sagittal sinus. Sinus thrombosis leads to increased venous pressure which impairs absorption of CSF and hence increased intracranial pressure. Because obstruction is beyond the subarachnoid spaces on the surface of the brain, hence the ventricles do not dilate and hydrocephalus does not complicate sinus thrombosis.

RISK FACTORS

- Head injury or obstetric delivery in a person with genetically increased risk.
- Risk of peripartum (last trimester) or postpartum sinus thrombosis is 12 cases/100,000 deliveries.
- Oral contraceptives (3rd generation containing gestodene or desogestril).
- Jugular vein catheterization or lumbar puncture (low CSF pressure after lumbar puncture (LP) causing downward shift of brain with traction on cortical veins).
- Headache following LP disappears when the patient lies down and resolves within a few days while headache due to sinus thrombosis does not change due to shift in posture and gradually increases over a couple of days.
- *Infections*: Otitis and mastoiditis (thrombosis of sigmoid and transverse sinuses), sinusitis, meningitis, systemic infectious disease.
- *Genetic prothrombotic conditions*: Antithrombin deficiency, protein C and S deficiency, factor V Leiden mutation and homocysteinemia. Acquired prothrombotic states—Nephrotic syndrome, anti phospholipids antibodies, pregnancy, puerperium.
- *Systemic diseases*: SLE, Wegener's granulomatosis, Sarcoidosis, inflammatory bowel disease (IBD), Behçet's syndrome, polycythemia (primary or secondary), thrombocythemia, leukemia. Cancer and dehydration.

CLINICAL SIGNS

Severe headache gradually worsens over a couple of days or thunder clap headache with vomiting mimicking SAH. Sometimes there are unilateral hemispheric symptoms (hemiparesis or aphasia), followed within a few days with symptoms from another hemisphere. Focal seizures or generalized sometimes in 50%. Thrombosis of straight sinus (deep sinus) causes bilateral thalamic lesions presenting as delirium, amnesia and mutism. Sometimes presents as coma with generalized seizures. Thrombosis of cavernous sinus causes headache, fever, proptosis, periorbital edema, chemosis and paralysis of eye movements due to involvement of 3, 4 and 6th cranial nerves. Isolated intracranial hypertension presents with headache, papilledema and sometimes diplopia due to 6th cranial nerve palsy.

DIAGNOSIS

It should be considered in young or middle age patient with recent unusual headache or stroke like symptoms in the absence of usual vascular risk factors with CT evidence of multiple hemorrhagic infarcts not confined to arterial vascular territories. MRI with MR venography shows hyper intense signal from thrombosed sinus (isodence before day 5 and after 30 days) and absence of flow. CT venography is also helpful. CT is useful to rule out other acute cerebral disorders if MRI is not available. Cerebral angiography is indicated if diagnosis is still uncertain after MRI.

TREATMENT

- Possible causes such as infection should be searched and treated.
- IV mannitol or surgical removal of hemorrhagic infarct or decompressive hemicraniotomy, for acute cerebral herniation. Combination of acutely raised intracranial pressure and large venous infarct is dangerous and patient may die within hrs.
- Heparin (fractionated or unfractionated) should be started as soon as the diagnosis is made even in the presence of hemorrhagic infarcts. Anticoagulants should be continued at least 6 months in the absence of risk factors. Endovascular thrombolysis with

urokinase only in poor prognosis group in centers using intervention radiology and thrombolysis in strokes. In patients with chronic intracranial hypertension after excluding space occupying lesion such as large infarct or hemorrhages, LP should be done to measure the pressure, to relieve headache and to reduce papilledema. CSF shows raised pressure, raised proteins and pleocytosis.

- Oral acetazolamide 500–1000 mg/day may reduce intracranial pressure.

Anterior Spinal Artery Thrombosis

Anterier spinal artery supplies the ventral 2/3 of spinal cord and medulla. Anterior spinal artery is a branch of vertebral artery.

Causes: Atherosclerosis, dissection of aortic aneurysm or vasculitis. Sudden onset of tetra or paraparesis with dissociated sensory loss of pain and temperature while sense of position and vibration is preserved (as posterior column is supplied by posterior spinal artery and is preserved while anterior and lateral columns are supplied by anterior spinal artery). There is also involvement of bladder. MRI is usually diagnostic.

Coma

HISTORY

Obtain as much information as possible from relatives, friends, ambulances crew and bystanders asking circumstances in which the patient was found. Also ask about alcohol consumption, diabetes mellitus, epilepsy, drug abuse and opioids, head injury, regular medication and past medical history.

CAUSES

- Coma with hyper ventilation (low $PaCO_2$)—ketoacidosis; diabetic or alcoholic; liver failure, renal failure, bacterial meningitis, poisoning with aspirin, CO, ethanol, ethylene glycol, methanol, paracetamol,

tricyclic's, stroke complicated by pneumonia or pulmonary edema and brainstem stroke.
- Coma with neck stiffness—bacterial meningitis, encephalitis, subarachnoid hemorrhage, cerebral or cerebellar hemorrhage with extension into subarachnoid space, cerebral malaria.
- Coma with focal neurological signs but no head injury or neck stiffness, with brain stem signs (deviation of eyes or abnormal pupils)—brainstem compression due to large intracerebral hemorrhage or infarction with edema, brainstem stroke, cerebellar stroke, basilar artery thrombosis.
- Coma without head injury or neck stiffness or focal neurological signs—hypoglycemia, poisoning with alcohol or tricyclics, anoxic brain injury, liver failure, respiratory failure, renal failure, diabetic ketoacidosis, myxedema coma, acute adrenal insufficiency, severe hyponatremia, severe hypercalcemia, after major tonic-clonic seizure.

Information from relatives, carers, ambulance personnel or GP is vital, remembering most common cause of nontraumatic coma in young is poisoning and in the elderly is stroke.

Two basic mechanisms to render a patient unconscious are damage to the reticular activating system in the brain stem and damage to the both cerebral hemispheres simultaneously.

ASSESSMENT USUALLY GCS <8

- *Airway*: Clear the air way, remove false teeth if loose, aspirate the pharynx, larynx and trachea with a suction catheter; if there is no reflex response (gagging or coughing) to the suction or RR is <8/min, ventilate the patient using bag-valve-mask system with 100% oxygen and cuffed endotracheal tube. If patient responds to suction and the respiratory rate is >8/min give 60% O_2 by mask (unless CO poisoning is suspected in which case give O_2 10 L/min by a tight fitting face mask). In trauma victims protect cervical spine.
- Breathing—assess and support.
  Slow and shallow—Drugs,
  Deep and rapid—pneumonia, acidosis, central neurogenic hyperventilation,

Irregular—brainstem lesion.
Cheyne-stokes—bilateral hemisphere disease.

- Circulation—check carotid and femoral pulse, if absent follow the guide lines for resuscitation.
- IV access.
    - Look for medic alert bracelet or necklace.
    - Tongue biting or urinary incontinence suggests (but does not prove) epilepsy.
    - Bruising or bleeding on back of the head suggests head injury.
    - Bleeding or CSF leak from ears or nose suggest basal skull fracture.
- Search pockets for clues, e.g. anticonvulsant tablets.
- Check temperature (hypothermia)
- Attach an ECG monitor, pulse oxymeter and take blood for glucose (immediate BM), U and E, arterial blood gases, FBC, toxicology and blood culture if indicated.
- Check for small pupils and slow respiratory rate (opioids over dose?).

DOCUMENT GCS

Eye Opening

- Spontaneous
- To voice
- To pain (eyes open to painful stimulus applied to trunk or limb)
- None.

Motor Response

- Normal, voluntary-obeys commands
- Localizes to pain-uses limb to locate or resist the painful stimulus
- Withdraws to pain
- Extensor response, decorticate posture
- Abnormal flexor response, decerebrate
- None.

Verbal Response

- Normal speech
- Disorientated conversation
- Words, but not coherent

- No words
- None

Coma is defined as GCS 8 or below, and reduced conscious level if score is 9–14.

Pupil size—
- Unilateral fixed dilated pupil—Uncal herniation, post-communicating artery (PCOM) aneurysm
- Mid position pupil and loss of light reflex—Mid brain lesion
- Bilateral fixed dilated pupil—severe damage, Tectal, very poor prognostic sign
- Bilateral small pupil with retained light reflex—opiates, pontine hemorrhage
- Unilateral Horner syndrome—damage to hypothalamus or lateral medullary syndrome
- Most comatose patients have up going planters regardless of etiology.

Investigations

- Blood glucose
- FBC, U and E, LFT, Calcium, ECG, EEG (selected cases).
- Focal/lateralizing signs (structural lesion likely)
- CT brain if patient not improving rapidly or diagnosis not clinically apparent looking for extradural, subdural, subarachnoid or intracerebral hemorrhage, signs of raised intracranial hypertension and focal ischemia.
- LP and blood culture in selected cases.

Management

- O_2 high flow keeping SaO_2 >92%.
- Endotracheal intubation in patients with GCS <8
- If systolic BP <90 mm Hg and no signs of pulmonary edema, give 500 mL of saline or colloid over 15–30 minutes.
- Exclude hypoglycemia and if blood glucose <5 mmol/L, give 50 mL of 20% dextrose IV and in chronic alcoholics give thiamine 100 mg IV before or shortly afterwards to prevent Wernicke's encephalopathy.
- Treat prolonged or recurrent fits with IV diazepam or lorazepam.
- If respiratory rate (RR) <12/min or pupils are pin point suspect opioid poisoning and give naloxone up to four doses of 800 μg IV every 2–3 minutes until RR is

15/min. If there is response, start IV infusion adding 3 mg in 500 mL dextrose and titrate it with RR. Naloxone has half-life of 4 hrs; if there is no response to naloxone opioid poisoning is excluded.
- Consider flumazenil if coma is due to therapeutic use of benzodiazepine; give 200 microgram IV over 15 sec.
- Look for signs of head injury.
- If alcohol intoxication is suspected, check blood alcohol level and coma is unlikely to be due to alcohol alone if level is <44 mmol/L; other causes must be sought.
- Further management on the cause of coma.

Hypothermia

Temperature <35°C use tympanic thermometer.

35–37°C—shivering, numbness of the hand, goose pimples, unable to touch thumb and little finger.

33–35°C—shivering, muscle in coordination, confusion, stumbling pace, looks pale and lips finger, ear, toes look blue.

Mild 32–35°C—difficulty in speaking, sluggish thinking, amnesia, stumbling, inability to use hands, unable to walk, skin blue and puffy, stupor.

Moderate 28–32°C (Amnesia, apathy, loss of fine motor skills, paradoxical undressing, reduced shivering, slurred speech, bradycardia, arrhythmias, stiff joints and hyporeflexia).

Severe <28°C (loss of consciousness, extreme bradycardia, slow RR, apnea, hypotension, impalpable pulse, cold edematous skin, areflexia and fixed dilated pupil).

Water temperature—10°C—death in 1 hr, water temperature—0°C—death in 15 min, water temperature—26°C—mild hypothermia.

CAUSES

Cold receptors in the skin → afferent fibers → preoptic nucleus of anterior hypothalamus → vasoconstriction of vessels. Also cold blood to hypothalamus through autonomic nerves causes immediate shivering.

Predisposition to thermoregulatory failure (CVA, CNS trauma, infections, multiple sclerosis, Parkinson's disease, CCF, diabetes with autonomic dysfunctions, Wernics encephalopathy) precipitated by minor insult.

- Cold exposure, inadequate clothing, old age, wet clothing, altered level of consciousness.
- Immobility/falls, debility, exhaustion.
- Cognitive impairment, malnutrition, hypothyroidism, hypoadrenalism, hypopituitarism, hypoglycemia, sepsis, shock and uremia.
- Alcohol, vasodilators/drugs, sedatives, narcotics, antidepressants.

EXAMINATION

Hypothermia causes generalize slowing of enzyme activity, peripheral vasoconstriction and uncoupling of O_2 dependent metabolism, so affects all organ. There is catechol amine release initially causing tachycardia, raised BP and cardiac output later on negative inotropic and chronotropic effect of hypothermia sets in causing decreased blood volume, diminished cardiac output and tissue perfusion.

- Check airways, breathing, circulation.
- Glasgow coma score (GCS).
- Reagent stick test for blood glucose.
- Check pupils if small with slow respiratory rate (Opoids overdose?).
- 37°C—N, 36°C cold, 35°C shivering, 34°C clumsy, irrational, confused and appears drunk.
- 33°C muscle stiffness, 32°C shivering stops and collapse.
- 31°C semiconscious and muscular rigidity, 30°C unconscious and no response to painful stimuli, 29°C slow pulse and slow breathing, 28°C cardiac arrest.
- Bradycardia with hypotension, partial pressure of O_2 (PaO_2) and $PaCO_2$ should be corrected for hypothermia.
- Look for aspiration pneumonia or pulmonary edema.
- Focal/lateralizing neurological signs indicate stroke.
- Patient may be confused or ataxic with incoordination.

INVESTIGATIONS

- FBC, U and E, LFT, TSH, glucose and chest X-ray to look for pneumonia and pulmonary edema.
- ECG may show sinus bradycardia with A-V block, pronged QT interval, wide QRS, inverted T-wave and J-wave (broad slurred deflection that is superimposed on the distal limb of QRS complex when temp <32°C).

- Cold heart is highly irritable and any physical stimulation may lead to VF. Severe hyperkalemia is common in profound hypothermia. K must be monitored during rewarming.
- Infections such as pneumonia, UTI and cellulitis are present in 90% of hypothermic patients and infection may be precipitant or consequence of hypothermia.

COMPLICATIONS

- Initial cold diuresis later acute tubular necrosis, metabolic acidosis, hyperkalemia, hyponatremia, hyperglycemia, hyperphosphatemia, rhabdomyolysis, gastric dilatation, ileus, pancreatitis, sever hepatic dysfunctions, hemoconcentration, increased blood viscosity, thrombocytopenia, leucopenia and consumptive coagulopathy.
- GI—Intestinal motility decreases, <34°C ileus so N/G, oral or N/G route avoided as absorption impaired.
- Gastric erosion, punctate hemorrhages, shallow gastric ulcers, increased gastric acid production, reduced duodenal secretions of bicarbonates leads to gastric ulcer.
- Decreased clearance of lactate leads to lactic acidosis and impairs liver functions of conjugation and detoxification and increases the half-life of many drugs including alcohol. 50% have pancreatitis due thrombosis of microcirculation leading to micro infarcts. Same mechanism operates for micro infarcts of brain, gut, liver and myocardium.
- *Hematology*: There is 2% increase in viscosity, fibrinogen and hemocrit for every 1°C decrease in temperature.
- Increased vascular permeability causes hypovolemeia.
- Marrow suppression and marrow failure.
- Cold also inhibits enzymes for intrinsic and extrinsic pathway leading to coagulopathy and DIC.
- There is increased cryofibrinogen with increased viscosity and wide spread micro infarcts.
- Heparin can polymerize cryofibrinogen in the presence of cryofibronogenemia and cause hyper viscosity, so heparin should not be used as DVT or PE prophylaxis.
- *Neuromuscular*: Symptoms as described above and cerebral blood flow (CBF) decreases by 6–7% with 1°C of hypothermia.

- Synovial fluid more viscous at low temperature so stiffness of joints and muscles. There is progressive reduction in conduction velocity and postural hypotension. So sitting position avoided in transferring patients.
- *Respiratory*: Impaired ciliary function leads to aspiration pneumonia. At 30°C, decreased O_2 consumption and increased CO_2 production by 50%, respiratory and metabolic acidosis, increased pulmonary resistances, V-Q mismatch, hypoventilation and pulmonary edema. There is risk of metabolic alkalosis on rewarming.
- *Cardiovascular system (CVS)*: Initially increased heart rate (HR), peripheral vasoconstriction and increased cardiac output, later decreased in HR (refractory to atropine), increased vascular resistance, prolonged QRS, P-R, Q-T interval, inverted T-wave, ST depression, and J-wave on the descending limb of QRS (also seen in SAH, cerebral injuries and myocardial ischemia).
- Some times asystole, VF or A-V block may appear on rewarming.
- Ventricular fibrillation is resistant to DC shock <28°C unless warming is done and bretylium or magnesium sulfate should be used in that situation.
- *Renal*: Cold diuresis is due distal tubular resistance to antidiuretic hormone (ADH) and there is decreased absorption of Na. Tubular capacity to secret H decreases, so acidosis.
- Basal metabolic rate (BMR) decreases 6% per 1°C. If resistance to rewarming then give hydrocortisone and thyroxin in case of occult hypothyroidism and hypopituitarism. No benefit of routine steroids. Insulin resistance in hypothermia and if hyperglycemia persists on rewarming then consider diabetic ketoacidosis (DK) or pancreatitis and insulin given if temp >30°C.

MANAGEMENT

- Treat hypoglycemia (if BM low) and opoid overdose if suspected.
- Replace wet clothing.
- Rewarm (mild hypothermia)—slowly in warm room covered with blanket (Do not use foil blanket), avoid rubbing. Core of the body should be warmed 1st (hot drinks helps).
- O_2 (warm) to keep PaO_2 >92%.

- IV access and ECG monitoring.
- If hypotensive or dehydrated then IV warm dextrose/0.9% normal saline slowly (increased risk of LVF). Antibiotics-Broad spectrum, e.g. cefotaxime 1 g 12 hourly.

If temperature <33°C, admit ITU, then re-warm rapidly using both external and internal.

- Apply heat to body surface, e.g. hot water bottle/warmed IV bags (not too hot and bearable against your own skin) in groins and axilla and warmed blankets.
- Give warmed humidified O_2 (42°C-43°C).
- Gastric, colonic, bladder and peritoneal lavage with warmed 0.9% saline (43°C) if core temperature not rising 0.5–1°C/hr.
- Forced-air rewarming blanket.
  - Avoid the use of catecholamine, digoxin. For VF use either magnesium sulfate (8 mmol of magnesium IV over 10–15 minutest) or bretylium 5–10 mg/kg IV over 15–30 minutest. Avoid lidocaine, epinephrine and procainamide in hypothermia as risk of accumulation. Death cannot be diagnosed until the core temperature is >30–33°C.
  - *Prevention*: No cotton fabric as cotton retains water and conducts heat away from body.

Meningitis

In bacterial meningitis there is 1st colonization of nasopharynx with pathogens, then followed by hematogenous spread to other sites and meninges while in viral meningitis viremia is acquired mostly by fecal oral route? Viral meningitis is usually in young people. Entero viruses (46%), herpes simplex type 2 (31%), varicella zoster (11%) and herpes simplex type 1 (4%).

HISTORY

- *Early*: Malaise, headache, fever, vomiting, diarrhea.
- *Later*: Increasing severe headache, photophobia, drowsiness and in very late stages convulsions and coma.
- Specifically ask for contact with meningitis.
- History of immunodeficiency.
- Pregnancy (increased risk of listeria).
- Previous history of meningitis.
- Travel history.

Suspect in any patient presenting with fever, headaches, meningism, (photophobia, neck stiffness, headache, Kernign's sign (resistance to extension at the knee when the lower limb is flexed at the hip), neurological signs (cranial nerve palsies in 20%), seizures, decreased level of consciousness and petecheal rashes in meningococcal septicemia.

EXAMINATION

- After checking heart rate (HR), RR, BP, look for petechiae/purpura in the skin, conjunctivae/palate (characteristic of meningococcal disease).
- After confirming signs of meningism, look for signs of infection (pneumonia, otitis media).
- Look for papilledema, cranial nerve lesion (particularly 5th).
- Factors associated with poor prognosis
  - Severity of disease at presentation, old age, prolonged symptoms
  - Shock/organ failure
  - Low GCS, seizure or focal signs suggest encephalitis
  - Suspected encephalitis warrants antiviral empirical treatment with IV acyclovir
  - Delay in antibiotic administration after arriving in the hospital (2 hrs in UK),

INVESTIGATIONS

- FBC, U and E, LFT, ABG in severe cases, glucose, clotting screen, blood culture, throat swab and stools for virology, blood sample (in EDTA) for PCR and swab from throat and skin lesion (if any) and urine for pneumococcal; antigen. Written consent for LP.
- Lumber puncture contraindications
  - Reduced level of conscious, GCS <12 or falling (>2 points fall since admission).
  - Lumbar puncture or CT should not be allowed to delay giving antibiotics in patients in whom bacterial meningitis is suspected.
  - Bradycardia/hypotension
- Focal neurological signs (cranial nerves, long tract or posterior fossa)
  - Papilledema.
  - Seizures, platelets <80,000, INR >2.
  - Age >60.
  - History of head trauma

- Anticoagulation or bleeding diathesis.
- Clinical suspicion of spinal cord compression.
- Inability to answer two consecutive questions correctly or follow two consecutive commands correctly.
- Arm or leg drift on motor testing.
- If no contraindication LP should be performed without delay. Normal CSF 500 mL, 100 mL produced every day.
- Measure and record CSF opening pressure, if >40 cm (severe cerebral edema, give mannitol 0.5 g/kg IV over 10 minutes plus dexamethasone 12 mg IV), and inform neurosurgeons.
- Send CSF for cell count, protein, glucose (fluoride tube), PCR for viruses, gram's stain.
- Zeihl-Neelson stain and India ink stain if immune compromised to exclude TB or *Cryptococcus meningitis*.
- If CSF is cloudy, start antibiotics immediately after taking blood cultures (X2). Blood stained CSF may be traumatic or sub arachnoid hemorrhage (SAH), collect 3 consecutive tubes and check RBC count in first and third and also check for xanthochromia in the supernatant. Xanthochromia is present from 12 hrs to 2 wks after SAH.

Likely organism—
- <50 yrs *Streptococcus pneumoniae, Neisseria meningitids*.
- >50 yrs *Streptococcus, Neisseria*, Gram negative bacilli, *Listeria monocytogenes*.

CSF	Pyogenic	Viral	TB	Cryptococcus
Cell count/cmm	>1000	<500	<500	<150
Cell type	Polymorphs	Lymphocytes	Lymphocytes	Lymphocytes
Proteins g/L	>1.5	0.5–1.0	1.0–5.0	0.5–1.0
CSF: Blood glucose	<50%	>50%	<50%	<50%

High polymorph count is typical of pyogenic meningitis, but may occur in viral meningitis. If the patient has low CSF glucose, start antibiotic therapy; but if the CSF glucose is normal and there are no feature suggestive of bacterial infection, hold off antibiotics and repeat LP in 12 hrs. By this time an increasing proportion of cells will be lymphocytes in viral meningitis.

High lymphocytes count may be seen in many conditions and distinguishing between viral and partially treated bacterial meningitis may be difficult; if in doubt, start antibiotics awaiting results of culture of CSF and blood.
- If eosinophils in the CSF ring microbiologist ASAP.
- *Poor prognosis*: >60 yrs, falling GCS, multi organ failure, focal neurology. GCS <8, 88% poor outcome, GCS >12, 88% good outcome.
- *Pre-hospital antibiotics*: Reduce blood culture positive but nasopharynx and CSF cultures positive just the same. PCR positive for 48 hrs.

Initial management: In suspected meningococcal meningitis/septicemia, give antibiotics immediately before referral to hospital and in hospital before LP
- Careful examination for neurological signs and rashes.
- Check for vital signs and if shocked give O_2 and IV fluids.
- LP if not contraindicated.
- Start antibiotics while waiting CT scan.

Antibiotics
- Give antibiotics within 30 minutes ceftriaxone 2 g IV bid if <50 and >50 add amoxicillin 1 gm tds.
- Parenteral penicillin or cefotaxime or chloramphenicol is the standard practice for suspected meningitis before sending the patient to the hospital.
- If gram stain of CSF does not suggests pneumococcal infection, and <50 yrs ceftriaxone 80 mg/kg IV every 12 hrs for first 3 doses then 80 mg/kg (maximum 4 g) daily.
- If LP is not done or gram stain shows pneumococcal infection, and <50 yrs cefotaxime 2–4 g, 8-hly IV and vancomycin 60 mg/kg IV daily in divided doses.
- If >50 yrs cefotaxime, vancomycin and ampicillin 200–400 mg/kg daily IV in 4 divided doses should be used.
- Risk factors for *Streptococcus pneumoniae* are head injury, sinusitis, CSF leak, elderly and alcoholism.

Further management: Analgesia, IV fluids and notify public health if meningococcal or hemophilus influenzae infections. They will contact tracing and arrange prophylaxis. Thromboprophylaxis and H2RA or PPI.
- NG to empty the stomach if GCS <8.
- *ICU*: If patient has shock, not responding to IV fluids, respiratory failure (arterial PaO_2 <8 kPa) and GCS <11.

- Prophylaxis for immediate contacts should be done from the hospital. Give prophylaxis to all who have prolonged contacts (>6 hrs), house hold, close contacts or kissing contacts; it is not given to non-household contact. Risk is <1:200 and increased for 6/12.
- For meningococcal—rifampicin 600 mg oral twice daily for 2 days (children <1 yr 5 mg/kg bid, >1 yr 10 mg/kg bid for 2 days), or ciprofloxacin 750 mg orally as single dose and immunize if serogroup C or A.
- Prophylaxis is not required for staff unless mouth to mouth resuscitation has been given. For hemophilus—Rifampicin 600 mg oral OD for 4 days.
- HIV+ patient (CD4 count 437) ten days of headache and fever.
- Opening pressure 33 cm H_2O, protein 1.9 g/dL, glucose 1.8 mmol/L (plasma 5.3), mononuclear cells 34/mm^3, Red cells 28/mm^3, Gram's stain negative. What is the most likely diagnosis?
  - *Cryptococcus meningitis*
  - Herpes simplex viral meningitis
  - Primary HIV illnesses
  - Tuberculosis meningitis.

Viral Encephalitis

May be due to several viruses but herpes simplex is the most important as it causes most severe damage which can be limited by acyclovir.

Presents as fever, headache, meningism, personality change, abnormal behavior, and alteration in conscious level, convulsions, focal neurological signs, hallucinations and temporal lobe seizures.

Investigations and management is same as meningitis with following additions.
- If patient needs CT, do not delay antibiotics and acyclovir. Steroids sometimes used for post vaccine encephalomyelitis. IV mannitol for severe intracranial hypertension.
- Send CSF for culture, bacteria, viruses and for PCR.
- CT scan may show general brain swelling with loss of cortical sulci and small ventricles, but may be normal. There may be areas of low attenuation in the frontal or temporal lobes.

- EEG is usually abnormal in two-thirds with spike and slow wave pattern localized to the area of brain involved.

TREATMENT

Antibiotics as per meningitis IV and acyclovir 10 mg/kg tds for 10 days depending on renal functions.

Differential diagnosis: TB, vasculitis, brain abscess, Para meningeal infection, septic emboli, partially treated meningitis, fungal, spirochete, parasites, leptomeningeal malignancy and rickettsia.

ICU: If raised intracranial pressure, depressed conscious level, shock or respiratory failure (PaO_2 <8 kPa).

Coning and Tentorial Herniation

Causes

- Raised intracranial pressure
- May occur post lumber puncture. It is rapidly fatal.

Diagnosis

- Suspect after recent lumber puncture in meningitis or SAH.
- Pupil(s) dilate abruptly, and fixed.
- Bradycardia with hypertension.
- Periodic respiration and coma.

Management

- Call neurosurgeon and transfer the patient to ICU.
- IV access and give mannitol 20% 200 mL along with furosemide 20 mg IV.
- Bag, mask, valve hyperventilate with high concentration of O_2.
- May require intubation and ventilation with anesthetic.

Acute Wernicke's Encephalopathy

HISTORY

- Alcoholism with nutritional deficiency and protracted vomiting.
- Confusion
- Difficulty in standing or walking.

Examination

- Ophthalmoplegia
- Horizontal or vertical nystagmus
- Weakness or paralysis of lateral rectus muscle
- Weakness or paralysis of conjugate gaze
- Ataxia affecting stance or gate often without intention tremor
- Confusion, confabulation
- Consider also acute alcohol withdrawal, acute liver failure and chronic liver disease
- Red cell transketolase will show thiamine deficiency
- CT brain should be done in all cases.

Immediate Management

Intravenous Pabrinex high potency 2 ampoules tds for 3 days and then oral thiamine 100 mg tds daily and vitamin B complex strong 1-2 tab tds.

Subarachnoid Hemorrhage (SAH)

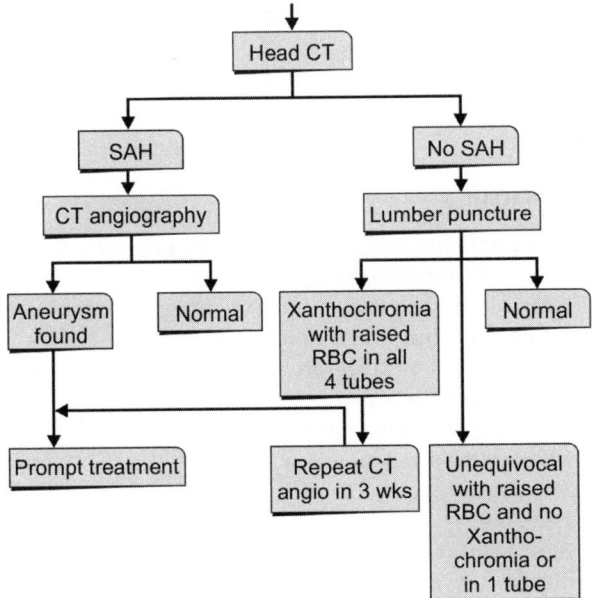

Acute bleed in the subarachnoid space, 70% from aneurysm, 5% from arteriovenous malformations, and 5% from various causes (tumor, vasculitis, bleeding diathesis) and in 20% no cause is found. Thunder clap headache is a headache which reaches 7 out of 7 (maximum) in severity in one minute.

Other causes of thunderclap headache apart from SAH are cervical artery dissection, cerebral venous thrombosis and reversible cerebral vasoconstriction syndrome (RCVS).

Incidence 6–10/100,000/yrs or 2–5% of all new strokes fatality 51% (mostly within 2 wks) and 33% of survivors need lifelong care.

Presentation

Acute onset, severe thunderclap headache +/− vomiting, photophobia. Headache is the worst ever and lasts over an hr, coma, seizure.

Risk Factors

Hypertension, smoking, alcohol (binge drinking), cocaine, cannabis, ecstasy use, mild trauma family history, adult polycystic kidney disease, previous episode of SAH, Ehler-Danlos syndrome type IV, Pseudoxanthoma elasticum and fibromuscular dysplasia.

Risk of rupture <7 mm aneurysm is nearly zero if no previous SAH, 7–12 mm risk is 14–25% and over 25 mm is 40%.

Examination

- Fever and meningism is uncommon in early stages but irritability is common.
- Cranial nerve signs 3rd nerve palsy (posterior communicating artery aneurysm).
- 6th nerve palsy (posterior fossa aneurysm or increased intracranial pressure).
- Neck rigidity, bilateral leg weakness (anterior communicating artery aneurysm).
- Dysphasia/hemiparesis (middle cerebral artery aneurysm).
- Subhyloid hemorrhages, hypertension with tachycardia.

- Consider SAH in any patient presenting with worst severe headache of sudden onset peak in one minute, stroke with neck stiffness or coma.
- 8% of cervical artery dissection present with thunderclap headaches.
- Conventional angiography may be useful if MRI, MRA, CTA are normal and headache persists or worsens or if other symptoms appear to search for occult intracranial arterial dissection, cerebral vasoconstriction syndrome or vasculitis.
- Reversible cerebral vasoconstriction syndrome (RCVS)—Thunderclap headache (acute and severe) with or without focal deficits or seizure, uniphasic course without any new clinical symptoms more than one month, segmental constriction of cerebral arteries on MRI or CT angiography, no evidence of aneurysmal subarachnoid hemorrhage, normal CSF protein <1 g/L, WBC <15 × 10^6, normal glucose and normal cerebral arteries on repeat MRI or CT in 3 months. Half the cases occur during the postpartum period or exposure to serotonergic agents or cannabis. Most patients have multiple thunderclap headaches that recur every day or so for few days to 4 wks. Pain lasts from five minutes to few hours. Usual triggers are sexual activity, emotion, exertion, coughing, straining, urination, bathing and showering. Sixty percent of sexual headaches are due to RCVS and the treatment is rest for few days to two wks.

Acute Hydrocephalous

- This may occur 24 hrs post-ictus and presents with sluggish pupillary response and bilateral downward deviation of eyes (sunset eyes) and 1 point drop in GCS scale. CT should be repeated and neurosurgical option should be sought.

MANAGEMENT

- *Airways*: Assess, maintain and give high concentration O_2.
- *Breathing*: Assess and support. Laryngoscopy and intubation causes severe hypertension and may precipitate rebleeding. So do not intubate unless the patient has arrested except by anesthetic technique.

- *Circulation*: Assess, support and gain intravascular (IV) access. Most patients will be hypertensive; do not attempt to lower BP.

Indications for Intubation

- Airway or breathing compromised.
- Hypoxemia not corrected by high concentration of O_2.
- GCS 8 or less.
- Hyperventilation with $PaCO_2$ <3.5 kPa.
- Hypoventilation with $PaCO_2$ >6 kPa.

GRADING OF SUBARACHNOID HEMORRHAGE (SAH)

- Grade 1—GCS 15 conscious patient with or without meningism
- Grade 2—GCS 13-14 drowsy patient with no significant neurological deficit
- Grade 3—GCS 13-14 drowsy patient with neurological deficit
- Grade 4—GCS 7-12 deteriorating patient with major neurological deficit
- Grade 5—GCS 3-6 moribund patient with extensor rigidity and failing vital centers.

PRIORITIES

- Resuscitate A (airways) B (breathing) C (circulation)
- Analgesia—Codeine phosphate 30-60 mg oral or IM or midazolam. Avoid aspirin.
- Intravenous morphine can be titrated with care preceded by metoclopramide 10 mg.

INVESTIGATIONS

- CT head, transport patient after stabilization and adequate monitoring with escort.
- LP should only be performed if CT is normal (as minor bleed may not be detected), and performed >12 hrs after the onset of headache unless meningitis is suspected (xanthochromia present in supernatant from 12 hrs-2 wks after the bleed).
- If confirmed inform the neurosurgeons.
- Other investigations U and E, FBC, coagulation screen, ECG and chest X-ray if aspiration pneumonia suspected.

PREVENTION AND TREATMENT

- Good fluid intake IV normal saline 3–3.5 L/day. Morphine 2–4 mg IV 2–4 hrly with metoclopramide or codeine 30–60 mg IM 4 hrly for pain.
- PPI, TEDS, Nimodipine oral or nasogastric (or IV through central line initially 1 mg/hr increased after 2 hrs to 2 mg/hr) 60 mg 4 hrly for 21 days (started with in 4th day of SAH).
- Nimodipine may cause hypotension, if systolic BP <110 mm Hg then decrease the dose or omit till BP recovers.
- Keep arterial SBP 90–140 mm Hg using IV labetalol or nicardipine.
- Laxatives for soft stools.
- Hyperglycemia and hyperthermia should be corrected. Ted stockings or sequential compression device should be used.
- Endovascular coiling in elderly, poor medical conditions and aneurysm of vertibro basilar artery. Clipping for wide base aneurysm, large parenchymal hematoma.
- Prophylactic anticonvulsants for 1 wk.
- Delayed neurological deficit/spasm usually occurs day 4–12.
- Rebleeding 4% in first 24 hrs and then 30% in the first month.
- Definitive treatment is to secure the aneurysm by clipping at craniotomy or by coiling when cerebral angiography is performed.
- Raised intracranial pressure (hematoma or hydrocephalous) is treated surgically.

NEUROLOGICAL DETERIORATION OR COMPLICATIONS

- Check U and E.
- Hyponatremia may occur due to cerebral salt wasting syndrome and not SIADH.
- If Na is normal get
- CT, possibilities are
  - Recurrent hemorrhage 10% in first 2 wks,
  - Vasospasm causing cerebral ischemia 25% day 5–14
  - Communicating hydrocephalous 15–20% from 1 wk to 8 wks after the bleed.

SCREENING

For unruptured intracranial aneurysms surgery is done in patients with two 1st degree relatives with SAH or in patients with adult polycystic kidney disease and a family history of SAH.

Small incidentally found aneurysms are at very low risk of rupture but aneurysms over 7 mm and in certain locations are at significantly higher risk of rupture as are those small aneurysms in patients with prior SAH from another aneurysm.

Epilepsy (Status Epilepticus)

- Drugs for status epilepticus
  Lorazepam 4 mg IV, oral, PR or diazepam 10 mg IV or PR, phenytoin or leveteracitam.
- Drugs for generalized epilepsy.
  Lamotrigine, topiramate and valproate.
- Drugs for refractory generalized epilepsy
  Clobazam, levetiracetam.
- Drugs for partial epilepsy
  Carbamazepine, gabapentin, lamotrigine, levetiracetam, topiramate and valproate.

FIRST EPILEPTIC SEIZURE

It is due to abnormal and excessive discharge of cortical neurons. Most epileptic seizures last <2 minutes and any fit lasting >5 minutes is treated as impending status epileptics. Epilepsy is defined more than on seizure.

Previous history of nonconvulsive seizure should be elucidate such as epileptic aura (rising epigastric sensation lasting seconds), psychic epileptic aura déjà vu (already seen) or jamais vu (never seen) a false impression that a present experience is familiar or nocturnal seizures (bed wetting, tongue biting, blood on the pillow, early morning headache or hangover with out alcohol), if any of these present then the diagnosis is epilepsy rather than first epileptic seizure.

Life time risk of seizure for normal population 8–10% and epilepsy 3%.

After single provoked (<7 days from insult) seizure relapse is 3–10%,

After unprovoked seizure the relapse is 44% in 1st 6 months and 32% in the next 6 months.

After 2nd unprovoked seizure the relapse is 70–80%.

Differential diagnosis: Tongue bite on the lateral side and post-ictal confusion suggests seizure. Tonic and clonic movements lasting >1 minute and deep cyanosis indicates likely seizure.

First seizure should be differentiated from vasovagal syncope and cardiac syncope by above mentioned two features (postictal confusion, tongue bite on the side, eyes are usually open and head or eye turning to one side). The mechanism of jerky movements is cerebral hypoxia originating from midbrain and convulsive movements are common in syncope.

Risk Factors for Recurrence

Fever, alcohol, withdrawal, preexisting brain damage, head injury, drugs, hypoglycemia, electrolyte disturbance, brain infection, stroke, intracranial hemorrhage, proconvulsive drugs (clozapine, maprotoline, tramadol, theophylline, baclophen, antidepressants, anticholinergics and prochlorperazine), sleep deprivation, tumors and focal neurological damage.

Driving after First Seizure

- Restriction of activities (swimming in deep water, taking bath alone, scuba diving and climbing).
- Noncommercial drivers stop driving for 6 months and commercial driver free of seizures for 5 yrs. After the 2nd seizure it will be 12 months for noncommercial drivers and 10 yrs for commercial drivers.
- Seizure is career ending in air pilots and HGV drivers, so 2nd opinion should be asked.
- History is the main diagnosis.
- EEG and MRI for unprovoked seizure. EEG shows abnormalities in 70% within 24-48 hrs and less after that.

MRI or CT scan is mandatory if:
- Focal seizure in onset
- Focal neurological signs
- >20 yrs of age or elderly
- More than one seizure
- Failure to recover

- Fever and other neurological signs or Todd' paresis (paresis of arms or legs or speech lasting less than 48 hrs after the generalized seizure).

Epilepsy

- Recurrent (>2) unprovoked epileptic seizures.
- Partial (focal), simple—No impairment of consciousness.
- Partial (complex)—Impairment of consciousness and secondary generalized.
- Generalized—tonic-clonic.
- Myoclonic and absence (petitmal).

Admit

- If >1 seizure in 24 hrs.
- Failure to recover fully after seizure.
- Pregnancy associated or postpartum seizure.
- Associated with rash, fever, severe postictal headache, confusion, hallucination, drowsiness, focal neurological symptoms and signs (of recent onset).

Causes

- Established epilepsy (sub therapeutic drug concentration, intercurrent illness, metabolic disturbance, progression of neurological disease). Exclude syncope as it can cause myoclonic, tonic/clonic movements and occasionally reflex anoxic seizures. Biting of the side of the tongue or the inside of the mouth is specific for seizures. Tip of the tongue can be bitten in syncope. Urinary incontinence merely reflects the bladder was full when patient lost consciousness.
- *Acute CNS disease*: Infection (encephalitis, meningitis, trauma, stroke including SAH, tumor progression and hypertensive encephalopathy).
- *Metabolic disturbance*: Poisoning (tricyclic antidepressants, cocaine and ecstasy), alcohol withdrawal, lack of sleep, hypoglycemia, hyponatremia, hypocalcemia, hypomagnesemia, uremia, liver failure and acute porphyria.

STATUS EPILEPTICUS

- Generalized tonic-clonic fits lasting more than 30 minutes or repeated fits without recovery of normal

alertness in between. Consider after 5 minutes of tonic-clonic seizures or anybody gets in the hospital and still fitting.
- In 58% of patients it is the first seizure. Prompt treatment is needed to prevent complications (cerebral hypoxia, neurogenic pulmonary edema, rhabdomyolysis, acute renal failure, hyperkalemia, temporal lobe cell loss, lactic acidosis, hepatic necrosis, DIC and death).
- *Differential diagnosis*: Blackouts (vasovagal syncope or simple faint), cardiac syncope, postural hypotension, hypoglycemia and pseudoseizures.

SYNCOPE

- Typical warning (unless cardiac cause), often external triggers, collapse usually short motionless, few sometimes myoclonic jerks can occur, incontinence can occur, rapid recovery without confusion.

Pseudoseizures or Nonepileptic Attack Disorder (NEAD)

Differentiate it from epileptic seizures, gradual onset, no cyanosis, asynchronous bilateral movements of the limbs, forced eyes closing, pelvic thrusting, thrashing, side to side movements of the head intensified by restraint and prevention of hand falling on the face. No incontinence or tongue biting. Normal tendon reflexes, planter response and no postictal confusion. Patient usually female (8 : 1), often childhood abuse and abnormal illness behavior.

Nonconvulsive Status (NCS)

Difficult to diagnose, complex-partial status presents as behavior change, long lasting stupor, staring, unresponsiveness and eye twitching. In patients with previous diagnosis of epilepsy, any prolonged change in personality, prolonged postictal confusion (>20 minutes) and recent onset of psychosis. Diagnosis relies on clinical suspicion and EEG. Treated with antiepileptic barbiturates, benzodiazepine and topiramate.

Management

- Recovery position, airways—assesses; maintain high concentration of O_2.
- *Breathing*: Assess and support.

- *Circulation*: Assess IV access.
- Check blood glucose, if low give 20% 50 mL dextrose IV. In chronic alcoholics or poor nutrition give thiamine (Pabrinex one ampoule IV) 250 mg before or shortly afterwards to prevent Wernicke's encephalopathy.
- Use 0.9% sodium chloride and avoid 5% dextrose if blood glucose is normal.

Drugs

Self-terminating, brief, single seizure do not require treatment unless pre-existing neurological disorder or an abnormal EEG or two or more seizures in 24 hrs at presentation. If oral route not available then RR, IV or NG enteral route should be considered.

- Lorazepam 4 mg (2 mg in elderly) IV/PO/PR, slowly or midzolam 5–10 mg buccal or diazepam 10 mg IV slowly or PR or diazepam emulsion (diazemules) IV 10–20 mg (5 mg/min).
    - Can be repeated once after 30 minutes or diazepam rectubes 0.5 mg/kg (0.25 mg/kg in elderly) rectally, repeated 12 hrly if necessary.
    - Can cause hypotension or respiratory depression. Flumazenil (benzodiazepine receptor antagonist) must be immediately available if using IV benzodiazepine.
    - Diazepam binds wkly to BDZ receptors, peak concentration 3–15 minutes post IV, rapid fall in plasma levels and after repeated dosing respiratory depression.
    - Lorazepam binds strongly to BDZ receptors more effective as rapidly as diazepam, long duration of action and little risk of accumulation.
- Phenytoin (pht) or Fosphenytoin (Fospht)—Fospht 1.5 mg = 1 mg pht 2nd line therapy if seizures continues 10 minutes after lorzepam or diazepam if the patient is not likely already loaded with phenytoin. Loading dose (adults) phenytoin 15 mg/kg (elderly 10 mg/kg) is given at the rate 50 mg/min. Give as IV infusions diluted to 100 mL 0.9% normal saline and flush the IV cannula with normal saline before and after the infusion. Fosphenytoin infusion does not need cardiac monitoring, equal efficacy, can be given IM and increased costs offset by reduced adverse events. Maintenance dose 100 mg tds.

- Levetiracetam IV 200-400 mg. Consider IV sodium valproate in hypotensive and elderly patients.
  - If the patient was taking phenytoin before, give phenobarbitone IV 10 mg/kg to a maximum of 1000 mg at the rate of 50-75 mg/min, diluted with water 1:10. Maintenance dose 1-4 mg/kg/day as IV or IM or oral.
  - *Drugs used in generalized epilepsy*: 1st line—valproate 200-400 mg bid, kepra 500 mg bid, lamotrigine. Ethosuxcimide (for absent seizures), carbamazepine 200-400 mg bid (may worsen absence seizures). Sodium valproate is teratogenic in pregnancy so carbamazepine is used in pregnancy. 2nd line—levetiracetam, clobazam, oxcarbazepine.
  - *Drugs used in focal onset epilepsy*: Carbamezapine (Oxcarbazapine), lamotrigine, valproate, topiramate. 2nd line—Phenytoin, levetiracetam, gabapentin.
- 3rd line refractory status call duty anesthetist for thiopentone or propofol.

Urgent Investigation

- Blood glucose, U and E, Ca, Mg, LFT, gamma GT, urine drug screen? FBC and coagulation screen and ECG to exclude cardiac arrhythmia.
- EEG for patients <25 yrs and no brain imaging if the diagnosis is idiopathic generalized epilepsy.
- CSF if CNS infections/SAH suspected.
- Brain imaging is recommended, if focal seizures, focal signs, middle age/elderly, >1 seizure and fever.
- Prolactin is not to be relied upon unless raised >3 times the normal then suggestive of generalized epilepsy.

General Measures

- Epilepsy cannot be diagnosed after a single seizure.
- For unprovoked 1st seizure, two-yr recurrence risk is 30-40%.
- Treatment is only indicated if there is underlying structural lesion or positive EEG spike and wave.
- Consider MRI or CT (if strong suspicion of structural lesion) either inpatient or outpatient.

Headache

MIGRAINE (6–18%)

Repeated attacks of unilateral pulsatile headache usually in <40 yrs or at menarchy, over frontal, temple with aura (80%) or without aura (20%), lasting 4–72 hrs. Headache begins within 60 minutes of aura symptoms and lasts more than 60 minutes.

- Normal physical examination
- No other reasonable cause for headache
- At least two of the following unilateral pain, throbbing pain, aggravation of pain by daily activity and moderate to severe intensity of pain
- At least one of the following:
  - Nausea or vomiting or photophobia or phonophobia.

Triggers

Stress, hormones, dehydration, lack of food, fatigue, lack of sleep.

Patients with following symptoms need neuroradiological investigations:

- Fundamental change in pattern or progression in headache
- New onset of headache after 50 and/or the worst headache (sentinel headache of intracranial aneurysm, SAH or carotid arterial dissection).
- New onset of headache awakening one from sleep or in the early morning. Personality change or worsening of headache with coughing, sneezing or straining.
- Abnormal physical examination results (neurological) unless longstanding.
- Neurological symptoms such as clumsiness or weakness lasting >1 hr.
- Onset of seizures or headache associated with systemic illness including fever.
- New headache in patients with cancer or immunosuppressed or pregnancy.
- Headache associated with alteration in or loss of consciousness.
- Headache triggered by exertion, sexual activity, or valsalva manoeuvre. Severity is a poor marker of secondary headache.

- Bilateral nonthrobbing headache without nausea and with no sensitivity to light (photophobia) or sound or smell should be investigated by scan.
  - *Basilar migraine*: Parasthesia in hands, ataxia and collapse in <50 yrs.
  - *Hemiplegic migraine*: Weakness of one side of the body, several attacks, fully reversibility and family history. If recurrent then for topiramate.
  - *Analgesic headache*: Analgesic intake >15 days/month. Treated by withdrawal of analgesics.
  - *Status migraines*: Attack of migraine with headache lasting more than 72 hrs despite treatment. Treated with sumatriptan 6 mg subcutaneous or 20 mg intranasal spray.
  - Migraine is head pain with associated features and biological features while tension headache is featureless head pain without biological features.

Treatment

- Triptan + NSAID or paracetamol
- Aspirin 600–900 mg or ibuprofen 400–600 plus domperidone 10 mg or prochlorperazine 3–6 mg or metoclopramide. Not codeine.
- Diclofenac suppository 100 mg+ domperidone suppository 30–60 mg.
- *Triptans*: Sumatriptan 6 mg subcutaneous or 20 mg nasal spray or rizatriptan 10 mg disintegrating tablet.

Emergency

Chlorpromazine IM 25–50 mg + metoclopramide 10 mg and IM diclofenac 75 mg.

Prophylaxis

Frequent attacks >2 attacks/month, frequent very long auras, not responding to acute drugs.
- Propranolol, metoprolol. Caution asthma, depression.
- Flunarazine
- Lisinopril, candesartan
- Amitriptyline 10–150 mg.
- Na valproate 600–2000 mg/day, topiramate 25–100 mg/d.
- Gabapentine 300–800 mg tds, methysergide 1–2 mg tds (caution retroperitoneal fibrosis).
- Beta-blockers plus amitriptyline is most effective.

CHRONIC TENSION HEADACHE

Tension headache is caused by activation of hyperexcitable peripheral afferent neurones from the head and neck muscles. Chronic recurrent pain usually in 40–50 yrs, bilateral, pressing or tightening of mild to moderate intensity, diffusely all over the head described as tight band or pressure over the head or as if my head is bursting. It is a daily occurrence lasting 30 minutes to 7 days worse in the evening, not aggravated by routine physical activities (walking or climbing), no nausea or vomiting and no visual symptoms. Pericranial muscle tenderness is common finding.

Treatment

Aspirin 500–1000 mg, NSAID, paracetamol (slightly better than placebo).

Preventive treatment: For more than 2 attacks a month amitriptyline 75–150 mg/day. Some benefit with mirtazapine, tizanidine and alpha agonist.

Medication headache: Patients taking opoids or combination analgesics for more than 10 days a month or simple analgesics more than 15 days a month.

Cluster Headache

Daily bouts of unilateral boring or stabbing or aching headache in clusters lasting 4–16 wks at a time, mostly in men (10 : 1) often at night 1–2 hrs after going to sleep lasting 45 minutes–1 hr. It may occur during the day at the same time. Ipsilateral blood shot and red eyes with profuse watering, blocked nostril and transient Horner's syndrome are seen in 25% of patients.

COITAL HEADACHE

- Type 1 male, bilateral dull pain, increases in severity as the sexual excitement, is due to tensing of face, neck and shoulder muscles.
- Type 2 vascular cause, onset at orgasm, fades by 2 hrs. 25–50% has migraine or family history (FH) of migraine. 4–11% of SAH occurs during sexual activity.

BENIGN INTRACRANIAL HYPERTENSION

- Young obese female, diplopia, mild bilateral 6th nerve palsy.

- Headache episodic in onset develops over wks to daily pains of moderate intensity, worse in the morning, physical activity and postural change, pulsatile tinnitus, transitory visual obscurations, nausea, blurred vision and diplopia.

Treatment: (Lowering intracranial pressure) Weight loss, acetazolamide, furosemide, topiramate and surgical options of shunting and optic nerve sheath fenestration.

Causes of Thunderclap Headache

Subarachnoid hemorrhage, cerebral venous thrombosis, carotid artery dissection, pituitary apoplexy, ischemic stroke, acute hypertensive crisis, colloid cyst of 3rd ventricle and infections.

TEMPORAL ARTERITIS (GIANT-CELL ARTERITIS)

Headache over the superficial inflamed temporal or occipital artery with raised ESR >50. Rarely below 50 yrs of age. It is more common in women than men. M : F 2 : 1. Visual disturbance 7–60% if untreated. Loss of vision can occur abruptly and hence this disease is treated as medical emergency.

Touching the skin (combing hair) causes pain and sometimes arterial pulsation is lost and artery becomes hard tortuous and thickened. Jaw claudication may be present. May have systemic symptoms like fever, weight loss, anorexia and malaise.

Instantaneous thunderclap headache followed by depressed consciousness is characteristic of sub arachnoid hemorrhage.

Temporal artery biopsy shows giant cell infiltration of the wall and the blood vessels are involved in a patchy pattern.

Treatment is high dose steroids beginning with 40–60 mg/day (60 mg/day if visual symptoms or jaw claudication otherwise 40 mg/day for 4–6 wks) on the earliest suspicion of the disease (even before the diagnosis is confirmed by biopsy) to prevent the blindness. Prednisolone dose is lowered after 4–6 wks (depending on ESR) by 10 mg every 2 wks till 20 mg and then 2.5 mg every 2–4 wks till on 10 mg/day and then 1 mg every 1–2 months. Treatment usually lasts 1-2 yrs. Chest X-ray every 2 yrs to exclude aortic aneurysm.

Malaria

- *Plasmodium (vivax, malariae, ovale, falciparum)* cause 300–500 million infections/yr.
- Most of the deaths (1–3 million) are caused by *Plasmodium falciparum*.
- Transmitted from human to human by anopheles mosquito bite.

CLINICAL FEATURES

- Travel history is important.
- Fever, chills, rigors and headache are usually present but not always.
- Unusual presentation such as diarrhea, vomiting, abdominal pain and cough are common in children.

SEVERE MALARIA

- Incubation period 7 days. Anemia, jaundice, renal dysfunction, hemostatic abnormalities, thrombocytopenia, pulmonary edema, shock, hypoglycemia and severe metabolic acidosis are common in severe malaria. Pregnancy increases the risk.
- Cerebral malaria is diagnosed when there is altered conscious state (which is not due to convulsions, sedatives, hypoglycemia or other nonmalaria cause). There is cyto adherence and cytotoxin along with excessive cytokines (TNFa) due to infection.

INVESTIGATIONS

Full blood count (FBC), thick and thin films, schizont in the film means high risk of cerebral malaria and poor prognosis. Leukopenia and thrombocytopenia are common. Rapid diagnostic Test (based on *Plasmodium falciparum* antigen histidine rich protein 2) has 93% sensitivity and 98% specificity.

TREATMENT

- No schizont, malaria count low and not vomiting.
- Quinine 600 mg tds for 3 days + doxycycline 100 mg daily for 7 days.
- Severe malaria Parasitemia >2% and temp >39°C requires IV treatment with quinine sulfate.

- IV quinine 10 mg/kg in 250 mL dextrose 4 hrly for 12 hrs. Loading dose increased to 20 mg/kg if increased parasitemia and IV artesunate if parasitemia >10%.
- Quinine can also be given rectally or deep intramuscular in anterior thigh but not intragluteal.

Spinal Cord Compression

HISTORY

- Leg weakness developing over days or hrs. Sensory symptoms with a level.
- Bladder symptoms.

CAUSES

- Back pain with intervertebral disc prolapse
- Malignancy
- Infections (TB)
- Transverse myelitis
- Anterior spinal artery thrombosis or dissection of aorta involving anterior spinal artery.

ANTERIOR SPINAL ARTERY THROMBOSIS

Common in thoracic area, acute paralysis with weakness below the lesion, dissociated sensory loss (loss of pain and temperature as lateral spinothalamic tract is involved while posterior column is supplied by the posterior spinal artery, so position vibration are intact), loss of sphincter function (urinary retention).

Urgent neurosurgical referral if rapid deterioration.

Examination

- Motor: Increased tone, hyper-reflexia and weakness.
- Sensory: Look for sensory level which can be suspended. Sensory loss in saddle area suggests cauda equina
- Is bladder palpable?
  Emergency chest X-ray, MRI spine, FBC, U and E, LFT, inflammatory markers, coagulation screen, immunoglobulin, protein electrophoresis and urine Bence-Jones proteins.

Treatment

- Nurse on pressure relieving mattress.
- Bladder care and catheterization if in retention.
- Surgical decompression in disc prolapse.
- For abscess drainage and antibiotics (Cephotaxime 1-2 g 12 hrly plus Flucloxacilline 1-2 g 6 hrly plus metronidazole 500 mg 8 hrly.
- For spinal cord injury—methylprednisolone 30 mg/kg IV over 1 hr followed by 4.0 mg/kg/hr for 23 hrs.
- Steroids if transverse myelitis suspected.
- Antibiotics for 4 wks if myelitis is suspected due to lyme disease, (doxycycline, amoxicillin in children, erythromycin in pregnancy, ceftriaxone, minocycline).
- Case History—45 yr old 2 wks history of progressive lower limb weakness and numbness.
- On examination—Distal limb weakness and reflexes retained. Diagnosis—myelitis, MRI central cord lesion, oligoclonal band in CSF, treated IV methyl-prednisolone and recovered.

Spastic Paraparesis

There is weakness, increased tone, brisk reflexes, clonus in both legs, plantars are extensors and there may be disuse atrophy and contractures in severe cases. There may also be signs of radiculopathy at the level of the lesion. Ask about sphincter disturbance and exclude acute cord compression which is acute with asymmetric weakness by MRI.

Guillain-Barré usually presents with distal tingling of lower limbs progressing upward with symmetrical weakness. Breathlessness in a Guinne-Barré patient suggest respiratory failure and can be progressive. Check stool and serology for campylobacter jejuni. CSF shows raised proteins and normal cells. Nerve conduction shows absence or impersistence of F-wave. There is presence of GQ1b antibody in the blood and it responds to IV immunoglobulin 0.4 gm/kg daily for 5 days.

Acute pain with weakness suggests herniated disc, spinal SAH or aortic dissection involving spinal arteries. Fever and rigors suggest infection, e.g. osteomyelitis, epidural abscess or TB. Anorexia and weight loss suggest malignancy. Check protein electrophoresis and Bence-Jones proteins to exclude myeloma.

Brown-Sequard Syndrome (Hemisection of Spinal Cord)

Spastic weakness (monoplegia or hemiplegia) with brisk reflexes (lesion through corticospinal tract) and loss of proprioception and vibration and fine touch (ipsilateral to lesion) and loss of pain and temperature on contralateral. Level of sensory loss gives lesion level. Ask about sphincter disturbances (bowel, bladder).

MRI spine is the image of choice

Causes: Same as for spastic paresis, spinal cord tumor, trauma, ischemia, infections, demyelination and degenerative vertebral diseases.

Acute Inflammatory Polyneuritis, Guillain-Barré Syndrome (GBS)

HISTORY

- Most common cause of flaccid weakness, macrophage stripping of myelin sheath which blocks nerve conduction and causes weakness.
- Sensory symptoms begin distally and ascend symmetrically.
- Mainly progressive motor weakness usually ascending but can be proximal, symmetrical. Sensory symptoms mild and only paraesthesia in hands and fingers.
- Muscle pain in lower back or inter scapular is common.
- Legs usually worse affected.
- Progression occurs over days (no longer than 4 wks)
- Patient often give history of acute URTI, diarrhea.
- Consider in any patient with paraesthesia in fingers and toes, weakness of arms or legs, respiratory failure, generalized areflexia and preceding history of infection (Epstein-Barr virus [EBV], cytomegalovirus [CMV], mycoplasma, campylobacter, HIV and Hepatitis B and C).

EXAMINATION

- *Motor*: Lower motor neurone muscle weakness distal > proximal, areflexia, reduced tone. Being unable to walk poor prognostic sign rarely facial involvement and opthalmoplegia.

- *Miller-Fisher syndrome*: Opthalmoplegia, ataxia, limb weakness and absent reflexes.
- *Sensory*: Glove stocking sensory disturbance often mild.
- Respiratory failure due to muscle weakness is avoidable by checking forced vital capacity (FVC) frequently.

CASE HISTORY

Twenty-six year old with 2 wks history of back pain preceded by URTI. Now presents with progressive lower limb weakness, Respiratory Rate 32, bilateral facial weakness, distal limb weakness and areflexia—diagnosis GBS.

Diagnosis

- High index of suspicion and areflexia.
- LP after 1/52 of symptoms looking for elevated protein >1 g/L but no increase in cells. If >10 cells/micro liter suggests alternative diagnosis (leptomeningeal malignancy, encephalitis or HIV).
- Anti GQ1B antibodies present 95% in Miller-Fisher syndrome.
- Nerve conduction studies—absent F waves.
- Peripheral demyelination starts proximally in the nerve roots, hence distal conduction velocities and motor latencies are often normal very early in the illness, even when there is profound weakness in distal muscles.
- Stool culture and serology for *Campylobacter jejuni*.
- Antibodies for atypical pneumonia.
- CSF for virology.

Monitor for vital capacity (at least 4 hrly), O_2 saturation, cardiac monitor, swallow test, TED stocking and blood test to include CK, ESR and immunoglobulins.

Differential Diagnosis

- Vasculitis, spinal cord disease, acute intermittent porphyria, low Na, K, Mg, Lyme disease and paraneoplastic syndrome.
- *Acute spinal injury*: Flaccid areflexia, absence of sphincter disturbance.
- *Complete cord compression*: Sensory loss, flaccid paralysis, areflexia initially (hyper-reflexia, spasticity, positive plantar reflex in days to months), <5% chance of recovery if no improvement within 24 hrs.

- *Conus syndrome*: Saddle anesthesia, dull ache, impaired sphincter function, bilateral foot drop, absent ankle jerk, large midline disc is the cause.

Management of GBS

- Monitor ECG and treat arrhythmia as appropriate. Consider elective assisted ventilation sooner than later if the patient is tiring.
- Vital capacity 4 hrly and watch for fatigue.
- ITU if VC 1-1.2L
- Avoid tracheal suction as it can trigger hypotension or bradycardia because of autonomic dysfunction.
- Watch for DVT/PE, constipation, urinary retention, arrhythmia, labile swings of BP.
- If gag reflex absent, stop oral feeds, for IV and early consideration of PEG.
- Nonsteroidal anti-inflammatory drug (NSAID) for pain and also consider amitriptyline or carbamazepine or gabapentin.
- TED stockings and enoxaparin for thromboembolism prophylaxis.
- IV immunoglobulin (IG) 0.4 g/kg/day for 5 days.
- Repeat course in 6/52 in fluctuant responding GB or 4-6 plasma exchange.
- IG contraindicated in renal failure or IGA deficiency.
- Significant weakness remains in 10% of cases.
- Steroids are not helpful.

Myasthenia Gravis (MG)

Fluctuating weakness, easy fatigability and diurnal variation causing ptosis, diplopia, weakness of jaw movements, swallowing, chewing and sometimes nasal regurgitation. Muscles that control breathing, neck movements and limb movements can also be affected. It is an autoimmune disease of neuromuscular junctions caused by decreased number of acetylcholine receptors (AchRs) due to antibodies and these IgG antibodies are T cell dependent.

An immune response to muscle specific kinase (MuSK) also results in MG by interfering with AchR clustering. In 85% weakness is not confined to ocular muscles but is generalized affecting asymmetric proximal muscles with preserved tendon reflexes. MuSK positive patients usually have bulbar weakness or generalized MG. Acetylcholine receptor (AchR) antibodies present in 85% but 50% in ocular MG. 40% of negative AchR antibodies have positive MuSK antibodies.

On EMG rapid decrement on repetitive stimulation (pyridostigmine stopped 6-24 hrs before). Tensilone test initial 2 mg IV if no response than 8 mg (if other tests AchR antibody and EMG do not give definite diagnosis) with full resuscitation equipment and atropine available.

For ocular or cranial MG CT or MRI of brain is done to exclude intracranial lesion. Myasthenic crisis can be precipitated by infection, reduction of medication and initiation of steroids. In this patient look for paradoxical breathing, bubbly cough and check FVC (make sure adequate lip seal) if <1.5 L call anesthetist, if <1.0 L then intubate. Ocular MG presents as diplopia and ptosis.

Congenital MG presents in infancy or childhood, negative for AchR antibodies and are due to genetic mutation and not autoimmune disease and responds to 3-4 diaminopyridine or quinidine but not to anti-AchE (acetyl choline esterase).

DIFFERENTIAL DIAGNOSIS

- Drug induced MG (penicillamine used for RA or scleroderma).
- Lambert-Eaton myasthenic syndrome (LEMS) presents with proximal muscle weakness, depressed or absent reflexes, diplopia and ptosis like MG but strength increases on repetitive use.
- Antibodies against P/Q calcium channels present in 85%.
- Present in oat cell carcinoma of the lung.
- Treated with 3-4 diaminopyridine or anti AchE or immune suppression like MG.
- 75% have thymic abnormalities including thymoma and are excluded by CT chest.
- Test for thyroid functions, thyroid antibodies, rheumatoid arthritis and antinuclear antibodies (ANA) should be done.

Treatment

Pyridostigmine (blocks breakdown of Ach), effect begins 15-30 minutes and lasts 3-4 hrs with the dose 30-60 mg

3 or 4 times daily. Side effects include stomach cramps, nausea and diarrhea. Atropine or loperamide can be given for these side effects.

Thymectomy: In all patients from puberty to 55 with generalized MG. Patients with MuSK antibodies positive MG do not respond to thymectomy.

Immunosuppression: (Steroids, Azathioprine, IV IG, plasmapheresis, cyclosporine, and tacrolimus) blocks the effect of antibodies, clinical improvement within from one to 3/12. Steroids initial dose 15-25 mg as a single dose, dose increased 5 mg every 3rd day, until marked clinical improvement or dose of 50-60 mg is reached. Dose is maintained for 1-3 months and then changed to alternate day regime over 1-3 months. Mycophenolate or azathioprine used to reduce the dose of steroids.

Plasmapheresis or IV IG can be used in MG crisis usually triggered by infections and patient should be treated like other immunocompromized patients.

DELIRIUM

Delirium is the most common cause of disturbed behavior and acute confusional state (1% <55 yrs and 42% >70 yrs), in medically ill, frail elderly, postoperative and terminally ill patients.

Diagnostic Features

- Lowered consciousness with variability from minute to minute and hour to hour in alertness (psychomotor agitation or retardation) and marked fluctuations (patient has disturbed behavior at night but quite lucid during daytime). It should also be considered when patients are described as confused, vague, poor historian or uncooperative. Patients with dementia may become delirious with minor physical problem like constipation.
- Impaired cognition (that cannot be accounted for evolving or established dementia) is central, affecting memory, orientation, attention and planning skills. Disorientation to time, place, day and person are common. Hence the history from 3rd party essential to differentiate from dementia (presence of rapid and

drastic decline). Impaired attentiveness can be tested at the bedside by asking to count backward from 20 or recall reverse days of the week or months of the year or draw a clock. Delusions are often fleeting and persecutory and hallucinations (visual and auditory) are strongly suggestive of delirium.

- Delirium develops over short period of time with fluctuations over day and night. A behaviorally disturbed patient with night time agitation and wandering around the ward is easy to recognize but apathy and hypo activity is equally common. A sudden worsening of confusion in a patient with established Alzheimer's disease may be due to superimposed delirium. Complete resolution of symptoms occurs in only 4% before discharge and 20% at 3 months.

Confusion assessment method (CAM) score:
- Acute onset and fluctuating course
- Inattention (difficulty in keeping focussed)
- Disorganised thinking (rambling speech, incoherent)
- Altered level of consciousness (hyper alert/drowsiness).

Delirium requires 1 and 2 + either 3 or 4. Two distinct subtype of delirium are recognized:
- Agitated variant with psychomotor over activity such as plucking at bed clothes or aggression.
- Quiet variant when patient appears apathetic and withdrawn. This is easily missed or misdiagnosed as depression.

There is cholinergic deficiency and dopaminergic excess in delirious patients. This explains the onset of confusion with anticholinergic drugs and its increased incidence in Alzheimer disease.

	Delirium	Dementia
Onset	Acute or sub-acute	Insidious
Course	Fluctuating, revolving over days or wks	Progressive
Conscious level	Often impaired, can fluctuate rapidly	Clear until late stages
Cognition	Poor short-term memory, poor attention span	Attention less affected
Hallucinations	Visual common	Often absent
Delusions	Fleeting	Often absent
Psychomotor activity	Increased or unpredictable	Can be normal

Neurological Emergencies

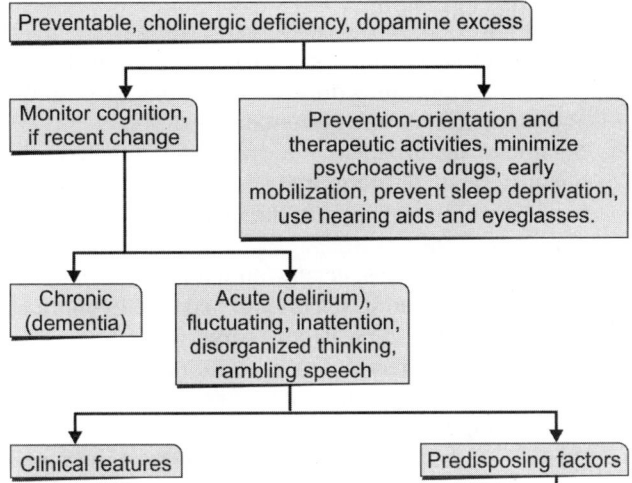

Its prevalence in hospitalized medically ill patients is 25–31%. Most at risk are elderly patients, postoperative and terminally ill patients.

Precipitating Factors

- Any acute severe illness, congestive cardiac failure (CCF), common infections (chest, urine, skin, joints and meninges) or urine retention.
- Metabolic disturbances, i.e. hypoxia, hypoglycemia, hepatic, renal or pulmonary insufficiency, hypo or hyper thyroidism, hypopituitarism and hypo or hyperparathyroidism.
- Any medication (especially anticholinergics), withdrawal of medication (alcohol or sedative hypnotics), any trauma (including elective surgery).
- Vascular disorders (TIA's, cerebral thrombosis, embolism and migraine, any anesthetic or environment change.

Prescribed drugs are implicated in 40% of cases and should always be considered 1st, particularly anticholinergics, sedating drugs (benzodiazepine) and narcotic analgesics. Withdrawal from alcohol or sedative hypnotics is the most common cause of delirium in hospitalized patients.

Diagnosis—Is cognitive impairment new or worse → No, evaluate as dementia ↓

Yes, has new medication started or old medication stopped or has localizing symptoms of infection.

On examination if focal or literalizing neurosigns → neuroimaging if meningeal irritation → Lumbar puncture, also exclude congestive cardiac failure (CCF), infection, dehydration and malnourishment.

DELIRIUM TREMENS

Associated with alcohol withdrawal, delirium with prominent anxiety and autonomic hyperactivity and these may be associated with metabolic disturbances and fits. Delirium with ataxia and opthalmoplegia should receive urgent IV thiamine to prevent Wernicke's encephalopathy.

MANAGEMENT

- Treat the underlying cause. Drug treatment should be used when essential.
- Haloperidol 0.5 mg or 1 mg or 1.5 mg plus lorazepam 1 mg tds for 3 days.
- Haloperidol and lorazepam can be given intramuscular (IM).

- Supportive care—Poor care promotes aggression.
- Calm carer, quiet well lit room with wall clock, calendar, promotion of self-care and freedom from restraint.
- Minimize polypharmacy.
- Family members taking shifts at bed side vigil.
- Correcting sensory impairments (providing hearing aids or glasses).
- Safe environment (removing objects with which patients could harm himself or others).
- Response should be monitored daily and when stable for few days then dose tapered and stopped.
- Prolongation of QTc on ECG and torsades de pointes can occur with high doses of neuroleptics if there is concomitant electrolyte disturbance.

Cerebellopontine Angle Syndrome

Any combination of cranial neuropathies involving trigeminal, facial and vestibulocochlear nerve may occur. Corneal reflex loss is often the 1st sign then facial sensory loss. Facial weakness is a late sign. There may be nystagmus and sensory neural deafness. Acoustic neuroma, meningioma may cause slowly progressive hearing loss or tinnitus.

Cerebellopontine angle (CPA) is a triangle between cerebellum, lateral Pons and Petrous bone. Cranial nerves 5–8 emerge through it.

Horner's Syndrome

It is due interruption of sympathetic chain anywhere.
- There is partial ptosis (levator palpebrae of upper lid is supplied partially with sympathetic nervous systems well as parasympathetic which travels with the 3rd nerve).
- Miosis (reduced pupil dilator activity).
- Anhydrosis in preganglionic lesions (sweat gland out flow is proximal to superior cervical ganglion).
- Enopthalmos (due to paralysis of upper and lower eye lid tarsus muscles).

Sympathetic fibers in posterior hypothalamus → spinal cord → ventral roots T1-2 → ascend through sympathetic chain → superior cervical ganglion → post ganglionic fibers ascend with carotid artery → ophthalmic artery → radial muscle of iris (dilator of pupil).

Causes

- *1st neurone*: Starts at hypothalamus brainstem—spinal cord C8 T1.
- Brain stem stroke (lateral medullary syndrome as sympathetic pathway lies close to spinothalamic tract).
- Demyelination in brainstem or spinal cord (other signs to look for are internuclear ophthalmoplegia, cerebellar signs, spastic para paresis and sensory disturbance.
- Syringomyelia/syringobulbia and spinal cord tumors.
- *2nd neurone or preganglionic neurone*: Sympathetic pathway from C8T1 to superior cervical ganglion (SCG).
- Pan coast tumor, cervical rib, a mediastinal mass, cervical lymphadenopathy, thyroid masses and complication of neck surgery.
- *3rd neurone*: Postganglionic sympathetic pathways travels from SCG in close proximity to carotid artery and innervates the pupil via long ciliary nerves.
- Carotid artery aneurysm and carotid dissection.

Ptosis

- Check for equal pupils, eye movements and whether ptosis is partial or complete, unilateral or bilateral.
- Complete (need to retract the lid), unilateral ptosis (dilated pupil and eye down and out) is highly suggestive of 3rd nerve palsy.
- Partial ptosis with small pupil, consider Horner's syndrome.
- Normal pupils with partial unilateral or bilateral ptosis consider myasthenia gravis, congenital ptosis and myotonic dystrophy.

Vertigo

It is an illusion of movement; balance depends upon visual, vestibular and proprioceptive inputs to the brainstem, cerebellum pathways and cerebral cortex.

Causes

Peripheral

Vestibular neuronitis, benign paroxysmal positional vertigo (BPPV), Meniere's disease, otitis media, cholesteatoma.

Central

Vertebrobasilar ischemia (ischemia of brainstem and cerebellum), demyelination and space occupying lesion affecting brainstem and vestibular connections.

Dix-Hall pike test: Patient sits on the couch in such a position that when recumbent, head will hang over the edge. With head rotated to 45° to one side, lie the patients back rapidly until the head is dependent. This induces nystagmus within 30 sec, which is self-limiting.

Vestibular neuronitis: Common in young and middle aged, previously well, usually after URTI and may be due to isolated degeneration of vestibular nerve. Hearing loss is unusual.

Marked vertigo usually in morning on waking up with nausea and vomiting. Horizontal or rotatory nystagmus may be present. Symptoms resolve in a few days as vestibular compensation occurs.

BENIGN PAROXYSMAL POSITIONAL VERTIGO (BPPV)

Recurrent episodes of vertigo provoked by change in head position, turning in bed, bending over or extending the neck. Nausea may occur but seldom vomiting. There is no hearing loss or tinnitus. It may be triggered by infection, vasculitis or trauma. Often there is no cause and is common in the 6th decade and Dix-Hall pike test is positive.

Vertigo in BPPV has short latent period, rapidly fatigued on repeat testing, short lived, self-limiting and usually causes nausea, while central vertigo is immediate, persists till underlying cause is treated and main symptom is severe imbalance.

MENIERE'S DISEASE

Vertigo, tinnitus and hearing loss, affects young people and cause is unknown. Differentiate between vertigo, presyncope (sensation of impending loss of conscious) and postural unsteadiness.

Peripheral Neuropathy

- Impairment of sensation to light touch, vibration, joint position and pinprick over stocking and to a lesser extent glove distribution. There may be distal wasting, weakness and a reflexia.
- If patient's signs and symptoms are motor only then consider motor neurone disease. In adults usually presents UMN and LMN dysfunctions.
- Autonomic dysfunctions (fainting, orthostatic light headedness, heat intolerance, bladder, bowel and sexual dysfunctions) in the absence of diabetes consider amyloidosis.
- If severe pain is the symptoms, then consider, diabetes neuropathy, GBS, peripheral nerve vasculitis, diabetic amyotropathy (sudden onset of back, hip and thigh pain and weakness).
- If there is severe loss of vibration and position and good power consider ganglionopathy (Para neoplastic, Sjögren syndrome, HIV).
- Sub-acute combined degeneration (SACD) due to B_{12} deficiency is symmetrical and also has UMN sign along with it.

Symmetrical proximal and distal weakness with sensory loss: Guillain-Barré (inflammatory demyelinating), and chronic inflammatory demyelinating.

Symmetrical distal sensory loss with or without weakness: Metabolic disorders, drugs, toxins, cryptogenic, amyloidosis and hereditary (Charcot-Marie-Tooth).

Asymmetrical distal weakness with sensory loss: Vasculitis, infections (Lymes disease, leprosy, HIV), compression neuropathy.

Asymmetrical proximal and distal weakness with sensory loss: Diabetes, carcinomatous, idiopathic and hereditary neuropathy.

Asymmetrical distal weakness without sensory loss:
- With UMN signs—motor neuron disease.
- Without UMN signs—progressive muscular atrophy, multifocal motor neuropathy.

Symmetrical sensory loss with distal areflexia and UMN signs—B_{12} deficiency.

Symmetrical weakness without sensory loss—with proximal and distal weakness—spinal muscular atrophy and with distal weakness-hereditary motor weakness.

Asymmetric proprioceptive sensory loss without weakness—Sensory neuropathy (ganglionopathy).

Causes

Take a drug history and full medical history to exclude, diabetes, alcohol, connective tissue diseases, chronic renal failure (CRF) liver and thyroid disease.

- Diabetes mellitus (look out for punched out foot ulcers), predominantly sensory.
- Drugs phenytoin, metronidazole, INH, ethambutol, vincristine, nitrofurantoin, gold, amiodarone, hydralazine, chloramphenicol and cyclosporine (predominantly sensory).
- Polyarteritis nodosa (PAN), RA, SLE, vasculitis, Guillain-Barré syndrome (these cause multiple mono neuropathy which require urgent immune suppressive therapy).
- Amyloidosis, AIDS, carcinomatous neuropathy, sarcoidosis, myxoedema, uremia.
- Carcinomatous neuropathy (cachexia, clubbing).
- Vitamin B_{12} deficiency, sub-acute combined degeneration (SACD) paraesthesia of feet, signs of peripheral neuropathy, absent ankle jerks, extensor plantar and Romberg's test positive (unable to stand with feet together and eyes closed).
- Vitamin B deficiency (alcoholics).
- Hereditary sensory motor neuropathy (HSMN 1) Charcot-Marie-Tooth disease. A severe predominantly motor with marked wasting (inverted champagne bottle legs), clawing of toes, pes cavus and marked bilateral high stepping gait due to bilateral foot drop. Ask for family history.

If symmetrical predominant motor neuropathy exclude Guillain-Barré syndrome. This can cause severe acute ascending paralysis involving legs, arms, chest and bulbar muscles.

Pathogenesis

- Autoimmune demyelination of peripheral nerves, secondary to mycoplasma infection of chest or *Campylobacter jejuni* of GI tract some wks previously.
- CSF protein is raised with normal white cells.
- IV immunoglobulin ± steroids hasten recovery.

Miller-Fisher syndrome: Variant of Guillain-Barré syndrome, areflexia, ataxia and ophthalmoplegia.

Demyelinating neuropathy: Usually motor, velocity is slowed but amplitude is preserved on nerve conduction studies. Chronic inflammatory demyelinating poly radiculopathy, HSMN 1, paraproteinemia (myeloma) and pressure palsies.

Axonal neuropathy: Sensory or mixed, loss of pain and temperature sense, burning or pricking neuropathic pain. Velocity is normal but amplitude is decreased on nerve conduction. Diabetes, alcohol, metabolic (Chronic renal failure, liver and thyroid disorders), SACD, vasculitis, carcinoma, drugs and toxins.

Investigations

Blood glucose, U and E, LFT, FBC, ESR, B_{12}, Folate. TSH, angiotensin converting enzyme (ACE), protein electrophoresis, ANA, ENA, ANCA, chest X-ray, Bence-Jones proteins, CSF proteins, oligoclonal band, Anti HIV antibodies, anti neuronal antibodies (HU, YO), antimyelin antibodies, antigliadin and nerve conduction studies.

Autonomic neuropathy presents as postural hypotension, constipation, urinary incontinence, sexual dysfunction.

Diabetic amyotrophy—Pain, wasting, weakness in one or both quadriceps in diabetes, caused by microvasculitis in lumbosacral plexus.

Median Nerve Palsy (Carpal Tunnel Syndrome)

Stout middle aged lady has pain, numbness and paresthesia in palm and fingers and this is worse at night. There is sensory loss over the 1st three and half fingers and wasting of thenar eminence. There is also weakness of abduction, flexion and opposition of thumb. She has median nerve palsy.

Presence of flexion of distal interphalangeal joint of thumb (noninvolvement of flexor muscles of forearm) suggests cause is carpal tunnel syndrome.

Signs

- Tinel's sign
  - Percussion over carpal tunnel (over the course of median nerve) produces tingling over distribution of the nerve.
- Phalen's sign
  - Flexion of both wrists for 60 sec produces exacerbation of paraesthesia, rapidly relieved by discontinuing flexion. Sometimes symptoms can be produced by hyperextension of the wrist. Both these tests are unreliable.
- Tourniquet test
  - Pressure above systolic pressure for 2 minutes produces symptoms.
- Nerve root supply to the median nerve C6-T1.

Causes

- *Idiopathic*: Obese middle age female with excessive use of hands.
- Pregnancy, contraceptive pill.

Myxedema

Thickened, coarse facial features, periorbital puffiness, skin rough dry and cold, hoarse and croaking voice, slow pulse, delayed ankle jerks, hard of hearing and thinning of hair.

Acromegaly

Large lower jaw, prominent supra orbital ridges, enlarged nose, tongue and ears, large doughy hands and voice is husky and cavernous. May also have bitemporal field defects.

Other causes are RA, OA of carpal bones or fracture of wrist, forearm or elbow, primary amyloidosis and tophaceous gout.

A nerve conduction study imperative before surgical decompression.

Ulnar Nerve Palsy

Hand shows generalized muscle wasting and weakness except the thenar eminence. Dorsal guttering (hollow 1st web space due to 1st dorsal interossie being affected) is noticed.

There is sensory loss over the 5th and adjacent half of 4th finger and medial side of hand (both dorsal and palmer side). Look for hyperextension at the metacarpal phalangeal (MP) joint due to paralysed lumbricals of ring and little finger with flexion at the interphalangeal joint due to intact flexor digitorum profundus (FDP) muscle group (ulnar claw hand).

Clawing of hand is usually seen in low ulnar nerve lesion. There is weakness of adduction and abduction of fingers and thumb. Nerve root supply of ulnar nerve is C8T1.

Causes

- As for all mononeuropathies consider diabetes, connective tissue disease and vasculitis.
- Fracture dislocation of elbow.
- Osteoarthritis of the elbow with osteophyte encroaching ulnar nerve, occupants constantly leaning on elbow.
- Mononeuritis multiplex diabetes, polyarteritis nodosa (PAN).
- *Churg-Strauss syndrome*: Eosinophilic granulomatous vasculitis similar to PAN but asthma, eosinophilia, raised IgE and pulmonary infiltrates are prominent and may present as asthma.
- RA, SLE, amyloidosis, leprosy, Sjögren's syndrome (dryness of mouth, keratoconjunctivitis sicca and autoimmune disease) or autoimmune liver disease or fibrosing alveolitis.
- Lyme disease (tick bite infection presenting as skin rash as large erythematous ring with central fading lasting 2 days to 3 months, malaise, cognitive impairment,

lymphadenopathy, arthralgia or erosive arthropathy, myocarditis, heart block, meningitis, neuropathy, cranial nerve palsy, amnesia. Diagnosed by serology and treated with doxycycline 100 mg 12 hrly or amoxicillin for 21 days or IV penicillin + ceftriaxone for neurological presentation).

DIFFERENTIAL DIAGNOSIS SYRINGOMYELIA

Dissociated sensory loss (loss of pain and temperature) extending beyond the ulnar zone, wasting and weakness of small muscle of hand, loss of arm reflexes and Horner's syndrome (sympathetic neurone C8/T1), nystagmus if lesion above C5 involving MLF (medial longitudinal fasciculus). Lower limb reflexes are brisk and planters are extensors.

C8 lesion-sensory loss involves the radial side of 4th finger.

Radial Nerve Palsy

Wrist drop and sensory loss over 1st dorsal.

Patient is unable to lift at the wrist or straighten out the fingers, but if wrist is passively extended the patient can extend the fingers at interphalangeal joints (interossei and lumbricals still work) but not at MP joints. Intact triceps reflex indicates lesion below the spiral groove. Absent triceps reflex implies high axillary or C7 radiculopathy. C7 root lesion causes weakness of shoulder adduction, elbow extension, wrist flexion and wrist extension while a radial nerve lesion does not affect shoulder adduction or wrist flexion.

Grasp is weak and adduction and abduction of fingers may appear weak but improves after extending the wrist passively.

Causes

- Saturday night paralysis (nerve compressed against the humerus. If the nerve is injured in axilla then triceps reflex is lost.
- Fracture humerus and fracture, dislocation at the wrist.

Foot Drop (Common Peroneal Nerve Palsy)

Wasting of anterior tibial and peroneal group of muscles and the patient cannot dorsiflex or evert the R/L foot. There is loss of sensation over the outer side of calf and gait is altered because of foot-drop.

Sciatic nerve has two branches, peroneal and tibial nerve. Ankle reflex is conveyed through tibial nerve (S1), and therefore spared in peroneal nerve lesion.

Common peroneal nerve has two branches superficial (supplying sensation to lateral calf, dorsum of the foot, peroneus longus and brevis) while deep supplying sensation to triangular area between 1st and 2nd toe dorsally, anterior tibial muscles and extensors of the toes.

Causes

- Injury to nerve at the head of the fibula by fractures or plasters, tourniquets, sometimes by squatting or crossing legs.
- Old polio, other causes of mononeuropathy, e.g. diabetes, vasculitis, autoimmune diseases.
- Charcot-Marie-Tooth disease (pes cavus atrophy of muscle of leg which stop abruptly half up the leg, weakness of extensors of toes and feet, absent ankle jerks and planters' no response, wasting of small muscles of hand and palpable lateral popliteal or ulnar nerve).
- Rarely lead poisoning.

If ankle jerks are absent along with foot drop then sciatic nerve lesion and S1 radiculopathy is likely and the cause is disc prolapse.

CERVICAL MYELOPATHY

Crepitus, restricted neck movement and neck pain without neurological symptoms is common over 50, but constant dull ache, numbness and paraesthesia in the forearm and wrist is common presentation of cervical myelopathy. Hands may feel weak and clumsy with weakness of legs.

Legs show spastic weakness, increased tone, brisk reflexes, clonus may be present, plantar extensors. Vibration and position sense may be lost in the lower limbs due to compression of dorsal column (DC), spinothalamic loss (pain, temperature) may sometimes occur. Sphincter functions are usually normal.

In the upper limb there is asymmetrical inversion of biceps and supinator jerks (when trying to elicit biceps and supinator reflexes (C5/6), there is brisk finger flexion when eliciting triceps reflex, despite absence of supinator and biceps reflexes. Triceps reflexes and finger flexion is usually brisk (C6/7) UMN signs below the lesion C5/6.

Cervical spondylosis usually affects C5/6 or 6/7 because of narrowing of the canal in this region. There is segmental wasting and weakness of muscles of hand if there is associated radiculopathy but no gross wasting as small muscles of the hand are supplied by C8/T1. There is often no sensory loss in the hands though sometimes patient may complain of unpleasant numbness and paraesthesia.

Lhermitte's phenomena (tingling or electric feeling or funny sensation passing down spine and lower limb on flexion of spine) or reverse (on extension of cervical spine) may suggest cervical myelopathy. Disk prolapse is common in young to middle aged adults causing radicular pain at C5/6 or C6/7.

Differential diagnosis: Spinal cord tumor, sub-acute combine degeneration (SACD).

Treatment

Conservative management with cervical collar and physiotherapy but sometimes surgery is required.

Absent Ankle Jerks and Extensor Plantars

This implies combination of upper motor neurone (extensor plantar) and lowers motor neurone (absent ankle jerks).

Causes

- Sub-acute combined degeneration (SACD) of the cord, loss of vibration, joint position and light touch (dorsal column); weakness and extensor plantar and brisk reflex (Corticospinal tract), absent ankle jerk due to peripheral nerve damage. Spinothalamic tract (STT) is not affected.

- *Taboparesis*: Dorsal column and cortical spinal tract signs as above and STT is not involved. Look for AR pupil, Charcot's joints and optic atrophy.
- *Friedreich's ataxia (recessive spinocerebellar degeneration)*: Dorsal column (DC), cortical spinal tract (CST) signs as above and absent ankle jerks. Spinothalamic tracts are spared. Look for pes cavus, kyphoscoliosis and bilateral cerebellar signs with wide base ataxia. It is caused by increased number of GAA trinucleotide repeat sequence at a gene encoding 9q13 on chromosome 9. Most patients have hypertrophic cardiomyopathy, skeletal abnormalities, diabetes, visual and hearing problems.
- *Motor neurone disease*: Spinal cord anterior horn cell degeneration, cerebral motor pathways and brain stem nuclei causes combination of upper and lower motor neurone signs with prominent fasciculation. The resulting muscle wasting leads to progressive weakness of speech, swallowing, limb movements and respiratory movements. Often presents in arm or leg with mixture of upper and lower motor neurone signs and early fasciculation. Bulbar involvement causes drooling, dysarthria and nasal regurgitation. There is never sensory impairment, cerebellar and extrapyramidal signs.
- Combination of cervical myelopathy (extensor plantars), with diabetes (peripheral neuropathy) or lesion of conus medullaris.

Cauda Equina Syndrome

Flaccid weakness of lower limbs with loss of knee and ankle reflexes and normal flexor plantars with sensory loss below L1.

Causes

- Neurofibromatosis, expanding conus lesion, and lumber disc disease.
- Lumbosacral disc prolapse common over L4/5 and L5/S1. L3/4 root involvement cause anterior thigh pain, quadriceps wasting and absent knee reflex. Pain in the distribution of L4/5 or S1 may be due to lumber

disc disease but higher lumbar disc disease or lower sacral root damage is unusual due to disc disease.

Spinal Stenosis

Neurogenic claudication: Pain on walking or on standing in legs or buttocks or back is relieved by sitting. There is incontinence of urine when there is radiculopathy. 75% acquired (degenerative disease of spine) and 25% congenital.

Multiple Sclerosis (MS)

- Symptoms are worse in hot weather, after hot bath, during fever or after exertion as conduction is blocked in demyelinated axon by the rise in temperature.
- Incidence M: F is 1:3, occurring commonly 20–40 yr of age.
- The 1st symptoms are weakness (40%), optic neuritis (22%), parasthesia (21%), diplopia (12%), disturbances of micturition (5%) and vertigo 5%.

OPTIC NEURITIS

- In acute stage blurred vision, decreased color and acuity of vision, pain in or around the eyes on movement (retrobulbar neuritis) and central or para central scotoma lasting few days.
- Pupil show afferent pupillary defect (pupil react sluggishly when light shown in affected eye but both react briskly when light shown in the normal eye). Decreased visual acuity, papilledema in acute stage and temporal pallor of the disc is suggestive of optic atrophy.
- Repeated episodes of optic neuritis are common.

CERVICAL CORD

Tingling, paraesthesia and numbness are usual symptoms with impaired sense of position and vibration (dorsal column) and less often pain and temperature (lateral spinothalamic) or Lhermitte symptoms (brief tingling in legs or trunk or upper arms on flexion of neck due increased sensitivity of dorsal column fibers in or around the plaque).

Lhermitte symptoms can also occur after trauma, cervical cord tumor or B_{12} deficiency. Bladder symptoms as urgency, frequency or sometimes incontinence or constipation or urgency with soiling or impotence or ejaculatory failure may be present.

BRAINSTEM AND CEREBELLUM

- Visual disturbances other than optic neuritis, diplopia with 6th nerve palsy or internuclear ophthalmoplegia (lesion in median longitudinal fasciculus, incomplete adduction on lateral movement with possible nystagmus in the abducting eye).
- Nystagmus with ocular palsy (trigeminal neuralgia, facial nerve palsy) is common.
- Vertigo due to lesion in vestibular nuclei, ataxia (trunk or limbs) and dysarthria due to cerebellar involvement. Dorsal column and pyramidal signs may also be present.

PAROXYSMAL SYMPTOMS

- Brief episodes of diplopia, facial numbness, trigeminal neuralgia, vertigo, dysarthria, ataxia, brief tonic spasms affecting one or both limbs on one side, disturbed sensations or power in limbs, lasting a minute or two and several times a day is due to brief discharges from demyelinated patch.
- Risk of relapse is reduced in pregnancy but increased in postpartum for 3/12.
- Later on depression, intellectual impairment and disinhibition are present due to cortical involvement. Disabling cerebellar tremor, facial myokymia and bulbar involvement (dysarthria, dysphagia and dysphonia) are late features.
- Lower motor neurons are rarely affected.

Pathogenesis

There are focal patches of inflammation and demyelination (breach in the integrity of blood brain barrier in a genetically predisposed individual with up regulated adhesion molecules on endothelial cells) in brain and spine that lymphocytes (type 1 helper T cells Th1 with inter leukin12 and 23) can traverse the vessel wall to enter white matter to cause inflammation in myelin antigen. There is edema, demyelination and remyelination on remission but remyelination does not compensate for myelin loss. Eventually there is scarring and axon loss.

Factors associated with axonal damage are cytokines, nitric oxide (NO), proteases, super oxides, CD8T cells and glutamate excitotoxicity.

Plaques single or multiple can be present in optic nerve, brain stem, cerebellum, periventricular and cervical spinal cord.

Slowing of conduction and axonal loss leads to permanent disability.

Diagnosis

- Magnetic resonance imaging (MRI)
- Oligoclonal band (gamma 4 and gamma 5) in CSF.
- These are synthesized locally and may be present also in neuro sarcoidosis or syphilis.
- Visual, auditory or somatosensory evoked potential.

Treatment

- Short course of high dose steroids (methyl prednisolone IV 1 gm daily for 3 days) speeds recovery from relapse.
- Interferon 1b in relapsing and remitting disease reduces disease activity by 30% and delays progression of disability.
- Natalizumab is recombinant humanized monoclonal antibody that antagonises A4B1-integrin. Indicated as monotherapy in relapsing/remitting disease, 2 or more relapses in 1 yr with one or more gadolinium-enhancing lesion on brain MRI or significant increase in T2 lesion load compared with previous MRI and has failed to respond to interferon.
- Dose is 300 mg IV every 4 wks for 2 yrs.
- Glatiramir (synthetic peptide mimicking myelin) may also delay progression.

Symptoms Control

- Fatigue (Planned rest, modafinil),
- Bladder symptoms (Oxybutynin or tolterodine or bladder botulinum toxin or catheterization).
- Spasticity (Baclofen or gabapentin or tizanidine or botulinum toxin), and sexual functions (Sildenafil).

Prognostic Factors

In 20% no disability after 5 yrs and in 75% runs a relapsing and remitting course. In 5% it is rapidly progressive. Average life expectancy is 20–30 yrs after the symptoms.

Older age, male sex, predominantly motor rather than sensory symptoms, increased number of relapses, incomplete remission and early disability carry unfavorable prognosis and should be treated aggressively.

Cord Compression

Sensory level, neck or back pain, no signs above the level. Sphincter function rarely disturbed. Often asymmetrical inversion of biceps and triceps reflexes. When attempt is made to elicit biceps or supinator reflexes, there is no response of supinator or biceps but there is brisk finger flexion and triceps jerk is brisk. This is because of pyramidal and lower motor neurone damage at C5/6 producing lower motor neurone signs at C5/6 level and upper motor neurone signs below.

Lhermitte's Phenomenon

- Tingling or electric feeling or funny sensations, which pass down the spine and lower limbs on bending head forward. It can occur in cervical cord tumor, cervical spondylosis with narrow cervical canal, SACD (subacute combined degeneration) and MS.
- Gross wasting of small muscles of the hand is uncommon due to cervical spondylitis as it mainly affects C5/6, 6/7 while small muscles are supplied C8/T1.

Motor Neurone Disease (MND)

- Clinical features are muscle fasciculation, weakness, wasting of muscles of hand, arms and shoulder and no sensory signs and never involvement of III, IV and VI cranial nerves (because of short axons). Reflexes may be exaggerated in upper limbs (Reflexes in MND may be increased or decreased or absent).
- There is spastic weakness in the legs with brisk reflexes, ankle clonus and extensor plantars (Amyotrophic lateral sclerosis).

- Progressive muscular atrophy (25%) where anterior horn cell lesion affecting distal muscles are affected (LMN) before proximal muscles.
- Patient also has nasal speech; fasciculating wasted tongue and palatal paralysis (progressive bulbar palsy 25%).
- *Cause:* Unknown
- *Diagnosis*: Think of MND in >40 with spastic gait or foot drop or weak grip or aspiration pneumonia. Look for involvement of upper and lower motor neurones signs in 2 or more limbs or limb +bulbar muscles.
- Motor neurone disease (MND) brains show high free radical damage and have excess glutamate levels and hence use of Riluzole in MND. It prolongs life by few months.

Other conditions where fasciculation can occur:
- Cervical spondylosis, syringomyelia, Charcot-Marie-Tooth (fasciculation less apparent, but atrophy stops abruptly in legs, pes cavus and palpable lateral popliteal and ulnar nerves).
- Neuralgic amyotrophy (pain, wasting and weakness of muscles in a shoulder C5/6 following a viral infection) and syphilitic amyotrophy (slowly progressive weakness of shoulder and upper arm with loss of reflexes and no sensory signs).
- After exercise in fit adults and benign giant fasciculation after tensilone test.

Syringomyelia

Syrinx (cavity) caused by a developmental anomaly (Arnold-Chiari malformation) or spinal cord injury yrs before, filled with CSF gradually enlarges compressing decussating spinothalamic fibers, anterior horn cells in ventral horn and corticospinal fibers.

Kyphoscoliosis, bilateral wasting and weakness of small muscles of hands (compression T1 nerve roots) and dissociated sensory loss (loss of pain and temperature) in the upper limbs and chest (spinothalamic tract) and usually is the earliest sign.

Reflexes are absent with hypotonia in upper limbs (anterior horn cells and nerve roots) with Horner's syndrome (sympathetic neurones C8/T1).

Dorsal column is usually spared so joint position; vibration and fine touch are preserved.

Scars on hands (from painless burns), spastic paraplegia with brisk reflexes and extensor plantar (rare involvement of cortico spinal tract).

There may be body asymmetry, hemihypertrophy or unilateral enlarged hands, podgy soft palms, stumpy fingers and coarse thickened skin (due to release of trophic factors).

Cold swollen dystrophic hands may occur due to autonomic vasomotor disturbances.

Charcot's joints in elbow or shoulder (Syringomelia), knees and hips (Tabes dorsalis) and toes and ankles (Diabetes mellitus).

Syringomyelia may extend to upper cervical and bulbar segments (Syringobulbia). Syringobulbia can present with nystagmus, ataxia, dissociated sensory loss and bulbar palsy (wasted fasciculating tongue, palatal paralysis, dysarthria, dysphagia, weakness of sternomastoid and trapezius.

Treatment after MRI is decompression of the cavity (syrinx).

Sub-Acute Combine Degeneration (SACD)

- Degeneration of posterior and lateral column of spinal cord due to vitamin B_{12} deficiency.
- Paraesthesia of feet with loss of touch, vibration and position sense over feet (and hands) and positive Romberg's sign.
- Legs may be weak.
- Brisk knee jerks (pyramidal disturbance), absent ankle jerk (peripheral neuropathy) and plantar extensors.
- Progressive lower extremity paraparesis with spasticity may occur in legs.
- Pupils are normal and no cerebellar sign.
- Vitamin B_{12} deficiency should be excluded in sensory neuropathy, spinal cord disease, optic atrophy and dementia.

Causes—autoimmune disease, partial or total gastrectomy, stagnant loop syndrome, ileal resection for Crohn's disease, vegan diet, fish tape worm, chronic tropical sprue and intrinsic factor deficiency.

Friedreich's Ataxia (Hereditary Spinocerebellar Degeneration)

- Usually autosomal recessive but in some families it is dominant, presenting as clumsiness in walking between 5-10 yrs of age. It is initially associated with loss of position and vibration sense, lower limb atrophy, loss of tone, absent reflexes and extensor plantar.
- Other features include pes cavus, high arched palate, kyphoscoliosis, ataxia, head shakes. Nystagmus, cerebellar signs and dysarthria.
- Cardiomyopathy (75%) leading to conduction defects and heart failure, optic retinal atrophy, diabetes mellitus and mild dementia are also seen.

	Friedreich's ataxia	*Ataxia due to MS*	*Ataxia due to Tabes dorsalis*
F/H	Major	Minor	None
Onset <15	Usual	Rare	Rare
Knee and ankle jerks	Absent	Brisk	Absent
Spine	Kyphoscoliosis	Normal	Normal
Feet shape	Pes cavus	Normal	Normal
Pupils	Normal	Normal	Argyll Robertson pupil
Plantars	Extensors	Extensors	Normal or decreased
Pain on deep pressure	Normal	Normal	Absent
Romberg's sign	Unequivocal	Negative	Positive

Taboparesis

Cause: Tertiary syphilis.
AR pupil
- Small irregular pupil, react to accommodation but not to light, bilateral ptosis.
- Wrinkled forehead due to compensatory over action of frontalis.
- Ataxic gait, Romberg's test positive.

- Loss of position and vibration sense and deep pain in Achilles tendon.
- Hypotonic and absent reflexes.
- There may be optic atrophy and risk of developing Charcot's knee and aortic incompetence.

Tuberous Sclerosis/Adenoma Sebaceum

Multisystem genetic disease causing hamartomas (nonmalignant) in the brain, kidneys, lungs, heart, eyes and skin. Papular salmon colored eruption (angiofibroma) in the face (butterfly area and nasolabial fold), appearing around age 4 and more prominent after puberty.

It is autosomal dominant and presents with epilepsy (75%) and mental retardation (50%), behavior problems, skin abnormalities, lung and kidney disease.

There are also shagreen patches (flesh colored lumpy plaques resembling studded leather on lower back), ungal fibromata (firm pink periungual papules under the nails), hypo pigmented macules as leaf shaped on the chest and buttocks.

Neurofibromatosis Type 1 (NF1, Von Recklinghausen's Disease)

There are multiple neurofibromatosis and café-au-lait spots (pigmented light brown macules, smooth edged, located on nerves) especially in the axilla or multiple skin lesions, sessile and pedunculated, fibromata and neurofibromata, soft and firm, single and lobulated felt as mobile subcutaneous lumps or nodules along the course of peripheral nerves.

Neurofibromin is a tumor suppressor gene whose function is to inhibit oncoprotein, the absence of which results in uncontrolled cellular proliferation and tumor development.

There are no more than five café-au-lait spots in normal persons.

It is usually asymptomatic, autosomal dominant and half of all cases are the 1st person in the family (*de novo* mutation due to variable expressivity) and penetrance is 100% by 5 yrs of age.

So children born to an affected parent if they have no cafe'-au-lait spots by five yrs then they have not inherited NF1.

NF1 gene on chromosome 17 encodes for protein neurofibromin.

Diagnostic criteria: Two or more of the following:
- Six or more café'-au-lait macules >5 mm in prepubertal and >15 mm in diameter in postpubertal. 10% of the population have 1-2 spots.
- Two or more neurofibroma of any type or one plexiform neurofibroma.
- Freckling in the axillary or inguinal region.
- Optic glioma
- Two or more lisch nodules (iris hamartoma).
- A distinct osseous lesion as sphenoid dysplasia or thinning of long bone cortex with or without pseudoarthrosis.
- First degree relative (parent or sibling or offspring) with NF1 by above criteria.

Clinical Features

Neurofibromas are of 2 types:
1. Dermal neurofibroma lie with in dermis and epidermis and move passively with the skin and the majority appear discrete nodules, soft to palpate and violatious color. Dermal neurofibromas rarely cause symptoms and are not at risk of malignant change but can cause considerable distress to patient.
2. Other type nodular neurofibroma (incidence 5-10%) arising on major peripheral nerve trunk are much firmer consistency and frequently cause neurological symptoms and need to be removed by neurosurgeons. Multiple nodular neurofibromas are at risk of developing malignant peripheral nerve sheath tumors (MPNST).

Common problems with NF1 patients are learning, behavior and coordination problems. 50% of patients never develop disease complications.

NF1 affects mortality at all ages, particularly <40 because of late complications.

As patient are reassured with sciatica only to present later as cauda equina compression, or headache with hypertension as warning sign of Pheochromocytoma and presenting later with intracerebral hemorrhage.

Complications

- Many of the complications occur in childhood, so children with NF1 should have annual review. Referral for genetic counseling for families when diagnosis is made is helpful.
- Because of lack of ability to predict severity and variability of the condition many couples decide to have a family without testing.
- Both preimplantation and prenatal diagnosis are available.
- Kyphoscoliosis, pressure effects of neurofibromata on peripheral and cranial nerves.
- Acoustic neuroma (Vth, VIth, VIIth, and VIIIth nerve lesion), nystagmus and cerebellar signs may be present which may be bilateral.
- Vth nerve neuroma
- Spinal nerve root involvement,
- Cord compression, muscle wasting, sensory loss (Charcot's joint), sarcomatous or other malignant change.
- Other intracranial tumors like gliomata (optic nerve and chiasma), meningioma and medulloblastoma.
- 5% of cases are associated with pheochromocytoma.
- NF2 is also autosomal dominant, gene is on chromosome 22, and bilateral vestibular schwannoma is a feature in all patients, is rare and causes significant morbidity and mortality. Presents as hearing loss due bilateral acoustic neuroma around the age of 20 yrs.

Lateral Medullary Syndrome (Wallenberg's Syndrome)

- Infarction of a small wedge of medulla by posterior inferior cerebellar artery.
- Presenting as acute vertigo, ipsilateral Horner's syndrome (descending sympathetic), decreased touch, pain and temperature over face (V and lateral spinothalamic tract), cerebellar signs, palatal paralysis (diminished gag reflex, dysphagia, hoarseness (IX and X), and contra lateral side trunk and limbs decreased pain and temperature (lateral spinothalamic tract).

- Involvement of tractus solitarius and nucleus (located along the length of medulla oblongata that carry and receive visceral sensation from facial VII, IX and X cranial nerves) may also cause hiccup and loss of taste.
- Usually there are no pyramidal signs (hemiplegia) unless vertebral or basilar artery is occluded.

Median Medullary Syndrome

- Occlusion of vertebral or lower basilar artery or its median branch.
- Contralateral hemiplegia sparing face, contralateral loss of joint position, vibration and ipsilateral paralysis and wasting of tongue.

Gait Disturbances

Cerebellar Ataxia

Wide based gait (patient cannot stand with feet together and eyes open) and arms are held wide. Patient cannot perform heel-to-toe test and tends to fall right/left (R/L). Other cerebellar signs are finger-nose test, nystagmus, staccato speech, dysarthria and impaired rapid alternate motion (dysdiadochokinesia).

Causes:
- MS (pyramidal signs, pale discs).
- Tumors (primary or secondary from carcinoma bronchus or breast).
- Nonmetastatic complication of malignancy from carcinoma bronchus (clubbing, cachexia, nicotine stain fingers).
- Alcoholic and other cerebellar degeneration.

Friedreich's Ataxia

Pes cavus, high arched palate, intention tremors, nystagmus, dysarthria, head shaking, kyphoscoliosis, absent ankle jerks, extensor plantar and diminished position and vibration sense in feet.

Spastic Paraplegia

Patient has stiff, scissors or wadding through mud gait. Patient leans forward, legs adducted and walks stiffly on toes.

Causes: MS, cord compression, hereditary spastic paraplegia and cerebral diplegia.

Sensory Ataxia

Gait is wide based, ataxic, stamping, and worse on poor light. Difficult to walk heel-to-toe and Romberg's test is positive.

Causes: SACD (brisk knee jerks, absent ankle jerk, extensors plantars).

Tabes dorsalis (A-R pupil, bilateral ptosis with wrinkle of forehead, loss of joint position and vibration sense and deep pain in tendon Achilles).

Cervical myelopathy, diabetes, Frederick's ataxia.

Parkinsonian Gait

Patient with expressionless faces, unblinking, stooped, hesitant, shuffling gait. Hands show a pill-rolling tremor, arms is held in flexed position and do not swing. Gait is festinate (appears to be continually about to fall forward as if chasing his own center of gravity). He also has cogwheel rigidity and glabellar tap sign positive.

Foot Drop

Patient flexes his R/L hip, lifting the foot off the ground and slaps down noisily. He is unable to walk on his R/L heel.

Causes: Lateral popliteal nerve palsy, Charcot-Marie-Tooth disease (pes cavus, atrophy which stops suddenly half way up the leg, wasting of small muscles of the hand, and palpable lateral popliteal nerve), old polio (affected leg short as affected in childhood) and rarely heavy metal poisoning (lead).

Hemiplegic Gait

Right/left (R/L) leg is stiff, with each step patient tilts the pelvis to other side trying to keep the toe off the ground and R/L leg moves in a semicircle with the toe scrapping the floor. R/L arm is held in flexion, fist is clinched and foot is inverted.

Myopathic Waddling Gait

Patient has lumbar lordosis, walks with broad base and waddling gait (trunk moving side to side and his pelvis dropping on each side as the leg leaves the ground and toe touching the ground 1st).

Causes: Duchess muscular dystrophy, polymyositis and osteomalacia.

Apraxic Gait

Patient is able to move legs normally while sitting or in bed but walks broad base, short steps (placing his feet on the ground like a person walking on ice), difficulty in turning and tendency for retropulsion increasing the danger of falling.

Causes: Frontal lobe signs (suck reflex with patients closed eyes gently touch the upper lip with index finger) and grasp reflex (distract the patient by asking to count backward slowly from 10, and gently run the index and middle finger across the palm).

Dementia, Sub dural hematoma, normal pressure hydrocephalous and tumor.

Parkinson's Disease

Described in 1817 by James Parkinson.

It is slowly progressive neurodegenerative disease (2nd most common, the 1st being dementia) of substantia nigra (60% neuronal loss at the time of presentation). Neuronal cytoplasmic protein alpha synuclein normally unstructured and soluble can aggregate to form insoluble fibrils called lewy bodies is present in the remaining neurones in the substantia nigra.

About 10-15% of affected Parkinson's patients will have affected 1st or 2nd degree relative.

Cause is idiopathic although some atypical cases have genetic origin, autosomal dominant LRRK2 (leucin rich repeat kinase 2) and recessive genes Park 2.

Oxidative stress and mitochondrial dysfunction is the main mechanism.

Accumulation of unwanted proteins exceeding the capacity of proteasomes to clear those results in proteolytic stress and Parkinson's disease.

There is disturbed processing of amyloid precursor protein (APP) and this contributes to mild cognitive impairment. There is a low alpha synuclein level in blood and plasma.

There is loss of melanin containing neurones in pars compacta of substantia nigra and also cell loss in locus coeruleus, dorsal nuclei of vagus, raphe nuclei and nuclei basalis of meynert and some others catecholaminergic brain stem structures.

About 3-4% of cells of substantia nigra contain lewy bodies irrespective of duration and lewy bodies are constantly forming and disappearing.

The amount of cortical beta amyloid is the key factor for cognitive decline in Parkinson's disease. Long course of Parkinsonism before the onset of dementia is dependent on low plaque frequency and cortical lewy body count.

Cardinal Features

Fatigue and stiffness, stiff face, masked expressionless faces, a flexion of one arm, lack of swing, monotonous speech, smaller and cramped writing after a sentence or two and flexed posture.

Cog wheel rigidity and bradykinesia, involves upper body 1st and fluctuates in severity. Only lower limb rigidity with brisk reflexes is due to vascular Parkinsonism.

Unilateral onset, rest tremor, persistent asymmetry, progressive disorder, excellent response to L DOPA is the main feature of the disease

Shouting out at night or falling out of bed during dreaming (REM sleep) is treated with clonazepam.

If falling backwards, urinary incontinence, delirium, amnesia, speech and swallowing difficulty with in 2 yrs of diagnosis indicates other diagnosis.

Freezing of gait for several seconds when starting to move or when entering in a room is sometimes present in Parkinson's disease.

Chewing or swallowing difficulty and drooling of saliva are common.

Risk of dementia is high in patients with gait and speech disorders and poor response to L DOPA.

Risk Factors

Nonsmokers, low coffee intake, head injury, rural living, middle age, obesity, lack of exercise, and exposure of herbicide or insecticide, MPTP, cyanide and carbon disulfide.

Tremor

Rest tremor, asymmetric, pill rolling of hand, 4–6 Hz, at rest, usually seen on walking or doing fine finger movements of the other hand. It is worse in emotional situations or cold weather. Essential tremor is worse on action while Parkinsonian tremor disappears on action.

Some times DaT scan can (a fluorodopa positron emission tomography scan) can help to differentiate between these two tremors.

Rigidity

Cog wheel rigidity increases with distracting maneuver like patient tapping knee. Anxiety and delirium in acute stage can give rise to rigidity called gegenhalten.

Bradykinesia

Slowness of the movement with decreased amplitude, fatiguable in amplitude and frequency (tested by opening/closing fist or finger tapping finger and thumb or large hand movements 20s).

Bradykinesia of the foot is tested by foot tapping or walking.

Lack of arm swing, diminished gesturing in conversation, expressionless faces, slowing of speech, difficulty in rhythmic movements (as stirring tea, cutting food or rapid alternate movements), micro graphia, and drooling from mouth are other features.

Bradykinesia is confirmed with slowness, progressive reduction of speed and amplitude on sequential motor tasks.

Gait: Difficulty in starting, loss of arm swing with a mild flexion of the arm at elbow, festinate shuffling gait, flexed posture, difficulty in turning, loss of righting reflexes, falls, freezing on-off. Foot dystonia is in young patients along with infrequent blinking and tendency to drag one foot when walking.

Vascular Parkinsonism usually presents with severe gait initiation difficulty, broad base shuffling gate, rigidity of arms, mild bradykinesia (lower half Parkinsonism) and usually absent rest tremor and sometime responds to L DOPA.

Fatigue, hypotension, depression, soft monotonous voice, greasy skin, excessive sweating and constipation are late features.

Loss of postural reflexes is tested by asking the patient to take several steps backward.

In patients suspected of Parkinson's disease failing to respond up to 1200 mg L DOPA for 12 wks MRI is needed to exclude supra tentorial tumors and normal pressure hydrocephalous and extensive subcortical vascular pathology.

Exclusion Criteria

- Cerebellar signs
- Corticospinal tracts signs
- Eye movements' abnormality, inability to look upward or downward suggests progressive supra nuclear palsy (PSP).
- Presence of dementia or severe autonomic changes (incontinence, postural hypotension, impotence) at presentation or in early disease.

Differential Diagnosis

ESSENTIAL TREMOR (ET)

Autosomal dominant, usually bilateral, 6–12 Hz, postural or action tremor involving hand or head or trunk, legs or larynx, improves with alcohol, treated with Beta blockers and DAT scan is normal.

Drug Induced Parkinson's Disease

It is caused by neuroleptic agents, antiemetics (Metoclopramide, prochlorperazine), calcium channel blockers (Cinnarizine), fluoxetine, manganese (Mn), carbon monoxide (Co), cyanide, methanol, reserpine, amiodarone, lithium, valproate and antipsychotic medication can cause Parkinson's disease, after days or wks. Oxybutynin often causes confusion as it crosses the blood brain barrier while trospium does not.

Vascular Parkinsonism

Small vessel infarcts bilateral and should be considered in differential diagnosis of any patient with vascular risk factors.

Presents as falls or akinetic rigid syndrome with rigidity in both legs, symmetrical, without involving face and upper arms. While in idiopathic PD usually face and upper limbs are involved initially.

There is no tremor, short mincing steps, brisk reflexes, dementia and CT showing multiple infarcts or basal ganglia lacunars infarcts with history of hypertension or diabetes.

PARKINSONISM PLUS

- *Progressive supranuclear palsy (PSP)*: Presenting as akinetic rigid in proximal and distal limbs, UMN with cerebellar signs, no tremor, falls, slowness, unsteadiness, supranuclear ocular movements affecting downward gaze. Patient has prominent stare and furrowed brow.
- *Risk factors*: Recurrent head injury, vascular disease.
- It is due to deposition of neurofibrillary tangles of Tauprotien (micro tubule-associated protein) associated with degeneration of brain stem, basal ganglia and cerebellum.
- Responds poorly to antiparkinsons drugs.

Cortical Basal Degeneration (CBD)

- Asymmetric apraxia (loss of ability to carry out learned purposeful movement despite having desire and physical ability), rigidity initially unilateral but soon becomes bilateral, dystonia, bradykinesia, myoclonic jerk.
- Alien limb is characteristic.
- Progressive aphasia and after 2–5 yrs paraplegia in flexion is common.

Multisystem Atrophy (MSA)

Alpha synuclein positive inclusion bodies are present.
- Patient has Parkinsonism with tremor present symmetrically.
- Upper motor neuron (UMN) signs (spastic legs), pseudobulbar palsy, myoclonus, autonomic failure signs (hypotension), urgency, retention, incontinence, fatigue, impotence and cerebellar signs.
- Poor response to L-DOPA.
- Drug induced dyskinesia typically involve face and neck rather than limbs as in PD.

- Response to L-DOPA disappointing but some response to amantadine.
- Lewy bodies are present in substantia nigra, olive, pons, cerebellum, brainstem and spinal cord while in DLB (Lewy body dementia) they are present in brain stem and cortex.

LEWY BODY DEMENTIA (LBD)

- Fluctuating cognition with marked variation in attention and alertness, recurrent visual hallucination well-formed and detailed.
- Some features of Parkinson's disease with action tremor rather rest tremor are present.
- Often L-DOPA induces sedation, myoclonus and hallucination.
- There is cortical atrophy as in Alzheimer disease, but there is loss of pigmented neurones with presence of lewy bodies in the remaining neurones as in Parkinson's disease.
- Lewy bodies are present in cerebral cortex.
- There is overlap with Alzheimer's disease with the presence of plaques and tangles.
- Lewy body dementia (DLB) has neuroleptic sensitivity and responds well to anticholinesterase (Rivastigmine).
- DaT scan is positive in Parkinson's disease (PD), lewy body dementia, multisystem atrophy (MSA), progressive supranuclear palsy (PSP) and vascular parkinsonism (PD) but is normal in essential tremor (ET).

Treatment

- *Non-drug*: Occupational therapy, physiotherapy, speech and language therapy and dietician.

Drug Treatment for Parkinsonism

- *Levo Dopa with dopa decarboxylase inhibitor*: Within 5–10 yrs 50% develop dyskinesia, dystonia and motor fluctuations on-off. Usually L-DOPA for >65 yrs.
  - Modified: Release L-DOPA used in nocturnal motor problems.
  - Wearing-off symptoms can be motor (tremor, rigidity, bradykinesia, on-off) or non-motor (fatigue, mood changes, anxiety, pain and sensory

problems). Wearing off some times can be helped by adding entacopone or raselegiline 1.5 mg/day.
- Patients nil by mouth can have either rotigotine patches or Apo morphine subcutaneous or infusion.
- Duodopa (continuous infusion of levodopa gel) directly into jejunum after gastrostomy. Costs £30,000/yr. Monotherapy with duodopa has been shown to reduce 'off' periods and improve motor functions and quality of life compared with conventional multidrug regime.
- Anticholinergics are only used in young patients with tremor and are avoided in elderly.
- Memantine for cognitive deficits.
- *Dopamine agonist (DA)*: For < 65 with normal mental functions, neuroprotective, delays dyskinesia but causes more hallucinations in elderly.
    - *1st generation*: Bromocriptine, cabergoline, pergolide (Ergot derivative).
    - *Side effects*: Retroperitoneal, pericardial or pulmonary fibrosis, so less often used.
    - *2nd generation non-ergot (preferred)*: Ropinirole, pramipexole, rotigotine and piribedil. Once daily preparations often used are ropinirole XL and rotigotine patch in early and advanced PD.
    - Pulsatile stimulation of dopamine receptors is the cause of motor complications. Thus Duodopa, rotigotine and ropinirole XL are nonpulsatile continuous stimulation of dopamine receptors.
    - *Side effects*: Excessive sleepiness and sometimes suddenly falling to sleep.

DOPA Dysregulation (DDS)

Gambling, hyper sexuality, binge eating, compulsive shopping or punding or cognitive dysfunction. Drivers should be warned.

Treatment is gradual withdrawal of DA.
- *Apomorphine*: Potent dopamine agonist used to reduce dyskinesia and off periods. Given as intermittent S/C injections for <6 off periods/day or infusion for more frequent. Need to be on antiemetic before and costs £10, 00/yr/pt.

- *MAO-B inhibitors*: MAO-B inhibitors limit the central metabolism of Dopamine. Selegiline 5 mg or raselegiline, zelapar 1.25 mg (oral, fast, melts in mouth, 1st pass metabolism in liver), so fewer amphetamine like metabolites. Rasagiline is as effective as COMPT or DA and can be used with L-DOPA or DA in later disease. SSRI should be avoided with MAO-B inhibitors as it causes serotonin syndrome.
- Catechol-o-methyl transferase inhibitors (COMPT): Reduce the metabolism of L-DOPA to 3-o-methyl-dopa, in periphery thus increasing the amount of L-DOPA crossing blood brain barrier and increasing half-life by 30–50%. Entacapone (Tolacapone withdrawn in 1998 because of hepatotoxicity) only used as 1st line. It reduces off time and improves motor symptoms. If patient still having on off swings then tolcapone can be used on named patient basis as 2nd line oral therapy and monitoring the LFT.
- Amantadine usually used for L-DOPA induced dyskinesia. Side effects are confusion, hallucination, ankle edema, livedo reticularis and tolerance on long-term use.

  There is some evidence that DA, MAO-B inhibitors and coenzyme Q10 may slow the progression of the disease.

  For refractory cases Apo morphine pump is helpful. Early use of domperidone, nurse support and skin hygiene are essential. Eosinophilic panniculitis of abdominal wall and orthostatic hypotension is the limitation. Hemolytic anemia is the rare complication.

  Parkinson's disease with confusion or psychosis use benzodiazepines or small doses of quetiapine.
- *Surgery*: Bilateral sub thalamic stimulation in refractory motor complications in L-DOPA responsive patients with no mental illness.

  Behavior problems abulia, depression, reduced verbal fluency, apraxia of eyelid opening and difficulty in social adjustment has been seen after surgery.

  Infection needing replacement of pacemaker, intracerebral hemorrhage and suicide has been reported.

Parkinson's Disease and General Surgery

- Continue taking medication till induction. Advance planning.

- Calculate total L-DOPA by calculating ordinary L-DOPA + controlled release L-DOPA X0.7.
- If taking L-DOPA + COMPT X1.3, ropinirole X20, pramipexole or cabergoline or pergolide X100.
- If <350 mg L-DOPA use rotigotine patch dose = L-DOPA/20, If >350 mg use Apo morphine with domperidone.
- Consider regional anesthesia if frequent medication.
- Antiemetics to be avoided are metoclopramide, cyclizine and prochlorperazine, but domperidone, and ondansetron can be used.
- If patient has deep brain stimulation (DBS) avoid electrocautery but bipolar diathermy can be used.
- Soluble Madopar can be used via NG during surgery if no ileus.

Neuroleptic Malignant Like Syndrome (NMLS)

It is an adverse reaction to either neuroleptic drugs (haloperidol, chlorpromazine) in patients or withdrawal/omission of dopamine agonist or PD treatment.

Neuroleptic malignant syndrome (NMS) presents as hyperthermia, muscle cramp, tremor, rigidity, autonomic instability raised creatine kinase (CK), neuropsychiatric manifestations delirium or coma, altered consciousness and cardiovascular collapse, dysphagia, metabolic acidosis and hyper salivation.

Treated with dantrolene 2.5 mg/kg + alkalinization of urine with 1.26% with sodium bicarbonate + restarting the PD treatment.

Dementia (De-Ment) Apart Brain

Cortical (Alzheimer's disease, vascular dementia, Lewy body dementia, fronto temporal, alcohol, Korsakoff and Wernick encephalopathy).

Sub cortical (hypothyroidism, low B_{12}, Huntington disease, Parkinson's disease, low thiamine, low folate, subdural hematoma, hypoglycemia, hypercalcemia, AIDS and syphilis).

It is progressive impairment in memory, language (dysphasia, dyspraxia, reading, writing, naming), visuo-spatial skills and personality. Other features are getting lost, lack of awareness, decline in activities of daily living, sleep wake cycle disturbances, apathy and no disturbance in consciousness.

Investigations

Blood test for ESR, FBC, U and E, LFT, TSH, B_{12}, Folate, calcium, glucose, serology for syphilis, Borrelia, HIV.

CT or MRI, PET or SPECT in selected cases where diagnosis uncertain. EEG if CJD or transient epileptic amnesia suspected. Rarely CSF for cell count, protein, glucose, raised total Tau, increased phosphorylated-Tau, decreased amyloid B42.

ALZHEIMER'S DISEASE AB (BETA AMYLOID) IS THE CAUSE

- Amyloid precursor protein (APP) in membrane wall → cleavage by secretase alpha, Beta and gamma to produce amyloid B1-40 AB 1-42 aggregates more readily, more fibrillogenic and produced by gamma secretase.
- Oligomer 2-12 more toxic
- Toxic AB → changes in TAU (microtubule associated soluble protein which normally stabilizes microtubule of the neurone) → hyperphosphorelated and forms insoluble tangles. This causes disintegration of microtubule and collapse of neurone transport system.
- Tangles are more closely associated with severity of dementia than AB plaques.
- Genes have 70% effect on dementia.
- PSEN (presenaline gene) 1, PSEN2 and APOE4 have effect on secretase or clearance of AB plaques.
- Amyloid precursor protein (APP) present in membrane for synapse repair → Amyloid B42 more toxic than AB40 (plaque).
- TAU (membrane associated protein soluble present in axons) normally stabilizes microtubules in the distal part of axon, on hyperphosphorelation no longer stabilizes → impairs axonal transport and synaptic loss, Tangles and Alzheimer's disease (AD).
- 30% are over 75 and 50% over 85.
- Sudden onset or focal neurological signs or seizures or gait disturbances early in the disease makes it unlikely.

There is degeneration of temporal parietal region particularly parahippocampal gyrus. Histologically there is extracellular deposit of amyloid (plaques) and intracellular neurofibrillary tangles. Plaque is composed of an amyloid B peptide, deposited in the cortex as well as wall of blood vessels. Some plaques contain dystrophic neuronal processes (neuritic plaques). Intraneuronal fibrillary tangles are present as flame shaped in the neuronal cytoplasm occupying much of the space in neuronal cytoplasm. Cortical nerve cell become dilated and twisted (neurophil threads) due to accumulation of the same filaments from tangles.

Chromosome 21 carries the gene for amyloid precursor protein (APP).

Apo E4 gene on chromosome 19 predisposes to Alzheimer's disease. Homozygous (3% in population) 90% risk of developing dementia while in heterozygous (25% of population) is at low risk.

Treatment

- Acetylcholinesterase inhibitors increase ACH in the brain.
- Choline esterase inhibitors.
- For mild to moderate dementia MMSE 10-26
  - Rivastigmine (1 capsule bid or patches) can be used for dementia in Parkinson's disease.
  - Donepezil (dispersible).
  - Galantamine
- For moderate to severe dementia
- NMDA antagonist
- Memantine.
- For aggression/agitation
- Choline esterase inhibitors (Rivastigmine in lewy-body), or quetiapine 25-100 mg or lorazepam 0.5-4 mg, citalopram 10-20 mg/day or carbamazepine.
- Insufficient evidence for use of trazodone.

VASCULAR DEMENTIA

- Common in men with hypertension, diabetes, smoking history with transient ischemic attack (TIA) or strokes.
- Step wise deterioration and focal neurological signs with brisk reflexes.
- Treat risk factors.

FRONTOTEMPORAL DEMENTIA

- Atrophy of both frontal lobes and anterior temporal lobes with intraneuronal inclusions (pick bodies).
- Resposible for 20% of early onset dementia.
- 50% have family history and linked TAU protein gene on chromosome 17.
- Difficulty in swallowing, pseudo bulbar palsy, frequent falls and Parkinsonian features may be present.
- Presents as altered social and personal behavior with disengagement, lethargy, disinhibition, social impropriety, decreased personal hygiene and executive functions. There are no hallucinations but 2-3% have delusions.
- Palmomenal reflex and palmar grasp reflex and rooting reflex are present.
- Acetylcholinesterase (ACH) inhibitors are not helpful.
- Sertraline or paroxetine may help behavior.

4

Metabolic, Renal and Endocrine

Acute Kidney Injury

In acute renal failure or acute kidney injury (AKI), an obstructive cause must be excluded 1st.
1. Acute kidney injury is an abrupt decline in renal function diagnosed by rapidly rising blood urea, or rise in serum creatinin 26 micro mols/L from the base line or within 48 hrs or urine output <0.5 mL/kg/hr for 6 hrs.
2. Oliguria is <400 mL/day or <30 mL/hr and anuria is <100 mL/day.

With the fall in BP (due to hypovolemia, vasodilatation or low cardiac output) there is gradual dilatation of preglomerular arteoles (mediated by angiotensin and NO) and vasoconstriction of postglomerular arterioles (by angiotensin II) maintaining the constant glomerular capillary hydrostatic pressure. There is interstitial inflammation independent of etiology.

NEPHROTOXIC DRUGS

Iodinated radio contrast agents—Nephropathy can be reduced by use of isotonic fluid Hartmann solution loading.

Nonsteroidal anti-inflammatory drugs (NSAIDs) or angiotensin-converting enzyme (ACE) interfere with auto regulation of renal blood flow and glomerular filtration rate (GFR) and can provoke acute pre renal failure particularly in patients >60 yrs with atherosclerotic cardiovascular disease with pre-existing chronic kidney disease (CKD) (serum creatinine >180).

Renal hypo perfusion is due to Na depletion, diuretic use, hypotension, heart failure, Nephrotic syndrome and Cirrhosis.

- Aminoglycosides
- Methotrexate
- AII angiotensin receptor blocker (ARB)
- Myoglobinuria in rhabdomyolysis
- Light chains in urine
- Recreational drugs.

Causes of AKI

- Pre-renal (70%) due to decreased renal perfusion. Hypovolemic—gastrointestinal hemorrhage, urinary or skin losses, low cardiac output, hypotension, sepsis, NSAID, ACE inhibitors, cardiac failure or decompensate liver cirrhosis.
- Renal 25%
  Causes: Ischemic 50%, Sepsis 35%, interstitial nephritis 10% (Eosinophil's in urine microscopy suggest interstitial nephritis), acute glomerulonephritis 5%.

  At risk are age >75 yrs, chronic kidney disease (CKD) eGFR <40 mL/minute, pre-existing renal impairment, hypertension, cardiac disease, peripheral vascular disease, diabetes and jaundice.

  Two components are involved in acute reduction of GFR
  1. *Vascular component*: Normally kidney receives 25% of the cardiac output but most of the blood supply is directed to renal cortex. Cortical pO_2 is 6.6–13.3 and because of counter current exchange there is progressive fall in pO_2 from cortex to medulla with pO_2 1.3–2.9 in proximal tubule and ascending limb despite their high metabolic activity (Na/K ATPase). In AKI renal blood flow is decreased by 30–50% and there is selective reduction in blood supply to outer medulla. There is also increased vasoconstriction of afferent arteriole caused by endothelin, angiotensin II, adenosine, thromboxane and sympathetic nerve activity.

     Impairment of endothelium attenuates the vasodilatation due to NO and prostaglandin. In sepsis there is release of tumor necrosis factor (TNF) alpha and endothelin causing renal vasoconstriction and leakage of fluid from the capillaries thereby further diminishing plasma volume.

2. *Tubular*: In hypoxia, integrin which mediates cell to cell adhesion, move from basolateral location to apical cell membrane leading to tubular cell desquamation and promote tubular cast formation and distal tubular obstruction. Damaged cells die not only from necrosis but also from apoptosis. Proximal tubular cells can undergo repair, regeneration and proliferation after injury in the outer cortex.

Glomerulonephritis (GN), disseminated intravascular coagulation (DIC), thrombotic thrombocytopenic purpura; hemolytic uremic syndrome, infections (Legionella, malaria, leptospirosis) and accelerated phase of hypertension are other causes of AKI.

- *Postrenal 5% (obstruction intrinsic or extrinsic)*: Urethral obstruction with palpable bladder, tumors, bladder neck obstruction by prostrate hypertrophy or carcinoma, neurogenic tumors, ureteric obstruction by stones, clot, sloughed papillae, tumors, lymphadenopathy, retroperitoneal fibrosis. Post obstructive diuresis (>4 L), hyperkalemia and renal tubular acidosis can occur after the release of obstruction. If hyperkalemia persists after reversal of renal failure then look for the presence of renal tubular acidosis (mild metabolic acidosis pH <7.35, bicarbonate <20 m moles/L, urine pH >5.3) treated by sodium citrate or sodium bicarbonate or potassium citrate.

Most Common Causes of AKI

- Acute tubular necrosis, pyelonephritis, myeloma, acute interstitial nephritis (AIN), Atheroembolic and rhabdomyolysis.
- Rhabdomyolysis is usually caused by major trauma, narcotic overdose, vascular embolism and drugs and treated by maintaining polyuria urine >300 mL/hr, urine pH >6.5 (alkalinization) and correction of compartment syndrome.
- *Less common causes*: Vasculitis, acute GN, lupus nephritis and good pasture's syndrome. If purpuric rash then consider systemic vasculitis, Henoch-Schönlein purpura, cryoglobulinemia, drug reaction (acute tubular interstitial nephritis) and cholesterol emboli.

Investigations

- Full blood count (FBC), U and E, CK and urinary myoglobin (if urine shows blood on dipstick and no RBC on microscopy) to exclude rhabdomyolysis. Serum creatinine depends not only on urinary clearance of creatinine but also on rate of production and volume of distribution.
- Chest X-ray, and renal ultrasound, ECG, blood and urine culture, autoimmune/vasculitic screen (ANCA, ANA, immunoglobulin, cryoglobulins, and anti-GBM) if clinically indicated.

Sterile Pyuria

- Partially treated UTI, renal calculus disease, analgesic nephropathy, interstitial nephritis, renal TB and rarely proliferative glomerulonephritis.
- Sediment without cast—Under perfusion or obstructive uropathy.
- Proteinuria, and hematuria with RBC cast—glomerulonephritis or vasculitis.
- Granular and epithelial cell casts with minimal proteinuria—ATN.
- Pyuria with white cells and granular casts—Tubular or interstitial disease.
- Pyuria alone—infection.

Management

- Stabilize the patient while trying to improve renal functions. Volume depletion is corrected and BP is restored. Use Hartmann solution rather than normal saline as IV infusion as chloride in excess causes renal vasoconstriction.
- Seek underlying reversible causes of AKI (history is most helpful in identifying the cause). Is it acute or chronic? Seek previous renal functions results and renal size on ultrasound (small kidneys indicate chronic disease). Exclude impaction and pelvic malignancy by rectal examination. Search for and aggressively treat infections.
- Immediate concerns are hypoxia, hypovolemia, hyperkalemia, metabolic acidosis and pericarditis.
- *Immediate treatment*: Correct hypoxia by high flow O_2 keeping SpO_2 >92%. IV access.

- Treat hyperkalemia >5.5 mmols/L (>6.5 mmols life threatening) with IV calcium gluconate 10 mL 10% IV over 2-3 minutes. ECG changes (tall T waves, broad QRS, prolonged QT interval, prolonged PR interval, flat P-wave) improve in 1-3 min, if persistent then repeat IV calcium gluconate.
- An infusion of glucose and insulin (15 U in 250 mL 10% glucose) over 15-30 minutes. This will lower K by 0.5-1.5 mmols for 4-6 hrs.
- Salbutamol nebulizer 5-10 mg will lower K 0.5-1.5 mmol or inhaler (reduces K 0.6-1.0 mmol/L with in 3 min of 1200 microgram via MDI and spacer).
- Correct hypovolemia (JVP clearly visible, no posture drop in BP). In oliguric patient give 400 mL Hartmann solution +previous days urinary output
- Catheterize and measure hourly urine volumes. Provide early nutritional support with dietary Na up to 2 gm/day and with low K.
- Dipstick urine: If proteinuria, hematuria, nitrite and leukocyte indicate infection.
- Stop ACE, NSAID, diuretics except in pulmonary edema and other nephrotoxins. Do not use furosemide and dopamine as renal protection. Magnesium containing antacids should be avoided.

Acidosis is common and if bicarbonate <15 and pH <7.2 then 500 mL 1.26% sodium bicarbonate can be given IV although potential for volume overload should be recognized.

Hyperphosphatemia should be treated with calcium carbonate. Fluid overload, pulmonary edema in AKI consider O_2, GTN infusion, CPAP and renal referral.

Indications for Urgent Dialysis or Hemofiltration

If oliguria persists or biochemistry worsens urea >30 mmols/L or creatinin >300 micro mol/L (hemodialysis or hemofiltration) is urgently required.

- Oliguria <200 mL in 12 hrs or anuria <50 mL in 12 hrs or pulmonary edema.
- Hyperkalemia persistent >6.5 mmol/L with pulmonary edema resistance to treatment.
- Severe acidosis pH <7.2.
- Uremic encephalopathy, pericarditis and neuropathy/ myopathy.

- Persistent plasma Na >155 mmol/L or <120 mmol/L.
- Pulmonary edema not responding to diuretics or CPAP.
- Drug overdose with dialyzable toxin.

There is no evidence that early or late dialysis influences the final outcome.

Continuous filtration is no better than intermittent dialysis though continuous therapy is preferred in cerebral edema and liver failure and intermittent in patients with increased bleeding risk. However, if dialysis is used it needs to be daily. If filtration is used it should be 35 mL/kg/hr or greater.

Hepato renal syndrome is mostly due to hypovolemia or cardiomyopathy caused by aggressive paracentesis, sepsis, diuretics or lactulose diarrhea. It is treated with IV albumin and terlipressin.

Adult Polycystic Kidney Disease

Adult polycystic kidney disease (ADPKD) is an autosomal dominant mutation on this short arm of chromosome 16. These are mutations of proteins (polycystin-1 and polycystin-2).

Incidence 1/2500 may be associated with polycystic liver disease with nodular enlargement of liver (LFT usually normal), berry aneurysm of cerebral arteries (10%), Mitral valve prolapse 25% (a systemic manifestation of collagen defect).

Patients with ADPKD 1/3 develop hypertension, 1/3 develops renal failure and 1/3 remains asymptomatic.

Presents as bilateral masses in the flanks which are bimanually ballotable. One can get above them and percussion may be resonant (colon lying over it). Usual presentations are hematuria after trauma, renal colic, renal failure, UTI or hypertension.

Hepatic, pancreatic, ovarian cysts and berry aneurysm are common. Liver cysts develop in 80% of patients and are more common in women.

Diagnosed by at least 2 cyst unilateral or bilateral <30 yrs, 2 cysts in each kidney 30–59 yrs, and 4 cyst in each kidney in >60 yrs.

Treatment

- ACE or ARB.
- Avoiding high impact sports (to avoid abdominal trauma, e.g. Rugby, Boxing).
- Low salt diet (6 g/day), protein 1 g/kg and sufficient intake of fluids (noncaffeinated beverages) to produce 2–3 L urine/day,
- Ideal weight and regular exercise (walking or swimming) are helpful.
- Patient is advised to inform the diagnosis to 1-degree relatives so that they can be screened.
- For screening individual should be >18 yrs old and expected to have children.
- Anticoagulants and low dose aspirin should be avoided.
- For UTI use IV fluroquinolone.
- Renal stones are X2 more common. There are usually uric acid stones.
- Exogenous estrogens and repeated pregnancies lead to cysts in the liver. Therefore, use minimal dose of estrogens.

Nephrotic Syndrome

- Normal urinary protein <150 mg/day.
- Micro albuminuria: 30–300 mg/day—early sign of diabetic nephropathy.

Nephrotic syndrome presents as proteinuria >3.0 g/day, low albumin and edema (pedal, sacral, facial or periorbital). Dyslipidemia, prothrombotic tendency (due to loss of proanticoagulant protein) and mild immune suppression due to loss of immunoglobulin is also a feature. They need renal biopsy to be treated effectively.

If proteinuria >2 gm/day + microscopic hematuria + renal impairment → need renal biopsy.

Causes

- Glomerulonephritis (GN), diabetes mellitus, myeloma, vasculitis (SLE, Wegener's granuloma), amyloidosis.
- *Minimal change GN*: Usually primary, selective proteinuria, effacement of podocytes on electron

microscopy, good response to steroids and occasionally associated with Hodgkin's disease.
- *Membranous GN*: Primary or secondary (Hodgkin's disease, lymphoma, carcinoma, diabetes, SLE, gold and penicillamine, amyloidosis, malaria, HBV, HIV and syphilis).
  - Associated with nonselective proteinuria, immune deposits in the basement membrane and may response to steroids/immunosuppressant. 30% improve, 30% static and 40% worsen.
  - *Poor prognostic factors*: Male gender, hypertension, heavy proteinuria, renal failure and interstitial inflammation.

Chronic Renal Failure (Chronic Kidney Disease)

- Albumin creatinine ratio (ACR) (normal <3 mg/mmol), 3–30 mg/mmol microalbuminuria and >30 mg/mmol proteinuria.
- ACR 25 mg/mmol equivalent to urine dipstick one plus protein.
- Hematuria—dipstick and microscopy—Glomerular hematuria has red cell casts and positive on dipstick.
- Hyaline casts formed of Tamm-Horsfall protein in fever or exercise and not indicative of renal disease.
- In chronic renal failure there is inability of the body to excrete K, water and acid causing hyperkalemia, acidosis and hypervolemia and these require emergency treatment.
- Kidney makes erythropoietin and vitamin D, the lack of which causes anemia and metabolic bone disease.
- Chronic kidney disease (CKD) is a marker of cardiovascular risk.
- Uremic symptoms are anorexia, nausea, vomiting, cramps, restless legs, peripheral neuropathy, cognitive disturbances, hiccups, itch, pericarditis and sexual dysfunctions.
- *Stage 1*: CKD with normal GFR—GFR 90.
- *Stage 2*: CKD with mild impaired GFR—GFR 60–89.
- *Stage 3A*: CKD GFR—45–59 and ACR <30 mg/mmol low risk.

- *Stage 3B*: CKD GFR–30–44 and ACR >30 mg/mmol high risk.
- *Stage 4*: CKD severely impaired GFR—GFR 15–29 Preparation for dialysis.
- *Stage 5*: CKD End-stage renal failure—GFR <15 dialysis, transplantation or conservative care.
- Spot urine samples are taken for ACR.
- GFR is calculated from Cockcroft-Gaut formula =1.23 × (140-age) × weight in kg divided by plasma creatinine (micromol/L). For females— × 0.85.
- GFR—140-age × (weight/SCr × 72) and for women × 0.85.
- Normal GFR >90.

Referral to Renal Unit

Patients with CKD with GFR <30 mL/min, ACR (albumin: creatinine ratio) >70 mg/mmol or ACR 30 mg/mmol with hematuria or poorly controlled hypertension or suspected renal artery stenosis should be referred.

Causes

- Hypertension (25%)
- Diabetes (40%)
- Autosomal dominant polycystic kidney disease (ADPKD) (4%)
- NSAID Glomerulonephritis (15%).

RENOVASCULAR DISEASE

Renal artery stenosis (RAS) is due to atheroma (90%) and fibro muscular disease (young women presenting with severe hypertension).

It is mainly in elderly associated with other atheromatous diseases, peripheral vascular disease, congestive cardiac failure (CCF) and ischemic heart disease (IHD).

RENAL ARTERY STENOSIS PRESENTATION

- Systolic hypertension with low diastolic pressure and resistant to treatment.
- Deterioration of renal function (>30% increase in creatinine in 10 days) after ACE.
- Flash pulmonary edema with no significant myocardial ischemia.

- Audible vascular bruite in epigastrium, renal or iliofemoral.
- Presence of atrophic kidney (>1.5 cm disparity) and presence of urinary proteins.
- Diagnosed by MRA if GFR > 15 mL/min, CT angiography (risk of contrast nephropathy) or duplex ultrasound.
- Stenting mainly in young with fibromuscular renal artery stenosis.
- In atherosclerotic renovascular disease (ARVD) stenting mainly in patients presenting as acute renal failure or flash pulmonary edema.

Management

- Ultrasound of abdomen to exclude urinary tract obstruction and autosomal dominant polycystic kidney disease (ADPKD).
- Stop smoking, salt intake <2–4 gm/day, weight <25 BMI, waist < 102 cm in men and <88 cm in women, exercise, BP <130/80, BM <7 mmols, for statin and aspirin and Hb 10–12 g/100.
- Metformin can be used up to stage 1–3, gliclazide and repaglinide can be used in stage 4.
- All type 2 diabetes mellitus (T2DM) and T1DM after 5 yrs should have annual albumin creatinine ratio (ACR).
- Metformin reduced by 50% if eGFR <45 mL/min and stopped if eGFR 30 mL/min.
- All CKD patients should have BP 120-139/<90.
- All CKD patients with proteinuria ACR >70 mg should have BP 120-129/<80.
- If ACR >70 mg/mmol combination of ACE and ARB is recommended in hypertensive or nonhypertensive.
- All CKD patients with diabetes and ACR >3 mg/mmol should have ACE inhibitors and should have BP 120–129/<80.
- All patients with diabetes and microalbuminuria should have ACE inhibitors even if BP is normal.
- Angiotensin converting enzymes (ACE) inhibitors should be considered if ACR >30 mg/mmol, if hypertensive, and in ACR >70 mg/mmol if nonhypertensive.
- Target BP—130/85 with ACE. Check urea and electrolytes 10th day and in a month, if rise in creatinine >30% then stop ACE.

- Reducing BP <100–110 mm Hg may be detrimental.
- *Low protein diet*: Effect is slight and less important.
- Infection—Recurrent UTI (search for anatomical cause, i.e. obstruction or calculi).
- All for lipid lowering and smoking cessation.
- Alpha calcidol and phosphate binder (calcium carbonate) to prevent hyperparathyroidism and renal bone disease.
- NSAIDs should be avoided.

ANEMIA

Target Hb >110 g/L, usually develops in CRF when GFR <30–45 mL/min.

Causes

- Iron-deficiency (absolute or relative), EPO (erythropoietin) deficiency, reduced half-life of RBC, occult blood loss, uremic inhibitors and B_{12} or folate deficiency.
- Iron deficiency anemia—Absolute—ferritin <20 μg/L or <100 μg/L in chronic renal failure (CRF).
- Functional—transferrin saturation (TSAT) <20% and ferritin 100–200 μg/L

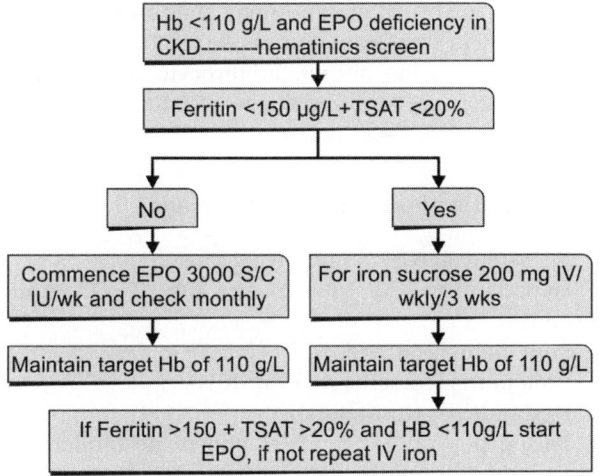

Monitoring on EPO

- FBC every 2 wks till target Hb then 1–3 monthly.
- Iron studies and TSAT 3 monthly.
- B_{12} and folate 6 monthly.

Side Effects of EPO

Hypertension 20–30%, hyperkalemia, myalgia and flu-like symptoms.

Mineral and Bone Disorder

- Increase in serum phosphate due to decreased excretion and decrease conversion to 1-25 (OH) D3 are the main reasons.
- 50% patients with GFR <60 have high PTH.
- Patients usually have high phosphate, low calcium and raised PTH.
- Monitor calcium, phosphate every 3/12 and PTH every 6/12.
- Prescribe phosphate binder if phosphate >1.5 mmol/L and active vitamin D analog one alpha.
- Pre renal failure—urine osmolality >500 mosm/L, urinary Na <20 and urine concentration normal while in ATN—Urine osmolality <350 mosm/L, urine Na >40 mmol/L and urine concentration dilute.
- cANCA—directed against proteinases and positive in Wegener's granulomatosis (WG) and microscopic polyarteritis (MPA).
- Chronic obstruction can impair the tubular function resulting in significant diuresis, so can be present even with good urine output. Erythrocyte sedimentation rate (ESR) may be raised due to CRF. Renal biopsy not indicated if kidneys are small.

Factors Causing Persistent Renal Damage

- Persistent activity of underlying cause.
- Hypertension, (BP >130/85 and BP> 125/75 in diabetics).
- Poor diabetic control.
- Proteinuria (consider ACE or ARBs).
- Dyslipidemia (for statins).
- Raised phosphate (consider phosphate binders and vitamin D one alpha).
- Restriction of K, phosphate and salt in diet.
- Anemia—Exclude the deficiency of Fe, B_{12} and folate and blood loss (EPO if Hb <11 g/dL except in ADPKD

where EPO is normal). Erythropoietin (EPO) is given subcutaneous 1–3 times weekly.
- Response to EPO is poor if inflammation is present.
- Hemodialysis—4 hrs three times a week, heparin is given to prevent clot formation. A-V fistula is created in the arm.

Complications of Hemodialysis

- Hypotension, headache, itch and muscle cramp may reflect rapid changes in blood volume and electrolytes.
- Infections including hepatitis B and C.
- Hemodialysis does remove large molecules (Beta-2 micro globulin) which accumulate and form amylodosis presenting as carpal tunnel syndrome.

Peritoneal Dialysis

Every 4 hrs patient connects the 2 L glucose bag, above the abdomen to allow the fluid to drain in and below to drain out. Most patient lasts only few years.

Patients with some residual renal functions only are considered for peritoneal dialysis, while those without any renal functions are considered for hemodialysis.

Complications

Infection of peritoneal cavity, skin and around the tube.

Renal Transplant

Kidney is removed with attached artery, vein and ureter from brain dead or recently dead or living donor and transplanted in pelvis of the recipient outside the peritoneal cavity; blood vessels are attached to iliac vessels and ureter to bladder. The donor and recipient are matched HLA-A, B and DR. Recipient is given immunosuppressive drugs (steroids, azathioprine, cyclosporine, tacrolimus, sirolimus and mycophenolate).

Alport's Syndrome

Genetically mediated, absence of alpha 5 chain from type IV collagen, presenting as sensory neural deafness, glomerulonephritis and end stage renal failure (ESRF).

Palliation in Advanced Renal Disease

Itching

High phosphate cause itching usually relieved by phosphate binders, calcium carbonate. Itching caused by uremia is relieved by low dose gabapentin or ondansetron.

Pain

Avoid morphine or codeine. Oxycodone is better tolerated and use lower doses if GFR low. If GFR <20 mL/min use buprenorphine or fentanyl patches or alfentanil syringe driver if higher dose needed.

Neuropathic pain: Amitriptyline 10 mg/d or Gabapentin or pregabalin.

Nausea: Haloperidol, ondansetron, granisetron or metoclopramide.

RHABDOMYOLYSIS

History

Rhabdomyolsis has muscle signs in 50%, myoglobin is absent in urine in 30% and should be considered in trauma, burns, epilepsy, coma with hypotension, falls and self-poisoning.

1. *Focal muscle damage*: Crush injury, high voltage electrical injury.
2. *Generalized muscle damage*: Excessive exercise (marathon running), prolonged seizure, acute dystonia.
3. *Infections*: Septicemia, viral myositis.
   Toxins: Statins, alcohol, barbiturates, opioids, ethylene glycol, Cocaine, amphetamine, ecstasy, snake bite, spider and co-poisoning.
   Heat stroke, hyperpyrexia, neuroleptic malignant syndrome and myopathies.

Clinical Features

Grossly elevated CPK (>10,000), myoglobinuria (when serum myoglobin >100 mg/dL), renal failure, hyperkalemia, hyperphosphatemia, hypocalcemia, metabolic acidosis and hyperuricemia.

Examination

- Look for swelling or tenderness of muscles or compartment syndrome.
- Pressure sores on back of head, spine, pelvis or heels indicate pressure damage to muscles.
- *Rash*: Septicemia or Dermatomyositis.

Diagnosis

- Urine dipstick positive for blood, but no RBC on microscopy.
- Creatine kinase >10,000 units/L.

Immediate Management

- AKI (acute kidney injury) is due to ischemia (intra renal vasoconstriction) and tubular obstruction by the casts and enhanced by volume depletion and acidic urine (urine pH <6.5).
- To prevent rhabdomyolysis leading to renal failure, fluids 10 L/day and if after 12 hrs urine pH <6.5 then alkalise the urine with 1.26% $NaHCO_3$.
- Restore intravascular volume alternating 0.9% NaCl with 5% dextrose.
- Urine output (>150 mL/hr) of alkaline urine (myoglobin more soluble at alkaline PH)
- 1.26% $NaHCO_3$ at 25 mL/hr to achieve high urine PH >6.5.
- If urine output remains low give mannitol 1 gm/kg as 20% solution IV over 30–60 minutes.

Hyperkalemia

- It is usually asymptomatic, but can cause tingling, paraesthesia, weakness, flaccid paralysis and bradycardia.
- Can cause cardiac arrest.
- Almost always occurs in the context of acute or chronic renal failure.

Causes

- Reduced renal excretion (ARF, potassium sparing diuretics spironolactone, amiloride, triamterene,

ACE inhibitors, NSAID, hypoaldosteronism, adrenal insufficiency).
- Shift of potassium from cells (rhabdomyolysis, trauma, burns, hemolysis, internal bleeding, acidosis, hyper osmolality, digoxin, Beta blockers, and insulin lack).
- Excessive intake.
- Pseudohyperkalemia (thrombocytosis, leukocytosis, leukemia, and hemolysis *in vitro* or sampling) delayed analysis.

  ECG changes: Tall peaked T-waves, flat P-waves and prolonged P-R interval, loss of P-wave and very wide QRS complexes and sine wave proceeding to VF.

Management

- Correct hypoxia.
- IV access
- Level > 6 mmol/L is dangerous.
- If ECG changes are more than peaked T-waves, give 10 mL of 10% calcium gluconate IV slowly over 5 minutes with continuous ECG monitoring, repeat as necessary until ECG changes are returning to normal.
- Calcium chloride is irritant to the vein and contains 272 mg of calcium while calcium gluconate contains 94 mg of calcium but is not irritant.
- Give 250 mL of 10% dextrose with 10 units of soluble insulin IV over 30 minutes. Check glucose after insulin/dextrose. This can be followed by 5% dextrose.
- Nebulized salbutamol 5 mg and repeated.
- Above measures will lower serum K by 1–2 mmol/L over 20–30 minutes.
- Ion exchange resins calcium resonium 15 g 8-hly orally or 30 g by retention enema should not be used as it can result in intestinal obstruction and will take at least 4 hrs to have an effect.
- Stop all drugs that might exacerbate hyperkalemia (Potassium sparing diuretics, ACE, ARB (angiotensin receptor blocker), trimethoprim and heparin.
- Hyperkalemia with normal renal functions, give IV fluids and furosemide to secure renal potassium loss.
- Consider hemodialysis or hemofiltration if K is still rising or persistent oliguria or pericarditis, severe acidosis or resistant pulmonary edema.

Diabetic Ketoacidosis and Hyperglycemic Hyperosmolar Syndrome (HHS)

	DKA	HHS
Blood glucose	>11 mmol/L	>33 mmol/L
Blood pH	<7.3	>7.3
HCO_3	<15 mmol/L	>15 mmol/L
Ketones in urine	+2	No ketones in urine
Ketones in blood	+3	No ketones in blood
Osmolality	Variable	Usually >330
Onset	Over hours/days	Slow onset over many days
DVT prophylaxis	Required	Essential
IV fluids	Normal saline 3 L in 1st 7 hrs	N saline 1 L/2–3 hrly
Antibiotics	Only if infection proven or strongly suspected	Essential as infection precipitant
Insulin	Fixed dose insulin 7 U/hr as per chart	1–2 U/hr after 12 hrs of IV N saline
Potassium	20 mmol/hr if K <5.5 mmol/L target 4–5 mmol/L	10 mmol/hr if K <5.0 mmol/L
Osmolality	2 (Na + K) + urea + glucose	Normal (280–295)

KETOSIS PRONE TYPE 2 DIABETES MELLITUS

There is glucose 6 phosphate dehydrogenase deficiency which may lead to reduced protection of Beta cell function in the presence of oxidative stress caused by acute hyperglycemia. People with ketosis prone T2DM fulfil same biochemical criteria and require same initial treatment and discharged on insulin as in diabetic ketoacidosis (DKA) in T1DM.

All non-white patients especially African-Caribbean presenting with ketosis should be considered as ketosis prone DM, who are generally older, more obese and have family history of T2DM. Patients with ketosis prone T2DM tend to have higher plasma glucose and glycated hemoglobin (HbA1c) than those with T1DM.

Once the acute hyperglycemia is controlled with insulin both B cell functions and insulin sensitivity improves good diabetic control can be maintained with oral agents like sulfonylureas and pioglitazones within three to six months.

Pancreatic autoimmune markers glutamic acid decarboxylase (GAD65) or islet antigen 2 (IA2) and B cell functions (fasting or glucagon stimulated C-peptide) should be assessed in 1–3 wks in a diabetic clinic after resolution of ketoacidosis. GAD65 and IA2 are not present in ketosis prone T2DM and distinguishes from T1DM. If autoantibodies negative and C-peptide levels sufficient and glycemic control is maintained then insulin can be safely down titrated so long as patient monitors home blood glucose and ketones testing. Once the patient is on oral agents, frequent C-peptide measurement (B cell function reserve) is advised.

- DKA is defined by metabolic acidosis venous pH <7.3, bicarbonate <15 and blood glucose >11 mmol/L and moderate ketonuria more than 2+ or ketonemia >3 mm/L. Degree of hyperglycemia is not a reliable guide for severity of DKA.
- It is present in type 1 diabetes (T1DM), rarely in non-overweight ketosis prone type 2 diabetes (T2DM) with severe inter-current illness or in acromegaly.
- Ketones—Acetoacetate: Beta hydroxy butyrate.

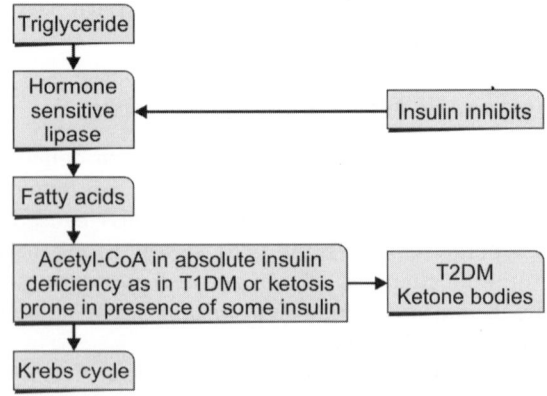

Most common cause is insufficient insulin, enhancing hepatic glucose production and fat breakdown causing increased serum free fatty acid which on metabolism produces ketones and metabolic acidosis.

Secondary insults, e.g. infections (respiratory, renal, GI, septicemia, meningitis), MI, stroke, surgery, non-compliance with insulin, cocaine and trauma produce DKA in susceptible patients.

Symptoms

Usually develops over hours or days. Thirst, polyuria, vomiting, abdominal pain and confusion are common. Consider DKA in any unconscious or hyperventilating patient.

Examination

- Rapid and deep sighing respiration.
- Smell of ketones.
- Volume depletion secondary to salt and water loss with reduced skin turgor.
- Tachycardia and hypotension.
- Conscious levels may be impaired in severe DKA.
- Careful examination of feet and skin for ulceration and sepsis.

Investigations

Blood glucose usually >20 mmol/L, FBC, U and E, creatinine, HCO_3, No arterial blood gases (ABG), venous samples instead for PH, ketonemia, total body hypokalemia (serum potassium may be high/normal/low) and urinary ketones.

ECG, Blood culture, MSU and chest X-ray.

Bedside capillary testing often not accurate with very high glucose concentrations and acidosis.

Management

- Correct hypoxia,
- IV access, No ABG, venous sample for pH instead. High-dependency unit (HDU) if blood ketones >6, PH <7.1, HCO_3 <5, systolic BP <90 mm Hg, GCS <12 and O_2 saturation <92% on air.
- NG tube if consciousness is impaired or protracted vomiting.

- *Intravenous fluids*: The fluids deficit in DKA is 6–10 L. Give 3 L of normal saline in 1st 7 hrs (1 L for first 1 h, 2nd L in 2 hrs 3rd L over 2 hrs and then 1 L 4 hrly for next 12 h), then individualized fluid replacement guided by clinical condition, urine output, measurement of JVP or CVP and blood glucose.

  Check U and E at 2, 5, 8, 12 and 24 hr and after that twice daily till bicarbonate in normal range. Avoid hypokalemia, Target K level 4.0–5.0 mmol/L.

  Maximum recommended rate is K (potassium) 20 mmol/hr therefore (nil if K >5.5 mmol/L or anuric) and 40 mmol/L over 2 hrs or two separate infusion lines if K <3.5 mmol/L.

  Patients with DKA and hypotension (systolic BP <100 mm Hg) should have volume resuscitation with colloid 500 mL over 15 minutes.

- When blood glucose <14 mmol/L switch saline to 5% dextrose and infuse 100 mL/hr until eating normally if using fixed dose of insulin as outlined below.

  Aim gradual reduction of blood glucose over 1st 12–24 hrs.

- *Insulin infusions*: Fixed dose insulin infusion is 0.1 unit/kg in 10% glucose 125 mL/hr when glucose <14.

  Make up an infusion of 50 units of soluble insulin (Humulin S or Actrapid) in 50 mL of 0.9% NaCl (1 unit/mL) and infuse using syringe driver. Flush 10 mL of prepared solution through the line before connecting to the patient (as some insulin will be adsorbed to the plastic).

	Varying dose insulin		Fixed dose insulin	
Blood glucose	Insulin	Fluids	Insulin	IV fluids
0–4	0.5 U/h	5% dextrose	7 U/h	10% glucose
4.1–7	1 U/h	5% dextrose	7 U/h	10% glucose
7.1–11	2 U/h	5% dextrose	7 U/h	5% glucose
11.1–15	3 U/h	N saline	7 U/h	5% glucose
15.1–19	4 U/h	N saline	7 U/h	N/saline
19.1–24 or >24	5 or 6 U/h	N saline	7 U/h	N/saline

If there is no fall in blood sugar in 2 hrs, confirm that the pump is working and the IV line connected properly and double the infusion rate.
- Bladder catheterization if no urine has been passed after 4 hours or the patient is incontinent, but not otherwise.
- Antibiotics only if infection is proven or strongly suspected. WBC commonly raised in DKA even in absence of infection. If there is soft tissue infection of the feet then treat with co-amoxiclav plus metronidazole IV (if allergic to penicillin, use clindamycin plus ciprofloxacin).
- DVT prophylaxes essential with subcutaneous heparin

Precipitant is infection in 50% DKA, all should get septic screen.

Continue insulin infusion and dextrose IV until ketoacidosis has resolved (plasma bicarbonate >20 mmol/L, urinary ketones negative) and the patient is well enough to eat and drink at least two meals. 30 minutes before stopping IV insulin, give subcutaneous long acting insulin like glargine or levemir insulin.

Half-life of IV insulin is 2–3 minutes. Estimate the daily insulin requirement from double the total dose given by infusion over the last 12 hrs, give 1/3 of the total daily dose as intermediate-acting at 22.00 h, divide the remaining 2/3 into 3 and give as short acting insulin SC before meals.

$NaHCO_3$ should only be used if pH <6.8 and patient remains cardiovascular unstable despite volume resuscitation, use isotonic 1.26% $NaHCO_3$ (150 mmol/L) dose 1 mmol/kg.

Causes of Mortality in DKA

- Arrhythmia secondary to hypokalemia.
- Aspiration pneumonia/ARDS.
- Cerebral edema due to over-rapid metabolic correction.

Special Cases

- Pregnancy can have full blown DKA with little hyperglycemia (check salicylates).
- Alcoholic keto acidosis in Type 2 DM.

- Para suicide in young Type 1 DM—Salicylate acidosis, hyperglycemia, unconsciousness.

HYPEROSMOLAR HYPERGLYCEMIC SYNDROME (HHS)

Consider the diagnosis in any patient with blood glucose >33 mmol/L, hypernatremia, uremia, no ketoacidosis (venous bicarbonate >15 mmol/L, arterial pH >7.3) and plasma osmolality >350 (normal range 280–295). This can be calculated from the formula = [2(Na + K) + urea + glucose].

- Common in frail, elderly, noninsulin dependent diabetics.
- Infection is precipitant in 50% of cases.
- Insidious onset often over many days.
- Consider HDU if GCS <12, O_2 <92%.

Investigations

- Venous blood glucose, bedside BM sticks.
- U and E, creatinine, HCO_3, ABG (arterial blood gases), FBC, urinary ketones.
- Chest X-ray, ECG, urine Gram stain and culture, blood culture and other infection screen.

Management

- Resuscitate intravascular space as in DKA with 0.9% saline 1 L 2 hrly, 1 L 3 hrly, 1 L 4 hrly and 1 L 6 hrly depending upon circulatory collapse. Caution in heart disease and elderly.
  Replace fluid losses gently over 24–72 hrs using 0.9% saline.
- Lower doses of insulin are required as compared to DKA, e.g. start with insulin infusion (50 mL normal saline with 50 U of actrapid) 1–2 units/hr and reduce if blood glucose falling >5 mmol/L/hr (target drop 2–3 mmol/hr).
  Monitor BM hrly finger prick initially.
  Check K 2 hrly initially.
  ECG monitors to exclude tall T-waves due to hyperkalemia.
  Slow metabolic correction is essential to avoid cerebral osmolar shifts of water.

Insulin sensitivity is greater in the absence of acidosis.

Continue insulin SC regime till total daily dose falls below 20 U, when oral hypoglycemic can be tried.

- *High risk of thrombosis*: Consider prophylactic LMWH until fully recovered.
- Broad spectrum antibiotics for infection.
- Total body K is lower, check the level after 30 minutes starting insulin and replacement rate of 10 mmol/h is adequate when K <5.0 mmol/L.
- Urethral catheterization has no place unless the patient is in retention with distended bladder.
- Unconscious patient should be nursed semi prone until a thin nasogastric tube can be passed and gastric contents aspirated.

Diabetic Foot

25% of diabetic patients have foot ulcer at some stage and 85% of amputations of lower limb are preceded by foot ulcer. Ulcers are caused by diabetic neuropathy (sensory, motor, autonomic), trauma (mechanical, thermal), infection, impaired blood supply, previous foot ulcer, improper or unobtainable chiropody services, poor metabolic control, tobacco smoking, improper foot wear and old age. Diabetic neuropathy is most important.

Claw hammer toe is due to motor neuropathy and muscle atrophy. MRI may help to distinguish between Charcot foot (neuropathic osteoarthropathy) and osteomyelitis.

Most common organism *Staph aureus, S. haemolyticus*, coagulase negative Staph.

ANTIBIOTICS

- Clindamycin or tazobactam or co-amoxiclav + Flucloxacillin + metronidazole for 2 wks with off-loading (total contact cast changed weekly) plantar wound.
- Topical antiseptic containing iodine or silver are helpful.
- For bone infection fluoroquinolone (Ciprofloxacin) plus clindamycin for 6 wks. Visible bone or high ESR suggests bone infection. Maggots are also helpful.

Diabetic Neuropathic Pain

After 25 years of diabetes mellitus (DM) 50% have diabetes peripheral neuropathy (DPN) in glove stocking distribution with absence of vibration sense (128 HZ tuning fork) and usually associated with autonomic neuropathy.

Presenting as numbness, paresthesia, burning pain, shooting pain down the leg or knife like stabbing pain, cramp like sensations or itchy feeling in the feet or hyperalgesia.

Reversible neuropathy: Cranial nerve or amyotrophy (femoral neuropathy) are due to poor glycemic control or rapid glycemic control. On present evidence duloxetine is probably most effective drug for diabetic neuropathy and pregabalin for post herpetic neuralgia.

- *1st line drugs*: Gabapentin (for peripheral neuropathic pain) or pregabalin (for peripheral and central neuropathic pain), tricyclics (amitriptyline) or serotonin and norepinephrine uptake inhibitors (Duloxetine, venaflexine).
- *Topical agents*: Topical capsaicin 0.075% (for postherpetic neuralgia), Capsaicin 8% (for peripheral neuropathic pain for nondiabetic patient) and topical lidocaine 5% patch (for postherpetic neuralgia)
- For trigeminal neuralgia carbamazepine or oxcarbamazepine.

Usually gabapentin 10 mg BD to 1800 mg/day or pregabalin 75 mg BD + either amitriptyline 10–75 mg/night or duloxetine 30–120 mg/day are better together.

Surgery and Diabetes

Good metabolic control BM 4–7 reduces the risk of infection and promotes wound healing in postoperative period.
- T1DM on insulin
    - If theater list in the morning, omit insulin, set up insulin dextrose drip sliding scale at 07.00 for the morning list and for after noon list omit insulin, light breakfast 07.00, and insulin/dextrose IV 08.00 for afternoon list.

- If one injection a day
  - On the morning do not take insulin and do not eat or drink and bring your insulin with you. Major or minor procedure set up sliding scale till patient is able to tolerate normal diet after the procedure. Monitor the BM and take half the normal insulin with normal eating.
- If 2 injection a day
  - On the day do not take insulin and do not eat or drink and bring your insulin. After the procedure monitor BM, if having lunch, take half the morning dose and normal dose in the evening with normal evening diet.
- If 4 injections a day
  - On the morning of the day do not take insulin and do not eat or drink and bring your insulin with you, after the procedure monitor the BM and take the usual insulin with the meal.
  - If persistent raised >7 preprandial and >9 postprandial contact diabetic team.
- If theatre list in the evening
  - *If 1 injection a day*: On the morning of the day do not take your insulin but have alight breakfast at 7.30
  - After the procedure monitor BM and take half your normal dose with evening meal and resume normal the next day.
  - *If 2 injections a day*: On the day do not take your insulin but have a light breakfast at 7.30.
  - Do not eat or drink until the procedure.
  - After the procedure, monitor BM; take usual dose of insulin prior to the evening the meal and resume normal regime the next day.
  - *If 4 injections a day*: Take normal dose of insulin the night before except glargine or lantus insulin, and then take half of usual dose. Starchy snack and milky drink at bed time.
- On the morning of the procedure do not take insulin and have light breakfast at 7.30 and bring your insulin with you.
  - After the procedure, monitor BM and usual dose of insulin with your next meal.

NONINSULIN DEPENDENT DIABETES MELLITUS (NIDDM)

- If theater list in the morning
  - *Minor procedure*: On the morning of the procedure, do not take tablet and do not eat or drink, if eating lunch, take half of morning dose or of normal lunch time dose and usual dose with the evening meal. Give oral hypoglycemic agents (OHA)/insulin as soon as normal diet is tolerated. Insulin infusion is not required.
- If theatre list in the evening
  On the morning of the procedure, do not take diabetic tablets and take light breakfast by 7.30
  After the procedure monitor BM and take usual dose of diabetic tablets with evening meal.
  - *Major procedure*: Keep sliding scale till normal diet resumed. Give usual OHA/insulin and check pre- and postprandial BM and if consistently >10 then contact diabetes department.

Sliding Scale

1st line—50 U in 50 mL saline in syringe driver and 2nd line 500 mL 5% dextrose to run over 5 hrs.

Less than 4 mmol/L—0, 4.1–6.5—1 U/hr, 6.6–8.9–2 U/hr, 9.0–11.0–4 U/hr, 11.1–17–5 U/hr, 17.1–28–6 U/hr, >28.0–8 U/hr.

Hypokalemia

Causes

- *Gastrointestinal (GI) loss*: Diarrhea, vomiting, villous adenoma of the rectum, laxative abuse, bulimia nervosa and ileostomy.
- Renal wasting (diuretics, alkalosis, hyperaldosteronism, Cushing's syndrome, ectopic ACTH, Barter's syndrome (hypokalemia alkalosis with high urinary K loss), Liddle's disease (hypertension with hypokalemia), antibiotics (Penicillin, gentamycin, amikacin), renal tubular acidosis.
- Decreased intake (urinary K <20 mmol/L)
- Beta-adrenergic stimulation, liquorice, theophylline overdose, glue sniffing.

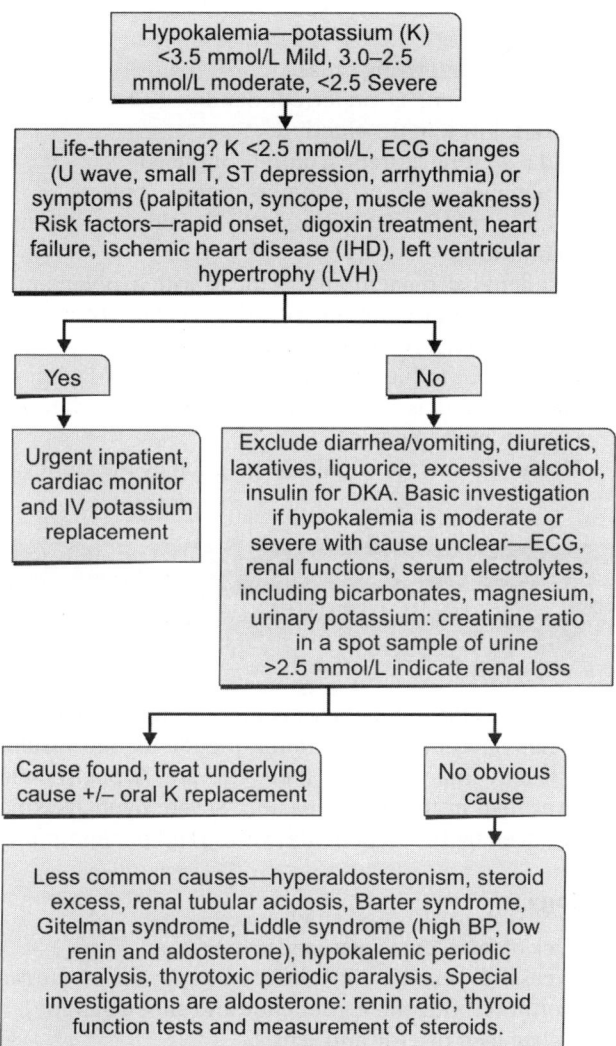

Symptoms

- Muscle weakness, hypotonicity, depression, constipation, ileus, arrhythmia, when plasma K <2.5 mmols/L muscle necrosis (rhabdomyolysis) may occur, <2 mmols/L ascending paralysis may occur resembling Guillain-Barré syndrome. Arrhythmia may occur when K <3 mmol/L.
- ECG may show flattening of T-wave, depression of ST segment and prominent U-wave.

Treatment

- Treat the underlying cause.
- Oral treatment is preferred; Sandoz K 2 tablets tds (avoid slow K in the elderly).
- Add K sparing diuretic if diuretic induced.
- In-patients with arrhythmias, target plasma K is 4–4.5 mmol/L. IV potassium should not exceed 40 mmol/hr.
- If patient has renal tubular acidosis with hypokalemia, then potassium citrate or potassium acetate is required.
- Mg depletion is common in K depletion.
- Intravenous in life-threatening arrhythmia. Maximum concentration is 40 mmol/L over 4 hrs and re check K. Use pre-prepared bags.
- Hypomagnesemia impairs K retention by the kidney.

Hypoglycemia, Diabetic Management and New Drugs in Type 2 Diabetes Mellitus

This complication of diabetes is most feared by patients. Mild hypoglycemia is common inpatients on insulin and usually managed by them. Severe hypoglycemia requires help from another person. Severe hypoglycemia experienced by 10% of patients' with T1DM per annum.

Etiology

- Lack of food, unaccustomed exercise.
- Excessive insulin, alcoholic binge, sulfonylureas (common with chlorpropamide and glibenclamide).
- Severe liver disease and sepsis.
- Insulinoma, hypopituitarism, adrenal insufficiency and salicylate poisoning.

Symptoms

- Sympathoadrenal stimulation (sweating, tremor, palpitation, pallor).
- Neuroglycopenic—confusion, drowsiness, weakness, visual disturbance.
- Presentation can be coma, convulsion, cerebral damage, impaired cognitive functions mimicking CVA or

TIA, arrhythmia, myocardial ischemia or myocardial infarction, vitreous hemorrhage or general accidents.
- Typically patient is pale, peripherally shut down with cold sweats.
- Obtain as much information as possible from others in attendance (relatives, friends, ambulance crew and bystanders) as patient may not be able to give any useful history.
- Look for evidence of diabetes by searching for Medic Alert bracelet/necklace, medication (insulin, oral hypoglycemic agents), glucose monitoring or outpatient clinic documents and sites of insulin injections.
- Awareness lost/impaired in 25% of patients with T1DM >20 yrs.

Management

Always confirm hypoglycemia if BM (blood sugar) <3.0 mmol/L by taking blood for blood glucose only in known diabetic patient, in others checking BM (blood glucose), serum insulin and C-peptide levels, to determine whether hypoglycemia is due to endogenous or exogenous insulin.

Other investigations include U and E, LFT, blood culture (if suspicion of sepsis) and tests for adrenocortical insufficiency, hypothyroidism and hypopituitarism if suspected.

Mild

Self-treatment with oral dextrose 20 gm (3 sugar lumps) or Hypo stop 10 gm/20 gm. Need long acting carbohydrate 15–20 gm afterwards.

Severe but Conscious

Assist with oral dextrose or Hypo stop gel.

Severe and Unconscious or Fitting

- IV dextrose 20% 100 mL (extravasation of 50% glucose can cause skin necrosis) or IV/IM/SC glucagon 1 mg.
- Administer oral dextrose once able to swallow.
- Glucagon may not work in sulfonylurea or alcohol related hypoglycemia.
- Dextrose 10% IV 1 L 12 hrly for 24 hrs may be needed if hypoglycemia caused by liver disease, sepsis, sulfonylurea excess or long acting insulin.

- Give oral dextrose with in 10 minutes of glucagon to replenish glycogen stores and prevent recurrent hypoglycemia.
- Reduce the dose of metformin (if GFR <45 and in intercurrent illness stop metformin to avoid lactic acidosis).

Targets for Diabetic Control on Oral Hypoglycemic Drugs or Insulin

Preprandial—4-6 mmol/L   Night time—6-8 mmol/L
Postprandial—6-8 mmol/L   2 hr postprandial—8-10

Pregnancy
Preprandial <5 mmol/L
Postprandial 2 hr-<8 mmol/L
Diet saturated fat <7%.

DIABETIC MANAGEMENT

Targets

- HbA1 <6.5—if on monotherapy or dual therapy. If >7.5 persistently then insulin.
- HbA1 <7.5—if on triple therapy or insulin.
- BP 130/75—all patients with diabetes without proteinuria.
- BP 125/75—all patients with diabetes with proteinuria treated with ACE (angiotensin-converting enzyme inhibitors) or ARB (angiotensin II receptor blockers).
- Keep cholesterol <4 mmol/L and LDL <2 mmol/L and treat with statin if >40 yrs or <40 yrs with high cardiovascular risk.

Intervention if HbA1 >6.5% → Life style measure
              If consistently HbA1 >6.5
              ↓

    Metformin (Gliclazide considered if not over weight or glucose levels high)
        Metformin reduced 50% if eGFR <45 or creatinine >130 mmol/L
        ↓ discontinue if eGFR <30 or creatinine >150 mmol/L
        ↓ if HbA1 >7.0

Metformin + Gliclazide (Exenatide subcutaneous if
BMI >35 better than pioglitazone, sitagliptin
↓ or glargine, no risk of hypoglycemia,
so better for drivers, bus drivers.
Intervention if HbA1 >7.5% pioglitazone or insulin
(Exenatide if BMI >35)
↓

Metformin + Gliclazide + insulin (Pioglitazone helpful if poor control with high dose insulin)

If ill or vomiting or diarrhea stop metformin. If GFR <45 reduce 50% metformin.

3rd agent for control of diabetes

- Metformin + gliclazide + exenatide SC (half-life 2.4 hr) liraglutide (half-life 13 hrs) when BMI >35 continue only if after 6/12 weight loss 3% and decrease in HbA1 at least 1%. Contraindicated if eGFR <30.
- Metformin + gliclazide + insulin
- Metformin + gliclazide + DPP4 inhibitors (Sitagliptin or Vildagliptin), when Pioglitazone contraindicated because of edema or weight gain (Sitagliptin 100 mg/day or Vildagliptin 50 mg/day) LFT before and every 3/12 for 1 yr.
- Metformin + gliclazide + pioglitazone.

Aspirin 75 mg/day >50 yrs with DM with normal BP (<145/75) or <50 yrs if high CV risk (CVD, microalbuminuria, metabolic syndrome, family history of CVD, hypertension, smoking).

Simvastatin for every one >40 yrs and <40 if at greater CV risk.

Risk of IHD

BM 3.9–5.6—No increase risk
    5.6–6.1—Risk increased by 11%
    6.1–7.0—Risk increased by 17%

Each 1 mmol rise in BM above 5.6 increases IHD risk by 12%.

- Add sitagliptine or thiazolidinedione if insulin unacceptable.
- Pioglitazone may be added if poor control on high insulin dose.
- Fenofibrate + statin slow diabetic retinopathy.
- Prevention of T2DM with small dose of metformin + small dose of pioglitazone.

NEWER AGENTS IN TYPE 2 DIABETES MELLITUS

- Consider adding DPP4 (Dipeptidyl peptidase-4) inhibitors (Sitagliptine) or thiazolidinedione (Pioglitazone) to metformin when HbA1 >6.5% or when serious risk of hypoglycemia with sulfonylurea or sulfonylurea not tolerated.

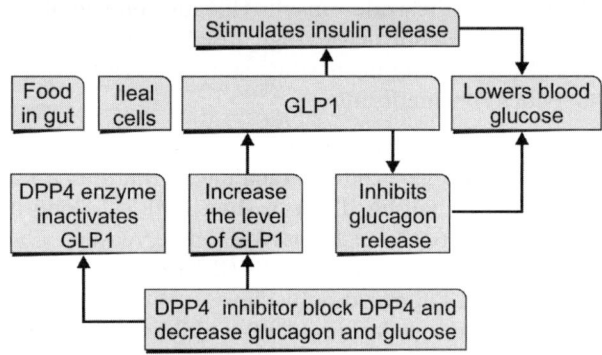

- *DPP4 inhibitors*: Inhibit the breakdown if endogenous GLP-1 (glucagon like peptide) and mimic many actions of GLP-1 secreted from intestinal cells on eating with half-life of 2 minutes. It stimulates insulin secretion; inhibits glucagon secretion and delays gastric emptying and cause weight loss.

  Consider adding DPP-4 inhibitors (Sitagliptine) or thiazolidinedione (Pioglitazone) to Sulfonylurea when HbA1 >6.5 and metformin cannot be used (creatinine >150 or eGFR <30) contraindicated or intolerance.

- Consider adding DPP4 inhibitors (Sitagliptine) or Thiazolidinedione (Pioglitazone) to sulfonylurea and metformin when HbA1 >7.5 and insulin is unacceptable or inappropriate.

- Continue DPP4 (Sitagliptine) or Thiazolidinedione (Pioglitazone) only if HbA1% reduction >0.7% in 6 months.

  Combine pioglitazone with insulin if previous good response with pioglitazone or patient on high dose of insulin. Pioglitazone contraindicated in CCF or risk of fracture.

  Glucagon like peptides (GLP-1) exenatide (short acting) and liraglutide (long acting). There is moderate hyposecretion of GLP-1 in T2DM. GLP-1 has direct effects

Metabolic, Renal and Endocrine

on hypothalamus to induce satiety and delay gastric emptying and both these factors induce postprandial fullness. So the physiological effects of GLP-1 are to improve B cell functions, reduce glucagon secretions and gastric emptying, induce satiety and facilitate weight loss.

Exenatide normal dose is 5 microgm SC bd with in 1 hr before meal for 4/52 and then 10 microgram bd. Liraglutide 0.6 mg once a day maximum is 1.8 mg/day.

GLP-1 if BMI >35, in BMI <30 when insulin has substantial problem with occupation.

Continue GLP-1 if HbA1 falls 1% and weight loss 3%.

Consider acarbose if unable to take other glucose lowering medication orally.

Avoid glitazones (DPP4) in peripheral vascular disease and coronary artery disease.

About 80% of T2DM end up on insulin and there is progressive failure of B cells and not prevented by aggressive therapy.

Hyponatremia

Investigations

- Plasma and urine osmolality, urinary Na, blood glucose and electrolytes.
- Chest X-ray.

Symptoms

- Headache, nausea, vomiting, muscle weakness, and confusional state, coma, respiratory arrest, and seizures may occur with severe hyponatrema.
- Symptoms and signs relate to the rate of onset more than the degree of fall in sodium.
- Gradual fall to 110 mmol/L can be well tolerated; acute fall to 127 mmol/L may be fatal.
- Na <120 mmol/L is associated with 50% mortality.

Management

- Depends on degree and rate of fall.
- Acute fall <12–24 hrs resulting in coma, encephalopathy and fits.
- With Na <120 mmoL/L in acute stage use hypertonic saline 3% 0.05 mL/kg/min in HDU aiming to increase

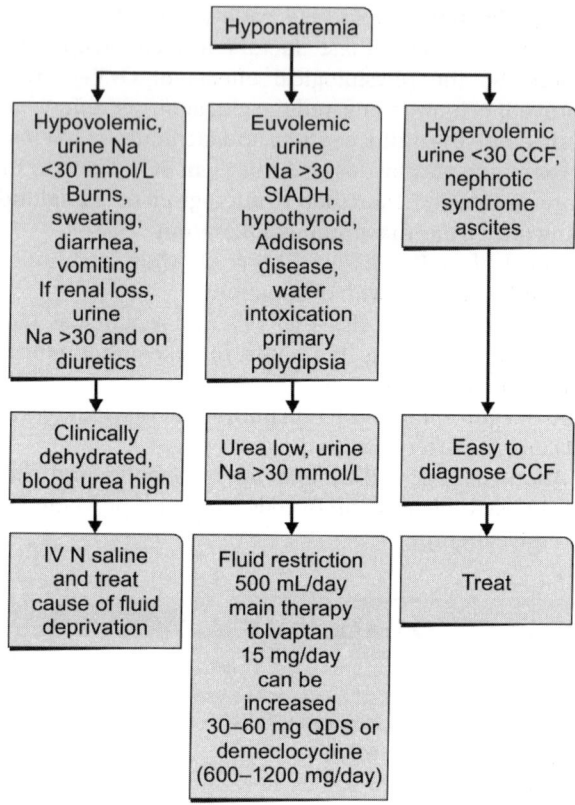

by 1 mmol/hour until Na is 120 mmol/L, not above 130 and by maximum 12 mmol in 24 hours and checking serum Na every 2 hrs.
- In chronic cases (>48 hrs) increase should not be more than 10 mmol L in 24 hrs. Rapid correction may result in pontine osmotic demyelization presenting as pseudo bulbar palsy, quardriparesis, mutism, respiratory arrest and fits.
- Treat fits with diazemuls.
- Remove cause.
- Fluid restriction in cirrhosis, nephrotic syndrome and cardiac failure. In volume depleted patients give 0.9% saline and correct hypokalemia.

Cerebral Salt Wasting Syndrome (CSWS)

- Presents as hyponatremia, hypovolemia (euvolemia in SIADH), and low urinary sodium (<30 mmol/L) usually

within one week after head injury or subarachnoid hemorrhage and treated with IV normal saline.
- Consider combination of IV normal saline + AVP receptor antagonist (Tolvaptan).
- Fluid restriction is not appropriate.
- Patient usually has polydipsia, polyuria, salt craving, muscle cramps, dizziness, vertigo and hypotension.

Syndrome of Inappropriate Antidiuretic Hormone Secretion (SIADH)

- Plasma NA (sodium) <130 mmols/L (mild), <120 mmols/L (severe).
- Urine osmolality >100 mOsmol/kg, plasma osmolality <275 mOsmol/kg.
- Urine NA >30 mmols/L.
- No edema and no signs of hypovolemia.
- Normal renal, adrenal, cardiac, hepatic, pituitary and thyroid functions.
- Patient is not taking any diuretics or purgatives, absence of edema, hypotension.

Causes

Malignant Diseases

Small cell carcinoma of bronchus, lymphoma, thymoma, mesothelioma, carcinoma of pancreas and duodenum.

Chest Disorders

Pneumonia, TB, empyema, asthma, pneumothorax and positive pressure ventilation.

Neurological Disorders

Meningitis, encephalitis, head injury, brain tumor, cerebral abscess, Guillain-Barré syndrome and intermittent porphyria.

Drugs

Antidepressant (tricyclics and SSRI), carbamazepine, Na valproate, cytotoxic, ecstasy, opioids, oxytocin, phenothiazine's (Haloperidol) and thiazides and bromocriptine.

Others: Postoperative state, adrenal insufficiency and HIV infections.

Clinical Features

- Cerebral signs are usually absent when Na >125 mmol/L.
- Headache, nausea, confusion, disorientation, coma and seizures are common when Na <120 mmol/L.

Treatment

- Treat the cause.
- Restrict fluid to 500 mL/24 hrs and this is the main treatment.
- Tolvaptan (AVP receptor antagonist) 15 mg OD and increasing it to 30–60 mg QID depending on response.
- Demeclocycline (600–1200 mg daily in divided doses) maximal effect may take 2 wks to achieve. Contraindicated in chronic renal failure.
- If sodium is corrected by IV 0.9% saline then serum sodium must not rise more than 4–6 mmol/L in 24 hrs.
- In hyponatremia of rapid onset with cerebral symptoms treat with hypertonic saline 3% 0.05 mL/kg/min in HDU to increase serum Na 1 mmol/L/h until serum Na 120 mmol/L is attained.
- If seizures are present then either mannitol 20% or hypertonic saline will be effective.
- Normally with symptomatic hyponatremia (Na <120 mmol/L) patient has both water excess (6–8 L) and Na deficiency (200–400 mmol).
- Monitoring of CVP is required during IV hypertonic saline administration.

Primary Adrenal Failure (Addison's Disease) and Secondary Adrenal Failure

- Primary failure of adrenal cortex is due to adrenal disease (autoimmune 75%, 20% TB) and 70% have autoimmune adrenal antibodies.
- Secondary failure is due to pituitary (failure of ACTH), hypothalamus or withdrawal of chronic glucocorticoids therapy.

- Mineralocorticoid action of adrenal steroids is Na (sodium) retention and K (potassium) excretion.
- Waterhouse-Friderichsen syndrome is acute adrenal crisis due to adrenal hemorrhage in meningococcal infection.

Signs and Symptoms

Tiredness, anorexia, nausea, weight loss, pigmentation (high ACTH) in skin exposed to sun light and pressure and irritation, lips, gums, cheeks, palmar creases and scars, abdominal pain, vomiting, diarrhea, salt craving, fatigue, postural hypotension, shock and vitiligo. Loss of axillary and pubic hair in women is suggestive of Addison's disease.

Secondary Adrenal Insufficiency

- Signs are pale skin without anemia, amenorrhea, decreased libido, scanty axillary and pubic hair, small testis, secondary hypothyroidism, headache, visual symptoms and diabetes insipidus.
- Personal or family history of autoimmune/endocrine disease, TB and recent flank pain should be elicited.
- Consider the diagnosis in patients with unexplained hypotension who has been taking steroids >5 mg daily or has clinical features suggestive of adrenal insufficiency.
- *On investigations*: Low Na, high K, metabolic acidosis, high urea, hypoglycemia and hypercalcemia.

Causes

- Rapid withdrawal of corticosteroids therapy.
- Sepsis or surgical stress.
- Autoimmune adrenalitis, TB.
- Bilateral adrenal hemorrhage, fulminant meningococcal sepsis, coagulation disorders, heparin or warfarin therapy.
- *Pituitary causes*: Posterior pituitary necrosis (Sheehan syndrome), necrosis or bleeding into a pituitary macro adenoma, pituitary surgery or after pituitary radiotherapy.
- Head injury (sometimes with diabetes insipidus).

Management

- If Addison's disease is suspected take blood for cortisol, ACTH and give hydrocortisone 100 mg IV 6 hrly for 24–48 hrs afterwards orally gradually reduced to 15 mg in the morning and 10 mg in the evening or 10 mg, 5 mg, 2.5 mg and fludrocortisone 50–100 microgram oral per day (primary adrenocortical failure).
- Check FBC, U and E, glucose, calcium, TSH, chest X-ray, adrenal CT, plasma renin (high in primary and normal in secondary adrenal insufficiency).
- If blood glucose <3.5 mmol/L give 50 mL of 10% dextrose.
- If systolic BP <90 mm Hg, give colloids 500 mL IV, if BP >90 mm Hg give normal saline 1 L 6–8 hrly till fluid deficit has been corrected.
- Start antibiotics if source of sepsis is evident, if WBC is <3,000 or >20,000 or the temperature is <36 or >38°C.

Short Synacthen Test

- To confirm the diagnosis, do short Synacthen test by taking blood for cortisol before and after 30 minutes of IM or IV 250 microgram synacthen.
- Base line cortisol >400 mmol/L excludes the diagnosis.
- Normal response is a 30 minutes cortisol >460 mmol/L.
- If the patient is already on hydrocortisone change to prednisolone (5 mg mane, 2.5 mg nocte) for two days and perform the test in the morning before the morning dose of prednisolone.
- Do not do Synacthen test in the very ill.
- Patient should be advised to wear medi-alert bracelet and carry a steroid card.

Patients on long-term steroid therapy when the dose should be increased.

Mild infection: Double the usual dose.

Minor surgery: 100 mg hydrocortisone IV 6 hrly for 24 hrs starting with the premedication, and then return to usual dose.

Severe infections or major surgery: Give hydrocortisone as minor surgery but continue for 72 hrs or until taking oral fluids. After this give same dose orally (and restart fludrocortisone) and gradually taper over 2 wks to usual maintenance dose.

ADRENAL CRISIS

- Shock resistant to fluids and vasopressor
- Random cortisol and ACTH should be requested
- Correct BP with normal saline and hydrocortisone 100 mg IV stat and 50–100 mg IM 6 hrly.

Hypocalcemia

Causes

Spurious hypocalcemia, that is failure to correct for low albumin (add 0.02 mmol/L to the total calcium for each g/L albumin below 40 g/L.
- Hypoparathyroidism.
- Renal failure.
- Vitamin D deficiency.
- Hypomagnesemia, hypermagnesemia, alkalosis, hypophosphatemia and rhabdomyolysis.
- Acute pancreatitis.
- Pseudo hypoparathyroidism.

Clinical Features

- *Early features*: Anxiety, nervousness, dysrhythmia around mouth, toes and fingers.
- *Late features*: (Calcium, 1.9 mmol/L).

Central Nervous System

Muscle cramps, tetany, proximal myopathy, tremor, ataxia, depression, psychosis, convulsions, muscle twitches, Chvostek's sign + (gental tapping over facial nerve causes facial twitching), Trousseau's sign + (inflation of sphygmomanometer cuff above diastolic BP for 3 minutes causes tetanic spasm of fingers and wrist) and papilledema.

Cardiovascular

Prolonged QT interval, T-wave inversion, loss of digoxin effect, hypotension and arrhythmia.

Respiratory

Apnea, laryngospasm and bronchospasm.

Investigations

U and E, calcium, phosphate, albumin, magnesium, vitamin D, PTH and alkaline phosphates.

Treatment

Acute severe hypocalcemia usually <1.875 mmol/L with tetany, fits or arrhythmia.

- Give 10% of 10 mL calcium gluconate IV over 5 minutes follow-up with infusion of calcium gluconate 10 ampoules of 10% in 1 L 5% dextrose infused at rate of 50 mL/hr (1 mg Ca/mL) till serum calcium is >1.9 mmol/L. Continuously monitor ECG.
- Failures to increase ionized calcium after oral calcium consider underlying Mg deficiency.
    Introduce oral calcium and vitamin D as soon as possible.
- Magnesium should be corrected IV 8-10 mmols magnesium sulfate diluted in 100 mL 0.9% NaCl and infused over 20 minutes or orally (if no dysrhythmia or tetany) 24 mmols/day. Hypomagnesemia is caused by chronic alcoholism, malabsorption, diuretic therapy, prolonged parenteral therapy, refeeding syndrome and use of PPI.

Hypercalcemia

Causes

- Primary hyperparathyroidism.
- Malignancy, tumors with secondaries to the bone, carcinoma of breast, bronchus, lymphoma and myeloma. These account for 80% of cases.
- Sarcoidosis, total parenteral nutrition, prolonged immobilization with rapid bone turn over (children, multiple fractures, Paget's disease), thyrotoxicosis, primary adrenal failure (Addison's disease), pheochromocytoma, milk alkali syndrome, vitamin D/A analogues, antiestrogens, lithium, familial hypocalciuric hypocalcemia and thiazides.
- An average total of 1-2 kg calcium is present of which 99% is present in bone and of the remaining 9/10 is present in the cell and 1/10 is present in extracellular

fluid. Of which 50% is bound to plasma proteins and so corrected with plasma protein levels 40-albumin levels (0.02). Mg is required for PTH secretion and end organ responsiveness.

Symptoms

- May be asymptomatic.
- *Acute hypercalcemia*: General malaise, anorexia, thirst, polyuria, constipation, abdominal pain, depression and confusion.
- *Complications*: Peptic ulceration, acute pancreatitis, muscle weakness, psychosis, drowsiness, coma, and corneal calcification and short QT interval.

Signs

Dehydration (reduced skin turgor, dry mucus membranes), postural hypotension and evidence of malignancy.

Investigations

- Calcium, phosphate, alkaline phosphates, FBC, ESR, U and E, LFT, ECG, chest X-ray, PTH and myeloma screen.
- Calcium may be normal if vitamin D deficient and hypercalcemia becomes apparent after correction of vitamin D deficiency. Similarly PTH may be normal in hypercalcemia and vitamin D deficiency.
- Specific investigation (Technitium bone scan, TFT (thyroid function test), serum ACE (angiotensin converting enzyme), and 24 hrs urine for calcium.

Treatment

- Surgery for hyperparathyroidism if Ca >2.85, renal impairment, renal calculi, osteoporosis T < 2.5, age <50 yrs.
- Medical treatment with cinacalcet is expensive treatment in asymptomatic hypercalcemia.
- Emergency treatment is required if corrected Ca >3.5 mmol/L.

Between 3 and 3.5 mmol/L may not require emergency treatment, but depends on signs and symptoms. For each gram of albumin <40 add 0.02 nmol/L to the uncorrected Ca.

- *Fluids*: Urgent fluids replacement with 0.9% saline 1 L 4–6 hrly (3–6 L/24 hrs) will lower Ca and enhance renal clearance (add KCL as required). Insert urinary catheter to monitor urinary output. Always give bisphosphonates after rehydration.
- A single infusion of bisphosphonates will lower calcium levels within 3 days and will last for 21 days. Zoledronic acid 4 mg IV over 15 minutes. Or pamidronate 60–90 mg given IV after dilution over 120 minutes if renal function are normal, if creatinine clearance <30 mL/min then administer over 4–6 hrs.
- *Never used thiazides*: If patient is on digoxin discontinue, as its effects are potentiated by hypercalcemia.

  Steroids should not be used routinely; there are help full in myeloma, sarcoidosis, lymphoma and hypervitaminosis D. If glucocorticoid deficiency is suspected then give hydrocortisone 100 mg IV 6 hrly until the diagnosis is excluded.

  If hypercalcemia persistent then consider urgent surgery after parathyroid MIBI scan and ultrasound scan.

Hyperthyroidism or Thyrotoxicosis

- Autoimmune thyroid disease is more common in smokers.
- Raised thyroid stimulating IgG antibody which bind to TSH receptors and causes Graves's disease.
- Toxic nodular goiter is common where there is iodine deficiency and its remission is rare and thyroid antibodies are absent.
- Thyroiditis causes transient thyrotoxicosis in 10%, low or absent uptake on thyroid scan, raised ESR and CRP (C reactive protein) and painless lymphocytic thyroiditis. Thyroid antibodies are positive.
- In postpartum thyroiditis (<1 yr), thyroid functions 1st hyper- and then hyporeturning to normal in 18 months. Hyperthyroid state is treated with propranolol and hypothyroid state is treated with thyroxin.
- Essential to have normal TSH before and during pregnancy.

Metabolic, Renal and Endocrine

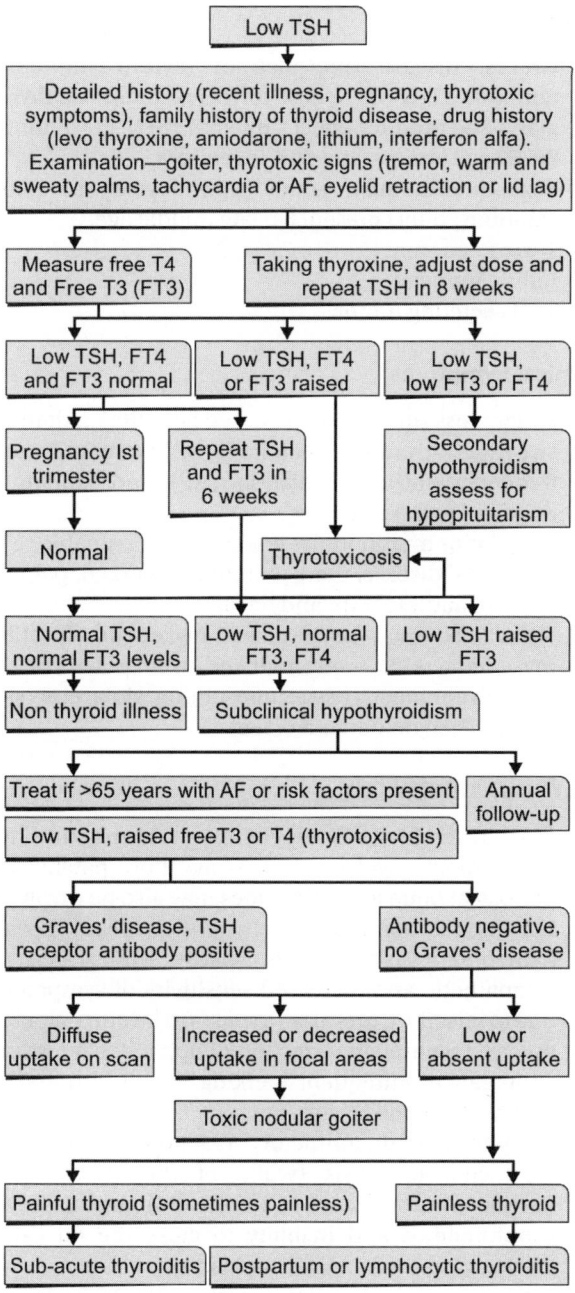

Causes

- Graves' disease (presence of thyroid stimulating antibodies IgG which bind to TSH receptors on thyroid gland and produce effect similar to TSH), presenting in 20-60 age groups, and 90% in females.
- Toxic multinodular goiter (may develop in a long standing goiter) presents in late middle age.
- Toxic adenoma.
- Iodine induced.
- TSH secreting tumor.

Clinical Symptoms

- Weight loss (in spite of increased appetite), irritability, sweating, tremors, palpitations, increased stool frequency, atrial fibrillation (AF) and sometimes proximal myopathy.
- Nodular or multinodular goiter may be palpable.
- In Graves' disease, there is smooth enlarged, palpable thyroid, audible bruit and lid lag.
- There also may be localized myxedema (pretibial myxedema 1-2%)—pronounced over growth of skin and sub cutaneous tissue, non-pitting, violaceous skin, usually seen on dorsum of feet.

THYROID ACROPACHY

- <1%—resembles finger clubbing, thumb and fore finger often involved and X-ray show patchy subperiosteal bone formation, toes may also be involved.
- Lid lag is common in hyperthyroidism. Levator palpebrae superioris is partly innervated by sympathetic and increased sensitivity of sympathetic due to raised T4, produces a spasm in levator palpebrae muscle resulting in retraction of upper eye lid, staring appearance, infrequent blinking, white of the sclera visible above the cornea.
- Autoimmune inflammatory reaction involves orbit producing proptosis (white of the sclera visible between cornea and lower eyelid) and if severe exophthalmos and inability to close the lid causes corneal and conjunctival edema.
- Tethering of extraocular muscles caused by inflammation leads to opthalmoplegia.

Investigations

- FBC, FT3, FT4, TSH and thyroid antibodies.
- Ultrasound if palpable thyroid nodule or goiter.
- T3 done when TSH is suppressed and T4 is normal for T3 toxicosis.
- In Graves' disease thyroid antibodies are positive.

Management

All patients are treated medically to make them euthyroid even if surgery or radioactive iodine selected.

Medical

- Carbimazole 40–60 mg/day for 4–6 wks and then 5–15 mg/d for 12–24 months. Some continue higher dose and thyroxin added after 4–6 wks.
    Side effects are agranulocytosis and rashes. Patient is told to stop carbimazole if they develop rash or sore throat and see doctor urgently.
    People with large goiter or HLA-DR3 tend to relapse.
- Propylthiouracil is used in 1st three months of pregnancy and then carbimazole.
- Propranolol 40–80 mg 6 hrly used for palpitation in early stages as it reduces conversion T4 to T3.

Surgery

- Large goiter.
- Patient unable to take drug therapy or relapse after drug therapy.
- Patient should be euthyroid before surgery and some surgeons use potassium iodide for 10 days before surgery to reduce vascularity.
- Recurrent laryngeal nerve palsy and transient hypocalcemia (10%) are complications.

Radioactive Iodine Therapy

- Difficult to control hyperthyroidism with drugs and recurrence after surgery.
- Patient is made euthyroid before and antithyroid drugs Carbimazole is stopped for 2 days before or Propylthiouracil for 2 wks before administering radioiodine to allow the gland to take up the dose and restarted after 7 days.

SUBCLINICAL HYPERTHYROIDISM

- Low TSH <0.1 and normal T4, T3 (absence of hypothalamic, pituitary disease, drugs and nonthyroid illness).
- TSH <0.5—X 3 times risk of AF.
- TSH <0.1 increased risk of hip fracture in postmenopausal women.
- If TSH <0.1 and T4 T3 normal—consider treatment.
- If TSH 0.1–0.5 and T4 T3 normal repeat in 3/12.

Thyrotoxic Crisis

- Known thyroid disease.
- Symptoms of weight loss, palpitation, heat intolerance, sweating, diarrhea, tremor, anxiety/extreme restlessness, irritability, confusion and psychosis. In elderly congestive cardiac failure (CCF), GI disturbance and apathy/depression.
- Consider the diagnosis in any patient with fever, abnormal mental state, sinus tachycardia or atrial fibrillation with signs of thyrotoxicosis. If the diagnosis is suspected, antithyroid treatment must be started before biochemical confirmation.
- *Precipitants*: Infections, surgical stress, trauma, radioiodine therapy, amiodarone, pulmonary embolism or myocardial infarction, thyroid surgery and child birth.

Diagnosis

Temperature: 38.5–41°C, atrial fibrillation (AF), heart failure, agitation and psychosis. Check for thyroid bruit, goiter and ophthalmopathy. Signs may be masked in the elderly and by the illness. Immediate treatment on clinical suspicion.

Urgent Investigations

TSH, free T3, T4, calcium, cortisol, CK, U and E, FBC, blood glucose, blood culture, urine microscopy and culture, chest X-ray and ECG.

Treatment

- Give oxygen keeping SaO_2 >92%, ECG monitor. IV fluids for GI loss and insensible loss. Cooling packs and paracetamol but not aspirin.

- *Nutrition*: High calorie, water-soluble vitamins and thiamine.
- Propranolol 40–80 mg 6 hrly PO, aiming to reduce heart rate <100/min. Diltiazem 60–120 mg 6 hrly PO can be used if beta-blockers are contraindicated because of asthma.
- *Anti-thyroid drugs*: Start propylthiouracil 600 mg Oral stat then 100 mg 6 hrly PO (or rectally if severe vomiting), when stable then switch to carbimazole 20 mg 6 hrly (inhibiting synthesis).
- Iodine (Lugol's iodine 5% or KI 10% in purified water) 4 hr after starting antithyroid drugs, (inhibiting secretion of thyroxine) 5 drops orally 6 hrly. Never before the patient is on antithyroid drugs for at least 4 hrs.
- Hydrocortisone 200 mg IV over 1 minute then 100 mg 8 hrly.
- Treat sepsis with antibiotics and reduce fever by tepid sponging or fanning or paracetamol (avoid aspirin).
- *Anticoagulation*: Therapeutic dose of LMWH SC to patients with AF. Other patients should receive LMWH at prophylactic dose.
- Consider digoxin for atrial fibrillation and furosemide for pulmonary edema.

Goiter

- Multinodular goiter (MNG)—palpable R/L lobe, no lymph nodes palpable, no retrosternal extension, no bruit and patient euthyroid and thyroid functions (TFT) should be checked.
- Fine needle aspiration (FNA) at any time if any enlarging nodule or in doubt.
- Hoarseness suggests involved recurrent laryngeal nerve suggesting malignancy.
- CT or MRI, respiratory functions and barium swallow to assess the tracheal and esophageal compression by retrosternal goiter.

TOXIC MULTINODULAR GOITER

Treated with radioactive iodine, antithyroid drugs with propranolol and surgery. Radioactive iodine will reduce the size by 50%.

Diffusely Enlarged Nontoxic Goiter

Simple Goiter

- Asymptomatic, euthyroid (no bruit, tremor, sweaty palms, lid lag), female, puberty or pregnancy. In iodine deficient areas, in goiter TSH is normal.
- If asymptomatic and no recent increase in size, no further investigation or treatment needed but 6 month/1 yr follow-up to confirm no change in size.
- Pembertons sign, faintness, congestion of face, external jugular obstruction, distended veins over face and head when both arms are raised above the head in Retro sternal goiter.
- Respiratory functions and CT or MRI to assess obstruction.
- If low TSH then thyroid peroxidase antibodies should be done to exclude sub clinical thyrotoxicosis. Urinary iodine <10 µg/dL supports iodine deficiency.
- Thyroid scan (unnecessary) may show increased uptake and ultrasound not done unless nodule is palpable.
- Maximum regression in 3–6/12.
- Surgery some times for cosmetic or retrosternal symptoms, after surgery give T4 to prevent re-growth of goiter.

Treated Graves' Disease

Exophthalmos, +/− bruit, patient may be euthyroid or hypothyroid.

Hashimoto's Disease

Goiter usually fine micronodular, firm, symmetrical and hypothyroid faces, pulse and ankle jerks. Pain in goiter with compressive symptoms and little enlargement is due to thyroiditis.

Viral Thyroiditis (De Quervain's Disease)

Thyroid tender, may have constitutional symptoms, absent radioactive iodine uptake, raised thyroxine and suppressed TSH.

SOLITARY NODULE

Thyroid adenoma (scan may show normal, decreased or increased uptake.

- Toxic adenoma (increased uptake on scan with tachycardia, sweaty palms, lid lag and tremor. Hot nodules are almost never malignant.
    So FNA unnecessary. Treated by radioactive iodine or surgery.
- Thyroid cyst –1/3 of palpable nodules
- Thyroid carcinoma (palpable lymph nodes, hard, recent change in size, cold on the scan). Papillary thyroid cancer (PTC) accounts 70–90% of all differentiated thyroid cancers.

Most thyroid nodules should have thyroid functions, thyroid ultrasound (to assess size and no of nodules, cystic or solid) and fine needle aspiration (FNA) to establish cytology.

Thyroid scans are performed less often and are useful only in thyroiditis (cold), thyroxin abuse (cold) and toxic adenoma (hot). If nodule is hot, it is not malignancy but if it is cold then it may be.

In an elderly patient if nodule has been present for a long time then wait and watch.

Most thyroid lumps are asymptomatic and euthyroid. Sometimes may have pressure symptoms (dysphagia, dysphonia, and stridor) or pain (bleeding in to adenoma with pain radiating to ear).

- Normal TFT → fine needle aspiration (FNA) if <1 cm or difficult biopsy or non-diagnostic 17% then ultrasound guided biopsy.
- Low TSH → Thyroid scan—cold → FNA, if hot treat medically.
- FNA—Benign 69%, repeat biopsy once for benign nodules and surgery if further growth or suspicious cytology.
- FNA—cysts—consider ultrasound guided biopsy and surgery if regrowth or suspicious cytology.
- FNA—suspicious follicular or malignant cytology → surgery.

Surgery

- Concern about malignancy,
- Pressure symptoms (dysphagia, dysphonia, pain and stridor).
- Enlarging lump.

Thyroid Functions in Pregnancy

1. Rise in hCG in 1st trimester stimulates TSH-Receptor but it is a weak binding, causing some times hyperemesis gravidarum presenting as severe nausea and vomiting. Parenteral fluid replacement is needed and anti-thyroid drugs rarely needed.
2. Increased urinary iodide excretion, so women with precarious iodide intake (<50 µg) are at risk of developing goiter during pregnancy, so iodine should be supplemented to prevent fetal and maternal hypothyroidism.

SICK EUTHYROID SYNDROME (SES)

- In severe nonthyroid illness—T4 normal, FT3 low, normal TSH—due to decreased conversion from T4 to T3 due to cytokines and severity of illness.
- In very severe illness—low T4, Low TSH and low FT3.

Amiodarone Effect

Amiodarone (half-life 60 days) contains 39% iodine leading to 40 fold increase in plasma and urinary iodine levels and as amiodarone is stored in fatty tissue, so high levels persist >6/12 after discontinuation.

Its metabolites are weak antagonists of thyroid hormone and it interferes with conversion of FT4 to FT3 and also inhibits deiodinase activity.

- At initiation there is transient decrease T4 because inhibitory effect on T4 release. Soon after most people escape from iodine dependent thyroid suppression and thyroid hormone receptor activity becomes prominent leading to raised T4, low T3 and transient raised TSH (up to 20 mµ/L) lasting 1-3/12 and after that normalizes.
- Hypothyroidism occurs in 6-13%, common in women or in people with thyroid peroxidase antibodies (TPO). Thyroxin can be used, so no need to discontinue. Monitor TSH as T4 is raised because of increased thyroid hormone receptor activity as above.
- Thyrotoxicosis (AIT)—2-10%.

Type 1: Associated with underlying thyroid abnormality (pre-clinical Graves' disease or multinodular goiter), T4 synthesis becomes excessive because of iodine exposure, Thyroid scan shows increased vascularity and increased uptake. Stop the drug after discussion with the cardiologist, high doses of antithyroid drugs can be used but often ineffective.

Type 2: No previous intrinsic thyroid abnormality, drug induced lysosomal activation leading to destructive thyroiditis with histiocytes.

Thyroid scan shows decreased vascularity.

Mild form resolves spontaneously or can lead to hypothyroidism.

Potassium perchlorate 200 mg 6 hrly or sodium ipodate 500 mg/d or sodium tyropanoate 500 OD or bid can be used.

Steroids are of variable benefit. Lithium blocks thyroid hormone release and is of modest benefit.

Sub-total thyroidectomy is effective long-term solution for type 1 and 2.

Case: Patient on amiodarone for AF has TSH 0.4 (.4–5), FT4-30 (11–23), FT3-4.2 (2.8–7.1). This patient is not thyrotoxic as TSH is suppressed because of non-thyroid illness and FT4 is raised because of amiodarone interference in conversion from FT4 to FT3. So in amiodarone FT3 should be measured.

Hypothyroidism

Results from decreased production of thyroid hormone caused by primary disease of thyroid or failure of TSH production from pituitary or thyroid releasing hormone (TRH) from hypothalamus.

Causes

Iodine deficiency, autoimmune thyroid disease or previous treatment for hyperthyroidism (postradioactive iodine therapy 50% in 10 yrs, postpartial thyroidectomy 30% in 10 yrs).

Clinical Features

- *Nonspecific symptoms*: Weight gain, cold intolerance, tiredness, constipation, aches and pains, poor

memory, mental slowness (depression, dementia), puffiness around the eyes and thickening of lips and tongue (infiltration of mucopolysaccharides).
- Husky speech, changes in skin and hair (alopecia, dry skin and hair), carpal tunnel syndrome, slow relaxing reflexes.

Investigation

Low T4 and raised TSH, if TSH is normal with low T4—secondary hypothyroidism due to pituitary or hypothalamus.

Subclinical Hypothyroidism

- T4 normal and raised TSH and peroxidase thyroid antibodies positive in 50% (absence of hypothalamic, pituitary disease, drugs and non-thyroid illness).
- Probability of hypothyroidism in 20 yrs.

TSH	Thyroid antibody	
2	−	2%
2	+	11%
5	−	11% check 3–5 yearly
5	+	42% check yearly TSH
10	−	32%
10	+	74%

- Levo thyroxine once TSH is 10 or more unless pregnant or growth phase then earlier.
- Half-life of thyroxine is 7 days, so improvement is seen in 2–3 wks.
- Chest X-ray may show pericardial and pleural effusion and ECG—bradycardia and low voltage complexes.

Treatment

- Thyroxine should not be started if there is suspicion of secondary hypothyroidism. 1st exclude pituitary or hypothalamic disease (ACTH reserve) otherwise thyroxin alone will precipitate glucocorticoid insufficiency.
- Thyroxine started 50 µg (25 in elderly or IHD) and increased monthly by 25.

Pheochromocytomas and Paraganglioma

- These are tumors of adrenal medulla which secrete catecholamines (adrenaline and noradrenaline). 10% extra adrenal (sympathetic chain), 10% malignant and 10% bilateral.
- Occur commonly in inherited conditions (25%).
- Episodic severe hypertension after abdominal palpation.
- Phechromocytoma is associated with neurofibromatosis (autosomal dominant, chromosome 17, sub cutaneous fibromas, Cafe-au-lait patches) and phechromocytoma (0.5–1%).
- Von-Hipple-Lindau (autosomal dominant, chromosome 3, cerebellar hemangioblastomas, renal cell carcinomas, retinal angioma, pancreatic cysts) and Phechromocytoma (25%).
- Multiendocrine neoplasia (MEN) type II A adrenal (Pheochromocytoma 70% bilateral), thyroid (Medullary carcinoma, calcitonin producing) and parathyroid adenoma (60%).
- MEN IIB is IIA + marfanoid phenotype.
- MEN Type I parathyroid, pituitary and pancreas adenomas.
- Sporadic tumors are unilateral and <10 cm while those associated with familial syndromes are bilateral and 25% are malignant.
- Presents as sustained or episodic hypertension, resistant to conventional treatment and with sweating, heat intolerance, flushing or pallor and feeling of apprehension.
- Severe hypertension can cause MI and stroke.
- High adrenaline can cause VF
- Diagnosis is by 24 hr urinary metanephrine, plasma metanephrine at least twice (>2000 pg/mL diagnostic), CT or MRI, MIBG (Metaiodo benzylguanidine) isotope scan. PET scan is more useful in paraglangioma.

Management

- Elective alpha blockade.
- Phenoxybenzamine 10 mg bd increasing to 20 mg bd.

- Penoxybenzamine 0.5 mg/kg IV over 4 hrs daily for 3 days before surgery and anesthesia. Phenoxybenzamine is non-competitive antagonist, slow in onset and irreversible.
- Beta-blockers added to prevent tachycardia (propranolol 80 mg 8 hrly after alpha blockade).

Emergency Alpha Blockade

- Give 1 L saline IV volume replacement.
- Na nitroprusside or diltiazem are helpful to lower BP when phenoxybenzamine is not available. Labetalol (alpha: beta-blocker 1:7) is not helpful.
- Phentolamine or nitroprusside are useful in perioperative hypertension.
- IV phentolamine 0.5-4 mg slow push.
- Phentolamine is short acting (minutes-hrs), rapid in onset, reversible, competitive antagonist.
- Beta-blockers propranolol to prevent tachycardia.
- If mother has IIA MEN and had adrenal removed (bilateral pheochromocytoma), daughter had gene and had thyroid removed (100% risk of cancer) has 20% chance of developing pheochromocytoma and should be screened annually for it.
- Pheochromocytomas are usually big tumors >4 cm
- False positive raised catecholamine's
- Catecholamine's are raised after surgery, MI or levo dopa therapy, ACE inhibitors and in obstructive sleep apnea (OSA).

Pituitary Apoplexy (Infarction)

- Sudden onset of retro-orbital headache in someone with known pituitary tumor.
- Visual field defect, nausea, vomiting, meningism and altered conscious level.
- Diplopia with hypopituitarism or hyperprolactinemia presenting as lethargy, reduced libido, oligomenorrhea/amenorrhea, impotence or galactorrhea.

Examination

- Assess GCS
- Vision acuity and fields

- Eye movements looking for opthalmoplegia
- Signs of underlying pituitary disease (acromegaly).

Management

- O_2 keeping SaO_2 >92%.
- On clinical suspicion take blood for serum cortisol if <100 mmols/L (diagnostic), prolactin FBC, U and E, glucose, LFT, coagulation screen, TSH, LH, FSH and estrogen/testosterone.
- Assume anterior pituitary dysfunction and give hydrocortisone 100 mg IV 6 hrly
- Urgent MRI.
- If vision severely affected-urgent surgical decompression.
- If vision not severely affected consider surgical decompression within 1 wk. Normal prolactin <400 mU/L, if prolactin >1500 mU/L (prolactinoma). Prolactin can be raised in stress, pregnancy and hypothyroidism.
- Non-surgical approach,
- Treat with hydrocortisone 10, 5, 5 mg/day + thyroxine 100 µg/day + sustanton 250 mg/3 wks.
- Consider dopamine agonist (Bromocriptine initially 1 mg nocte, gradually increase to 2.5 mg tds or cabergoline) if underlying prolactinoma pituitary tumor suspected.

Cushing Syndrome

Excessive cortisol production by adrenal cortex in zona fasciculate layer.

CUSHING DISEASE

- Excessive ACTH production by the pituitary gland.
- Ectopic Cushing syndrome—Ectopic ACTH from lung carcinoma or other carcinomas or carcinoids.
- Cushing disease common in females, central obesity, buffalo hump (dorso cervical fat pad), protuberant abdomen, proximal myopathy, thin skin, purple striae, easy bruising, osteoporosis in young, back pain, depression, psychosis, hirsutism, acne and greasy skin.
- If severe virilization with clitoral enlargement then adrenal carcinoma highly likely.
- Many of these features may be due to alcoholism.

Investigations

Overnight dexamethasone suppression test:
- 1 mg dexamethasone at bed time and cortisol at 9 am >100 nmol/L suspect cushing and if <50 nmol rules out.
- Urinary free cortisol >250 nmol/L in men and >400 nmol/L in women. False negative 5–10%.
- If both tests are normal, this excludes Cushing syndrome.
- If positive then for low dose dexamethasone test 97% diagnostic of Cushing syndrome (0.5 mg 6 hrly for 48 hrs), cortisol levels are not suppressed in Cushing's disease and also there is loss of normal diurnal rhythm (high mid night cortisol).
- Plasma ACTH <5 ng/L indicates adrenal cause of Cushing syndrome.
- ACTH >15 ng/L suggests Cushing disease.
- ACTH 5–15 needs careful evaluation.
- Low K <3.2 mmol/L (100% in ectopic ACTH and 10% in pituitary dependent disease).
- Glucose intolerance
- High dose dexamethasone 2 mg 6 hrly for 48 hrs will suppress cortisol in 50–90% in Cushing disease but not in ectopic ACTH.
- Corticotropin-releasing hormone (CRH) test—exaggerated response in rise in ACTH in Cushing disease.
- CT chest and abdomen, MRI head and bilateral inferior petrosal sinus sampling (BIPPS) are helpful in diagnosis.

Treatment

- Trans-sphenoidal surgery in Cushing disease or adrenal surgery in Cushing syndrome or radiotherapy (if surgery fails to control levels of cortisol).
- If this fails then bilateral adrenalectomy and pituitary radiotherapy to prevent Nelson syndrome (increasing level of ACTH, skin pigmentation and enlarging pituitary tumor because of loss of inhibition from cortisol).
- Metyrapone 500–1000 mg qds, aminoglutethimide and ketoconazole 200-400 mg tds—useful when not sure whether Cushing disease or ectopic ACTH.

Polycystic Ovarian Syndrome (POS)

Common in women 20–40, obesity, hirsutism, oligomenorrhea.

Investigations

- Serum LH and testosterone raised in 40%.
- Hirsutisms with normal hormone levels have mild polycystic ovarian syndrome.
- Polycystic ovary on ultrasound
- 17-hydroxy progesterone levels are raised in congenital adrenal hyperplasia.
- If serum testosterone levels are >4 nmol/L, short history and severe hirsutism, androgen secreting tumor should be excluded.

Treatment

- *Hirsutism*: Responds to estrogen and anti-androgen (cyproterone acetate).
- *Menstrual disturbances*: Combined oral contraceptive pill.
- *Anovulation*: Oral clomiphene citrate or parental gonadotrophin.
- *Insulin sensitizing drugs*: Metformin or thiazolidinedione may lead to resumption of normal ovulatory cycles and amelioration of clinical features.

Acromegaly

- Excessive growth hormone secretion from anterior pituitary.
- If before epiphyseal fusion causes gigantism and after epiphyseal fusion causes acromegaly.
- *Features*: Changes in the face, enlarged hands, nose, lips, large tongue, interdental separation.
- Prognathism, prominent supraorbital folds and ridge, greasy skin, sweaty spade like hands.
- Carpal tunnel syndrome, increase in shoe size, arthropathy and proximal myopathy.
- Obstructive sleep apnea, hypertension, IHD and CCF.

Investigations

- Raised IGF1, high calcium (10%), diabetes mellitus (10-25%), MRI pituitary, ECHO and colonoscopy.
- Benign micro adenoma of the pituitary is the most common cause.

Treatment

- Transphenoidal surgery with preservation of pituitary. Radiotherapy is sometimes given as an adjunct to surgery.
- Dopamine agonist (DA) bromocriptine or cabergoline or somatostatins (Octreotide) can normalize IGF1 in 90% of patients.

Hypopituitarism

- Non-secreting pituitary tumors may present with hypopituitarism.
- Gonadotropins and growth hormones are affected 1st followed by TSH and then ACTH.

Causes of Hypopituitarism

- *Developmental*: Kallmann syndrome—isolated gonadotrophin deficiency in men with anosmia.
- *Infiltration*: Sarcoidosis, hemochromatosis, autoimmune hypophysitis.
- *Vascular*: Sheehan syndrome, acute pituitary infarction due to hypovolemic or septic shock as in meningococcemia or pituitary apoplexy due to sudden pituitary hemorrhage, presenting as headache, visual loss, diplopia, and cardiovascular collapse.
- Tumors (pituitary), injury (radiation, surgery, trauma), infections (meningitis, TB), anorexia, starvation, stress, exercise and depression.
- Signs and symptoms depend on the hormone affected and local effects of enlarging pituitary.
- Testing for visual field loss of bitemporal hemianopia.
- Pallor, fine facial skin.
- In women, decreased libido, amenorrhea, genital atrophy, decreased axillary and pubic hair, and decreased breast size.

- In men decreased libido, impotence, decreased size and softening of testes, azospermia and loss of body hair.
- ACTH deficiency results in pallor of skin (hypopituitarism with secondary adrenal failure). Symptoms are same as primary adrenal failure except pigmentation.
- Vasopressin deficiency (Diabetes insipidus): Large tumors (Craniopharyngioma) or trauma or sarcoidosis, may cause failure of normal vasopressin production resulting in diabetes insipidus.
- Symptoms are usually masked because of associated ACTH deficiency. It is when steroid are started that patient develops D I (polyuria and polydipsia).

Causes of Polyuria

- Diabetes mellitus, diabetes insipidus (D I), psychogenic polydipsia, hypokalemia, hypercalcemia.
- *Nephrogenic diabetes insipidus (DI)*: Pyelonephritis, renal obstruction, sickle cell disease, hypokalemia, hypercalcemia, and lithium toxicity, is due to resistance of renal tubules to vasopressin.

Diagnosis

- *Water deprivation test*: Normal concentration of urine >1000 mOsm/kg, if unable to concentrate urine—DI. Give DDAVP (desmopressin) responds (DI), non-responder (nephrogenic DI).
- Treated with DDAVP.

Acid-base Balance

- Any acutely ill patient should have O_2 saturation measured by oximetry (SpO_2) and if <90% then arterial blood gases (ABG) should be done.
- One cannot live for long with pH outside of normal range.
- Normal pH-7.35–7.45 (hydrogen ion concentration 35–45 nmol/L). Also note if pH in the normal range whether it is sitting at the acidic or alkalotic end of the normal range. In health we are driven to take our next breath by the $PaCO_2$ (arterial partial pressure of carbon dioxide) which is intimately linked to pH.

- pH <7.35 is acidosis and pH >7.45 is alkalosis.
- CO_2 is acidic gas (normal $PaCO_2$ is 4.7–6 kPa). Consider is the $PaCO_2$ is contributing to or attempting to compensate for the problem. If for example, the problem is acidosis and the $PaCO_2$ is low, then clearly the respiratory system is attempting to compensate the metabolic problem.
- Actual bicarbonate ($aHCO_3$) is bicarbonate measured in the blood and standard bicarbonate ($sHCO_3$) is the bicarbonate would be if $PaCO_2$ is normal. It is alkaline and normal values are 22–28 mmol/L.

Primary change in HCO_3 is metabolic and in $PaCO_2$ is respiratory. If pH and $PaCO_2$ lead to the conclusion that problem was primarily metabolic; then $sHCO_3$ (or base excess) will only confirm, that $sHCO_3$ being high in alkalosis and low in acidosis. If it is established that the problem is respiratory then BE (base excess normal value −3 to +3) can tell about the duration of the problem. If in a respiratory acidosis, $sHCO_3$ has shown no signs of responding (still with in normal range), explanation is there has not been time to respond (i.e. the problem is acute respiratory acidosis). In chronic respiratory acidosis perhaps pH in the lower half of the normal range and high $sHCO_3$ would indicate longer time course. A respiratory acidosis with low bicarbonate indicates combined respiratory and metabolic acidosis.

If pH acidic, is $PaCO_2$ abnormal if raised then respiratory acidosis, if $PaCO_2$ no change or opposite then compensatory. Similarly HCO_3 is low with metabolic acidosis.

Alveolar-arterial gradient (difference between alveolar partial pressure of oxygen (PAO_2) and PaO_2 (arterial partial pressure of oxygen)—$PAO_2 = PiO_2-(PaCO_2/0.8)$. In healthy young adult alveolar—arterial gradient (PAO_2-PaO_2) is <2kPa but if the patient is older or breathing higher concentration of O_2 or over breathing then 4 kPa. If the alveolar-arterial gradient higher than it should be, then type 1 respiratory failure is present implying V/Q mismatch either due to lungs or pulmonary vasculature.

PiO_2 is the partial pressure of oxygen in the inspired air (21 kPa when breathing room air and 24 kPa when breathing 24% O_2 on venturi mask.

When to check ABG—Cardiac arrest, severe hypotension, acute severe chest pain, acute breathlessness, coma, sepsis, severe poisoning, pulmonary edema, pulmonary embolism, pneumonia, severe asthma (SpO_2 <92%), exacerbation of COPD, renal failure and liver failure.

Causes of Metabolic Acidosis

- *Tissue hypoxia*: Shock with lactic acidosis, hypotension, and sepsis.
- *Non-tissue hypoxia*: Diabetes, alcoholic, starvation, ketoacidosis, poisoning with CO, ethanol, methanol, ethylene glycol, paracetamol, salicylates, tricyclic's, toluene (glue sniffing), renal failure, renal tubular acidosis (RTA) and loss of bicarbonate from gut (severe diarrhea). Anion gap $(Na + K) - (Cl + HCO_3)$ usually equals 10–18 mmol/L. If anion gap is high with acidosis, measure specific toxins in the blood. Normal anion gap acidosis is caused by severe diarrhea, RTA.

Causes of Metabolic Alkalosis

Loss of gastric acid (prolonged vomiting, gastric aspiration), diuretic therapy, prolonged hypokalemia, mineral corticoid and glucocorticoid excess.

Causes of Respiratory Alkalosis

- Pulmonary disorders with hyperventilation (acute asthma, pneumonia, pulmonary embolism and pulmonary edema).
- Primary hyperventilation (anxiety, pain, CNS disorders (stroke).
- Liver failure, sepsis and salicylate poisoning.

RESPIRATORY ACIDOSIS

- Inadequate pulmonary ventilation resulting in raised arterial PCO_2.
- CNS—stroke.
- Sedative drugs, COPD.
- Status epilepticus, encephalitis, cord compression, transverse myelitis, Guillain-Barré syndrome, SLE, myasthenia gravis, Eaton-Lambert syndrome.
- Hypokalemia, hypophosphatemia, rhabdomyolysis.
- Morbid obesity.
- Crushed chest.
- Severe kyphoscoliosis.

- Ankylosing spondylitis and upper airways obstruction.
- Bicarbonate should be used in metabolic acidosis if pH <7.0 or hydrogen ion concentration >60 nmol/L with hypotension. Give 50 mmol (250 mL of 1.6% solution $NaHCO_3$) IV over 60 minutes, recheck pH after a further 30 minutes.

Definitions

- Arterial hypoxemia PaO_2 <10.7 kPa.
- Respiratory failure (arterial PaO_2 <8 kPa).
- Type 1 respiratory failure is when $PaCO_2$ is normal or <6 kPa. Type 2 respiratory failure is when PCO_2 is high (>6 kPa).
- O_2 should be given when hypoxemia (O_2 saturation by oximetry <90%), or hypotension, respiratory distress or cardio respiratory arrest.
- Initial FiO_2 should be 40–60% except type 2 respiratory failure ($PaCO_2$ >6 kPa), who should start with 24% O_2.
- Arterial blood gases should be checked within 2 hrs of starting O_2 and FiO_2 adjusted accordingly. An adequate response is PaO_2 >8 kPa or SaO_2 >90%.

5

Musculoskeletal

Acute Arthritis

Consider whether the patient has arthritis or periarticular inflammation (bursitis, tendinitis or cellulitis)? Painful limitation of movement (active or passive) of the joint suggests arthritis. Gout and pseudogout are self-limiting diseases.

GOUT (SUPERSATURATION OF SERUM FOR URATE)

- 1st affected joint MTPJ (metatarsal phalangeal joint) > ankle joint > knee joint > upper limb, spine, hips and shoulders rarely affected.
- Presents as acute painful, swollen, red hot, erythematous, tender 1st metatarsal phalangeal joint and in 40% in other joints such as knee, instep, ankle, wrist or finger. Usually single joint is involved but can present as polyarticular in patients with hyperuremia and gout secondary to myeloproliferative and lymphoproliferative disorder or organ transplant recipients on cyclosporine A.
- Gout is usually precipitated by trauma (mechanical loosening), starvation, or allopurinol treatment (reduced crystal size and partial dissolution), hospitalization or surgery (local increase in cytokines), and less often due to alcohol consumption (beer, spirits), dietary excess (purines) or use of diuretics by volume depletion and increased reabsorption in proximal tubules.
- There may be low-grade fever and should be differentiated from septic arthritis by joint aspiration for MSU (mono sodium urate crystals).
- M > F, middle age, rare before menopause (estrogen cause increase excretion of urate from kidney). 10% are polyarticular.

- *Atypical onset*: Subacute in hands in PIPJ (proximal interphalangeal joints) and DIPJ (distal interphalangeal joints) in elderly women with renal impairment on diuretics. There is predilection for tophi to form over the Heberden nodes in patients with concomitant osteoarthritis of the hands.
- Locally elevated uric acid with repeated joint microtrauma, prior degenerative change, reduced temperature in poorly perfused distal joint may predispose to gouty inflammation.
- Resolution occurs in days or wks. If left untreated, recurrent attacks are frequent resulting in chronic arthropathy and tophaceous deposit. Chronic tophaceous gout presents as irregular firm nodules on extensors surfaces of fingers, hands, forearm, olecranon bursa, achilles tendon, 1st metatarsal (MT) phalanx and ear helix. Organ transplant recipients (renal or cardiac) treated with cyclosporine, on diuretics and with compromised renal functions are at risk of developing chronic tophaceous gout.
- Tophi can form in any parenchymal organ including meninges except brain and spinal cord.

Risk Factors

- Family history, excess alcohol (beer or spirits but not wine), obesity, diuretics, renal disease and history of previous attacks are risk factors. Uric acid (70% endogenous and 30% from dietary purines) is usually raised above 380 micromol/L and target after treatment is <360 micromol/L.
- Excess meat or fish consumption or sea food or fructose and sugar sweetened soft drinks are a risk factor but vegetables, cherries, dairy products. Vitamin C and coffee reduce the risk.
- Mono sodium urate (MSU) crystals are needle shaped, surface irregular, strong negative birefringence and are in abundance.
- Hyperuricemia (>0.42 mmol/L in males and postmenopausal females, and >0.36 mmol/L in premenopausal females) is a risk factor for hypertension.
- Risk of gout increases with increasing serum uric acid (>0.60 mmol/L in females and >0.7 mmol/L in males, the 5 yrs prevalence of gout is 30%).

- In general population 80–90% of gouty patients are under excreters. Uric acid is primarily excreted by the kidney.
- Certain medication (Thiazides, loop diuretics, low dose aspirin, cyclosporine, niacin, ethambutol, pyrazinamide) and renal insufficiency reduces the excretion of uric acid. In spite of aspirin being a risk factor, it should be continued and not stopped as cardiovascular protection.
- Alcohol, obesity and dietary excess (red meat, offal, game, sea food and legumes) lead to increased uric acid production.
- For uric acid stones, hyperuricemia, daily urinary uric acid excretion >6.5 mmol/L, low urine volume and low urine pH are risk factors.
- Chronic urate nephropathy presents as progressive azotemia and mild proteinuria. In urate nephropathy raised serum uric acid is out of proportion to renal insufficiency, i.e. urate >0.535 if plasma creatinine <132 micromol/L, urate > 0.595 with plasma creatinine 132–176 micromol/L and urate >0.714 with advanced renal failure.

Selective investigations—Gout = Serum urate (poor discriminator as 30% drop in blood levels in acute attack).

- Aspirate synovial fluid (avoiding skin affected by cellulitis) where ever possible and send for polarizing microscopy, Gram stain and culture.
- Venous blood culture × 3 if septic arthritis suspected.
- FBC, ESR, CRP and X-ray of the joint on admission. Rheumatoid factor if indicated.

Treatment of Gout

Acute Attack

- Splinting the joint and icing four times daily reduces pain.
- NSAIDs—Naproxen 500 mg twice daily, PPI's added if high risk of gastric ulcer or GI bleeds.
- Lower dose colchicine 600 micrograms 8–12 hrly can be used in acute gout when it is not possible to use NSAID. Colchicine is not recommended for long-term use (6–12 months after normal uricemia).

    Discontinue diuretics for hypertension. Use losartan and fenofibrate as both are uricosuric.

- Intra articular steroid triamcinolone 20 mg may be used after diagnostic aspiration if single joint is involved.
- Oral prednisolone may also be used 30 mg/day and tapered throughout 8 days, flare up may occur if tapered too soon.

  An alternative to oral steroid is single IM injection of 40 mg methyl prednisolone or ACTH 40 U IM 12 hrly 2 days and then once daily for a few days.

  Whenever a corticosteroid or ACTH is used low dose colchicine (0.6 mg bid) should be used to prevent rebound flare up of gout. Patients with renal failure and acute gout should not be treated with NSAID or colchicine; such patients should be treated with intra-articular or oral steroids.
- Many elderly patients develop diarrhea on colchicine 0.5 mg bid; satisfactory prophylactic is achieved with colchicine 0.5 mg daily or every other day.

  Do not use allopurinol until acute attack has settled for at least 2 wks and introduce slowly with either NSAID or low dose colchicine 0.5 mg bd. Adjust the dose if renal function impaired.

If asymptomatic hyperuricemia is present then secondary causes like lymphoproliferative and myeloproliferative disorders, psoriasis, vitamin B_{12} deficiency, pre-eclampsia, lead exposure, excessive alcohol (beer and spirits) and drugs should be excluded. Majority (80–90%) has excess dietary purine consumption (red meat and sea food) or decreased urate excretion. If hyperuricosuria (24 hrs urinary urate >5 mmol/L), 24 hrs urine should be repeated after 5 days of low purine diet. If hyperuricosuria is persistent then exclude overproduction due to various enzyme defects before treating as primary hyperuricemia.

Hyperuricemia asymptomatic is treated if recurrent acute gout attacks (2/yr) (discuss with the patient), then target is blood level <300 micromol/L with gradually increasing allopurinol by 100 mg every 4 wks and average of dose of allopurinol 300–500 mg/day (max 900 mg/day).

Uric acid stones and nephropathy are treated with potassium citrate or potassium bicarbonate for urine alkalinization but not allopurinol.

Patients allergic to allopurinol or cannot take allopurinol can be treated with febuxostat 80–120 mg/day. Uricosuric drugs (Sulfinpyrazone, probenecid (both weak) or benzbromarone (potent uricosuric) and pegloticase sometimes can be helpful after the acute attack if allopurinol or colchicine cannot be used. Lisinopril and fenofibrate also increase uric acid excretion.

Treatment is also required if tophi are present or very high uric acid levels (>0.77 mm/L in males and >0.6 mmol/L in females when heart failure excluded), uric acid stones, coexistence renal disease, recurrent acute attack (>2/yr), bone or cartilage damage on X-ray and over production of uric acid by tumor lysis or about to receive radiotherapy or chemotherapy.

Uric acid lowering drugs are used long-term after 2nd acute attack or previous history of recurrent attacks.

Asymptomatic hyperuricosuria >6.5 mmol/L/day has 50% risk of developing uric acid stones. Allopurinol should be used if low purine diet does not decrease excretion <4.8 mmol/L/day.

Diet with low red meat or sea food, fish, liver, sweet bread, decreased saturated fats and calorie restriction helps. Patient should be advised to cut down beer and distilled spirits. Loss of weight if overweight should be encouraged.

Uricosuric drugs (contraindicated if GFR <60) Probenecid or sulfinpyrazone are rarely used these days but losartan or fenofibrate or benzbromarone are useful if patient is intolerant of allopurinol and febuxostat. Benzbromarone is particularly useful in renal transplant patients treated with cyclosporine A and the dose is 25–150 mg/day. Urine must be kept alkaline and flow rate >1 mL/minute to prevent uric acid crystallization.

Losartan is only ARB found to have uricosuric properties and can be used when hyperuricemia due to diuretics. Finofibrates also have uricosuric property

PSEUDOGOUT

Pseudogout is chondrocalcinosis of hyaline or fibrocartilage or calcium pyrophosphate dihydrate (CPPD) crystal deposition disease.
- Middle aged or elderly (>55), knees, wrist and meta carpophalangeal joint (MCPJ) are commonly involved and can mimic gout, septic arthritis and flare up of OA.
- It can present as acute synovitis or chronic arthritis or be incidental.

Risk Factors

- Intercurrent illness, local trauma or surgery.
- It is the most common cause of chondrocalcinosis on X-ray and if presenting <55 or polyarticular then exclude, hemochromatosis, hyperparathyroidism, hypophosphatemia, hypomagnesemia, hypothyroidism, familial hypocalciuric hypercalcemia, acromegaly and Wilson's disease.
- Calcium pyrophosphate (CPPD) crystals are oval shaped, weakly positive birefringence and are scanty.
- Sometimes presents as pseudo RA as symmetrical arthritis with morning stiffness and positive RA factor (as in normal elderly people) but X-ray of the joint shows OA changes only.
- Diagnosis is made by the presence of weakly positive birefringent crystals by polarized microscopy or presence of typical cartilage or joint calcification on X-ray.
- Aspirate synovial fluid (avoiding skin affected by cellulitis) where ever possible and send for polarizing microscopy, Gram stain and culture.

Following blood tests should also be done in a patient with Pseudo gout. Serum calcium, phosphorus, magnesium, alkaline phosphatase, ferritin, iron, total iron binding capacity and thyroid-stimulating hormone (TSH).

Treatment of Pseudogout

- Bed rest, intra-articular steroid, NSAIDs and colchicine as in gout.
- Joint use restricted for 48–72 hrs after triamcinolone injection (40 mg triamcinolone + 1 mL lignocaine) in the joint. If oral medication is not possible or NSAIDs or colchicine are contraindicated then steroids or ACTH can be used as in gout.
- Prophylaxis with colchicine 0.5 mg bid when more than 3 attacks/yr.

SEPTIC ARTHRITIS

- Any age (common over 60 or under 3) acute red hot swollen joint which is extremely painful even to touch or move the joint passively with fever and malaise.

- Skin infection (boils, pustules) may be present and *Staphylococcus aureus* or Streptococci are the organism in adults and gram-negative bacilli in children.
- Gonococcal 20% often preceded by migratory tendinitis and poly arthralgia, sexually transmitted and have rapid response to penicillin. Skin pustules, genitourinary (GU) symptoms and abnormal LFT may also be present.
- Nongonococcal (80% gram-positive)—60% Staph, 15% Strep B hemolytic, 3% *Strep pneumoniae* and 18% are gram negative.
- If one or two joints are inflamed in RA then consider septic arthritis unless proved otherwise.

Risk factors: Previous OA, RA, diabetes mellitus, sickle cell disease, prosthetic joints, suppressed immune functions, sexually transmitted diseases, repeated intra-articular steroids, IV drug misusers, indwelling vascular lines or undergoing invasive procedures.

- Around 2% prosthetics joints become infected.
- Septic arthritis follows intra-articular corticosteroid injection in 1 in 1,7000–50,000 injections.
- Sometimes fever and malaise may be absent.
- Blood culture and aspiration culture and plain X-ray should be done.
- Being on warfarin is not a contraindication for aspiration.
- When infection develops in a prosthetic joint a year or more after surgery, the condition may progress gradually rather than acutely and the patient may present with slowly increasing joint pain.

Treatment of Septic Arthritis

- Rest the joint with the splint. Passive mobilization started 24–48 hrs after symptoms subside.
- IV flucloxacillin 1 gm qds (Clindamycin if penicillin sensitive) plus gentamycin.
- Inform the orthopedics, as the patient needs daily joint aspiration to dryness till no fluid accumulates. Adjust the antibiotics after the results of culture are available. Duration of antibiotics is 2 wks IV and 4 wks oral (12 wks oral in RA and in immune suppression). NSAIDs for pain relief (with PPI in elderly and previous history of peptic ulceration).

Continue antibiotics if no organism on Gram stain till blood and synovial culture is available.

REACTIVE ARTHRITIS

Young male > female, large joints (lower limb), usually more than one and can mimic sepsis. Enquire about gastrointestinal (GI), genitourinary (GU) infections and look for circinate balanitis, oral ulceration, keratoderma blennorrhagicum, nail changes, conjunctivitis and iritis. Urethritis usually predates arthritis and conjunctivitis. Conjunctivitis usually either follows or is simultaneous with urethritis.

Aspirate synovial fluid where ever possible and send for polarizing microscopy, gram stain and culture.

Stool for *Salmonella, Shigella, Campylobacter* and serology for *Chlamydia, Yersinia,* and *Campylobacter.* In Reiter's, swab culture from urethra, high vagina, rectum and throat.

Treatment

Bed rest, NSAIDs, intra-articular steroid and treatment of triggering infection.

OSTEOARTHRITIS

Flare-up of osteoarthritis (OA) can present as painful bony swelling, restricted joint movement and crepitus. Etiology is multifactorial, mechanical, genetics, metabolic, inflammatory, age, gender and obesity.

About 80% >65 yrs have X-ray evidence of OA but only 25–30% are symptomatic.

Balance of the system lies with inhibitors of matrix degrading enzymes tissue inhibitor of metalloproteinases (TIMP) and plasminogen activator inhibitor (PAI-1), which are synthesized by chondrocytes and limit the degrading activity of MMPs and plasminogen activator. When TIMP or PAI-1 is present in small concentration or absent, plasmin or stromelysen are free to act on matrix.

Initially there is enzymatic degradation of aggrecan and collagen in the cartilage by collegenases, aggrecanases and stromelysin 1 (metalloproteinases-3) resulting in chondrocytes multiplication and increased turn over to increase matrix component of cartilage. With increased turn over there is decrease in size of hydrophilic aggrecan molecules resulting in increased water concentration and swelling pressure in cartilage making cartilage vulnerable to load bearing injury and fissuring, localized chondrocytes death and decrease in cartilage thickness.

- If OA <45 following should be excluded, previous trauma or localized instability, prior joint disease (juvenile idiopathic arthritis), metabolic disease (hemochromatosis, acromegaly, hyperparathyroidism, hypothyroidism, onchronosis), avascular necrosis and neuropathic joint.
    - Joint pain present as deep ache after use, relieved by rest, later on as night pain in the hip or knee and joint stiffness after immobility lasting less than 20 minutes.
    - Pain is due to stretching of nerves over the periosteum or medullary hypertension or micro fracture of subchondral bone, stretching of joint capsule or muscle spasm or synovitis in late stages.
- Bone and soft tissue swelling, crepitus on movement of joint, deformity and decreased joint motion are clinical features.
- X-ray changes are joint space narrowing, subchondral sclerosis, cysts and osteophytosis.
- Aspirate synovial fluid (avoiding skin affected by cellulitis) where ever possible and send for polarizing microscopy, Gram stain and culture.

Following blood tests should also be done, serum calcium, phosphorus, magnesium, alkaline phosphatase, ferritin, iron, total iron binding capacity and TSH.

Treatment

- NSAIDs
- Intra-articular steroid
- Physiotherapy.

RHEUMATOID ARTHRITIS (RA)

It is auto immune disease, primary target synovial tissue, affecting small and large joints with extra-articular features.

Incidence 1–1.5% with 3 : 1 F : M (frequently beginning in child bearing years), with strong genetic susceptibility

HLA DR4 (HLA DR1 in Indians, Israelis, and HLA DR15 in Japanese).

Classification Criteria for Diagnosis as RA

A. Joint involvement
   1 large joint—0
   2–10 large joints—1
   1–3 small joints (with or without involvement of large joints)—2
   4–10 small joints (with or without involvement of large joints)—3
   >10 joints (at least one small joint)—5
B. Serology (at least one test result is needed for classification)
   Negative rheumatoid factor (RF) and negative ACPA (anti-citrullinated protein antibody)—0
   Low positive RF or low positive ACPA—2
   High positive RF or high positive ACPA—3
C. Acute phase reactant (at least one test result needed)
   Normal CRP and normal ESR—0
   Abnormal CRP or abnormal ESR—1
D. Duration of symptoms
   <6 wks—0
   >6 wks—1
   Score > 6 definite RA.

- With these new criteria of early diagnosis of RA early initiation of therapy with DMRD <12 wks of disease duration and prompt referral to rheumatologist should be considered.
- Primary target of for treatment of RA is clinical remission.
- Remission is no more swollen or painful joints, normal ESR or CRP or anti CCP.
- Global visual analogue scale <10 on 0–100 scale.
- In RA morning stiffness usually lasts >1 hr and synovitis usually involves the hand and wrist joints.
- Antibodies to anti-citrullinated protein antibody (ACPA) appear early with 90–98% specificity and 50–65% sensitivity helps to diagnose early and is a strong predictor of persistence.

Pathology

Synovitis which becomes hyperplastic which destroys the articular cartilage and underlying subchondral bone.

Synovitis is driven by proinflammatory cytokines such as TNF, IL-6 (interleukin 6) and IL-1. Synovium in RA shows infiltration with lymphocytes (CD4), macrophages and plasma cells, hence current immunotherapy targets B-cells, T-cells, TNF and IL6.

Clinical

Acute onset with florid morning stiffness, polyarthritis and pitting edema is common in the elderly and should be differentiated from polymyalgia rheumatica.

Symmetrical swelling of metacarpophalangeal (MCP) and proximal inter phalangeal (PIP) joints is common. These joints are considered to be actively inflamed if they are tender on pressure and have stress pain on passive movement. Deformities of the hands (ulnar deviation of fingers, wasting of small muscles of hands, swan neck deformity of fingers) and foot (subluxation of MTP joints) are common chronic manifestation of the RA.

Extra-articular Manifestations

They are common in long standing seropositive RA patients.
- *Rheumatoid nodules*: These are subcutaneous nodules at the sites of pressure or friction (extensor surfaces of forearm, achillies tendon, sacrum and toes).
- Vasculitis includes nail fold infarct, pyoderma gangrenosum and skin necrosis, mesenteric, renal or coronary artery occlusion. Rheumatoid arthritis leg ulcers have also underlying vasculitis.

Chest

- Rheumatoid arthritis patients are susceptible to chest infection due to subclinical pulmonary disease. They can also develop pleurisy or pleural effusion, interstitial lung disease, rheumatoid nodule in the lung and bronchiectasis.

Ocular

- Dry eyes due to keratoconjunctivitis sicca or Sjören's syndrome (dry eyes, dry mouth), scleritis, episcleritis and scleromalacia.
- Usually treated with steroids and cyclosporine or cyclophosphamide.

Heart

- Pericarditis, myocarditis, endocarditis, myocardial infarction (MI), conduction defects, coronary vasculitis and granulomatous aortitis and increased risk of atherosclerosis are reported due to RA. There is increase in cardiovascular events by 30–60% in RA.

Neurological

Cervical cord compression due to atlanto axial subluxation (due to erosion of transverse ligament around the posterior aspect of odontoid peg), presenting as new occipital headache with paraesthesia or electric shock in the arms.

Median nerve, ulnar nerve, lateral popliteal nerve compression, tarsal tunnel syndrome (entrapment of posterior tibial nerve in flexor retinaculum causing burning, tingling and numbness in distal sole and toes) or carpal tunnel syndrome and peripheral neuropathy can be extra articular presentation in RA.

Rheumatoid arthritis can also cause anemia microcytic (cause NSAID?), normocytic (active disease), muscle wasting, fatigue, osteoporosis, bursitis, pleural effusion, nodules, bronchiolitis, fibrosing alveolitis amyloidosis with nephrotic syndrome and Felty's syndrome (splenomegaly with neutropenia).

Investigations in Acute Arthritis

- Aspirate synovial fluid if large joint (avoiding skin affected by cellulitis) where ever possible and send for polarizing microscopy, Gram stain and culture to exclude gout and septic arthritis.
- Venous blood culture × 3 if septic arthritis suspected.
- FBC, ESR, CRP and X-ray of the joint on admission, rheumatoid factor and antibodies to ACPA.
- Aspiration from prosthetic joint should be done in operating theatre by orthopedic surgeon.

Management of Rheumatoid Arthritis

- Rheumatoid arthritis is autoimmune polyarticular inflammation of synovial tissue causing pain swelling and stiffness of hand, wrist and feet.
- Rest (in acute stage), passive exercises, hydrotherapy and physiotherapy are essential.

- NSAIDs for 1st few wks while diagnosis is being considered then with DMRDs.
- Long-term NSAID can cause GI ulcers, perforations, fluid retention, renal impairment and exacerbation of hypertension. These complications are increased in old age, corticosteroids use and history of peptic ulcer.
- Cox-2 inhibitors have increased incidence of thrombotic events. Cox-2 inhibitors are no better in efficacy than NSAIDs.
- PPI's can be used with NSAIDs to decrease GI side effects.
- All patients supplement calcium and vitamin D and Bisphosphonate if osteopenic with T score <1.5 on DEXA scan.
- DMARDs—methotrexate (MTX), sulfasalazine, leflunomide and hydroxychloroquine.
- Efficacy of MTX, sulfasalazine, IM gold and penicillamine is similar.
- Antimalarials (Hydroxychloroquine) are less effective.
- MTX and sulfasalazine are 1st choice and should be started early within three months of symptoms.
- Penicillamine and Gold are rarely used because of toxicity.
- MTX 17.5–30 mg/wk is the effective dose and folic acid 1–3 mg/day, or folinic acid 2.5–5 mg given 12–24 hrs after MTX.
- MTX should be started 7.5 mg orally once/wk and increased by 5 mg each month.
- If still active disease then increase to 20–30 mg/wk, if still active disease then switch to subcutaneous injections.
- FBC, LFT, U and E, creatinine and albumin should be measured every 4–8 wks.
- In case of sulfasalazine FBC every 2–4 wks—1st 3 months and then 3 monthly.
- Dose of MTX should be decreased if aminotransferase (ALT) is raised and stopped if raised ALT is persistent.
- Leflunomide (a new synthetic DMARD) has similar efficacy as MTX and sulfasalazine.
- MTX and leflunomide are teratogenic, so reliable birth control is essential.
- If pneumonitis is suspected clinically or on chest X-ray then MTX should be stopped.

- Best tolerated DMARDs is hydroxychloroquine when used in doses <6.5 mg/kg/day with yearly visit to ophthalmologist to prevent rare retinal toxic effects.
- Minocycline (more efficacious then hydroxychloroquine) causes reversible hyperpigmentation (30%) on long-term use.
- Biological DMARDs are anti TNF-alpha (Infliximab, etanercept and adalimumab), anti-interleukin-1 (Anakinra) and anti-CD20 (Rituximab).
- Addition of prednisolone 5–7.5 mg to MTX for 28 wks causes early rapid suppression of disease activity.
- DMARDs should be started within 3 months of start of symptoms and combination of MTX, sulfasalazine and hydroxychloroquine should be considered if disease is still active on optimum dose of MTX for 3 months.
- If active disease persists after 3 months of DMARDs combinations as described above then addition of leflunomide or TNF alpha inhibitors to MTX should be considered.
- Usually TNF alpha inhibitors is given for 1 yr to induce remission.
- First three months → MTX, or (MTX + prednisolone 7.5–15 mg short-term + sulphasalazine) if MTX contraindicated then leflunomide or sulphasalazine or hydroxychloroquine or IM gold.
- Three to six months → If still active RA MTX + 2nd DMRD or steroids.
- Six to twelve months if still active RA then biologics with TNF inhibitors or IL6 inhibitors or B or T cell targeted therapy.
- Treatment with methotrexate (MTX) and one other DMRD is necessary prior to escalation to biologics. Patients on biologics needs require regular monitoring for efficacy and adverse effects as there is increased risk of serious infection (septic arthritis, pneumonia and infections of the skin) in the 1st six months of treatment, in older patient and those on steroids. One third of patients on biologics respond very well and one third do not respond at all. All patients for biologics are screened for latent tuberculosis before starting therapy.

Biologics

All biologics are given in combination with MTX.

TNF inhibitors (monoclonal antibodies): Adalimumab is first line therapy given as SC injection fortnightly in combination with MTX.

IL6 inhibitors: Tocilizumab is also first line therapy given as monthly IV infusion. It should be 1st choice biologic therapy for patients who cannot tolerate MTX.

B cell targeted therapy: Rituximab is 2nd line therapy given IV infusion 2 doses over 2 wks at disease flare and minimum duration between therapies is 6 months. It is more effective in RA patients with positive R factor or ACPA. Infusion reactions (fever, urticarial) are frequent and can be prevented with IV methylprednisolone before every infusion.

T cell targeted therapy: Abatacept is 2nd line therapy and given as monthly IV infusion following 3 loading infusions at 0,2 and 4 wks or wkly SC injections following the loading infusions.

Rituximab (anti-B cell therapy) which depletes the B cells should be considered in patients who fail to respond to one anti TNF alpha and are RA factor positive. Surgery for synovectomy of wrist and finger tendon sheaths may be required for pain relief and prevention of tendon rupture.

Poor Prognostic Factors

- Higher baseline disability, female sex, involvement of MTP joints, positive R factor, disease duration >3 months.
- All patients should have yearly influenza vaccination, pneumococcal vaccine at appropriate interval (before starting DMARDs).
- Before considering TNF inhibitors patients should be screened for TB.
- MTX should not be used if underlying renal or hepatic disease, who cannot stop alcohol, or who plans to become pregnant.

All the patients in these 7 studies were already taking methotrexate, to which the other medications were added. Responses were measured in terms of an improvement of at least 20% as per American College of Rheumatology (ACR20).

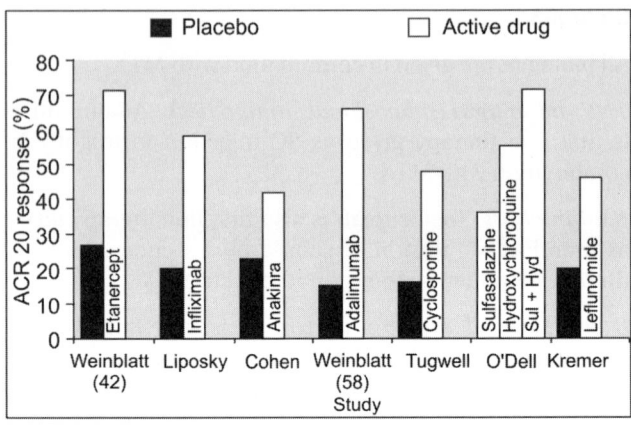

Fig. 5.1: Response to drug therapy in seven studies involving patients receiving methotrexate

Polymyalgia Rheumatica, Temporal Arteritis, Vasculitis

- Bilateral pain and stiffness around shoulder, pelvic or neck muscles with morning stiffness lasting >45 minutes over 50 yrs is diagnostic. It may be acute or sub-acute onset with bilateral upper arm tenderness.

Diagnostic criteria	Points without ultrasound	Points with ultrasound
Morning stiffness >45 minutes	2	2
Hip pain or limited range of motion	1	1
Absence of R factor or anti-cyclic citrullinated peptide antibodies	2	2
Absence of other joint pain	1	1
Ultrasound at least one abnormal shoulder and at least 1 abnormal hip		1
Ultrasound (synovitis and bursitis) both shoulder abnormal		1

- Score >4 diagnostic of polymyalgia rheumatica (PMR)
- Sometimes difficulty in getting up from chair or bed, raising arms above shoulder, combing their hair or turning in bed are the main symptoms. Symptoms are usually worse on waking up.
- Raised ESR >40 mm and raised CRP
- Age usually >75, F>M 3:1.
- *Differential diagnosis*: Rheumatoid arthritis (distal joints, positive R factor, anticyclic citrullinated peptide present, erosive joint disease on X-ray), RS3PE syndrome (remitting seronegative symmetric synovitis with pitting edema) peripheral hand and foot edema, temporal arteritis, large vessel vasculitis, crystal arthropathy and SLE, It is important to check for other causes of myopathy (statin induced or hypothyroidism) with normal creatine kinase.

Treatment

- *Steroids*: Prednisolone 15 mg/day for 6 wks, then 12.5 mg/d for 6 wks, 10 mg/d for 6-12 months and then reduce 0.5-1 mg every 4 wks. IM methylprednisolone 120 mg every 4 wks reducing 20 mg every 3 months for those who cannot take oral prednisolone. Excellent response >70% within 7 days with normal ESR and CRP in 3-4 wks. Total duration 1-3 yrs.
- Lack of response to 20 mg prednisolone (<70% improvement in symptoms) and lymphopenia can be a clue to other diagnosis like tumor, osteoarthritis or seronegative rheumatoid arthritis.
- Where there is doubt 'Steroid Sandwich' test of one wk prednisolone, 2nd wk vitamin C and 3 wk prednisolone can be done. In classic PMR symptoms resolve in 3 days and do not return till the dose of prednisolone is reduced or stopped. Raised CRP or ESR should normalize within two to four wks.
- *Temporal arteritis*: New onset of headache, jaw tenderness, temporal artery tenderness or decreased pulsation, visual symptoms and ESR usually >50. Temporal artery ultrasound or temporal artery biopsy should be considered to confirm the diagnosis.

For temporal arteritis prednisolone 60 mg/day for 4 wks then 50 mg/day for 4 wks, 40 mg/day for 4 wks, 30 mg/day for 4 wks, 20 mg/day for 4 wks and then decrease 1 mg/4 wks for 2 yrs.

Osteoporosis prevention cover with bisphosphonates and calcium and vitamin D is required.

Add MTX in relapse cases if not responding to increase dose of steroids.

Vasculitis

Presents as chronic unexplained illness, polymyalgia, polyarthralgia, fatigue, malaise, fever, headache, high ESR. Non healing skin ulcer, mononeuritis multiplex and antibiotic resistant pneumonia. ANCA +
- Urine protein and blood always present.
- Secondary causes of vasculitis.
  - *Drugs*: Hydralazine, propylthiouracil.
  - *Cancer*: Lymphoma
  - *Infections*: Hepatitis B/C, HIV, TB
  - *Autoimmunity*: Rheumatoid arthritis, Sjögren's syndrome.

CHURG-STRAUSS (ALLERGIC GRANULOMATOSIS)

Small/medium arteries autoimmune vasculitis, mainly involving lungs (asthma), gastrointestinal system and peripheral nerves with granulation lesion in tissues or wall of vessels. It may also involve skin, heart and kidney.
- Presents as fever, weight loss, malaise, asthma, allergic rhinitis, sinusitis, pulmonary infiltrate purpura and cutaneous or SC nodules.
- Presents in three stages.
- 1st stage involves sinuses and onset of allergies.
- 2nd stage involves onset of acute asthma. Normally person has not had asthma before.
- 3rd stage involves various organ systems.
- High ESR, raised eosinophil's in the blood and positive p-ANCA.
- Myocardial involvement frequent.
- *Criteria for diagnosis*: Four of these six must be present for diagnosis
- Asthma, blood eosinophil's >10%, presence of mono or poly neuropathy, non-fixed pulmonary infiltrate, para nasal sinus abnormalities and histological evidence of extravascular eosinophil's.

Treatment

Steroids + cyclophosphamide or azathioprine or rituximab.

- *Polyarteritis nodosa (PAN)*: Necrotizing vasculitis small/medium arteries of unknown cause, involves bifurcation of arteries. It is more common in people with hepatitis B infection. Men are more often affected than women between ages of 30 and 49.
- Symptoms result from ischemic damage to the affected organ often the skin, heart, kidneys and nervous system.
- Fever, malaise, fatigue, loss of appetite, weight loss. Muscle and joint aches are common.
- Skin-rashes, ulcers, livedo reticularis, palpable purpura.
- *Nervous system*: Peripheral neuropathy, strokes or seizures.
- *Kidneys*: Renal failure, hypertension, edema, oliguria, uremia.
- *Heart*: Heart failure, MI and pericarditis.
- Blood eosinophil's not high, raised ESR, raised CRP (C reactive protein), hepatitis B + (hepatitis B positive), raised gamma globulin, rarely ANCA +, and tissue biopsy.
- *Treatment*: Steroid + cyclophosphamide.

MICROSCOPIC ANGIITIS (NECROTIZING SMALL VESSEL VASCULITIS)

- Constitutional symptoms like fever, anorexia, weight loss, fatigue and renal failure. A majority may have hematuria and proteinuria, muscular/skeletal pain, hemoptysis, acute renal failure (ARF), anemia, raised WBC, raised platelets.
- Glomerulonephritis and pulmonary capillaries commonly involved. pANCA positive with myeloperoxidase.
- *Treatment*: Prednisolone + cyclophosphamide.

6
Cardiovascular

Acute Chest Pain: Acute Coronary Syndrome (ACS)

Cardiac monitor, O_2, intravenous (IV) access, opiates, aspirin + clopidogrel, low molecular weight heparin (LMWH), IV nitrates (if persistent angina, hypertension and LVF), insulin if BM >11 mmol/L + ACE inhibitors or angiotensin receptor blocker (ARB) + Beta-blocker for 2 yrs if no contraindication + statin.

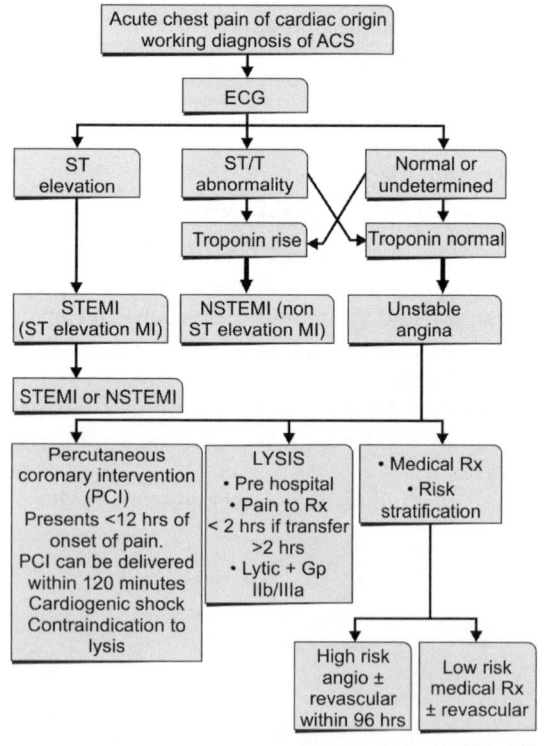

Contd...

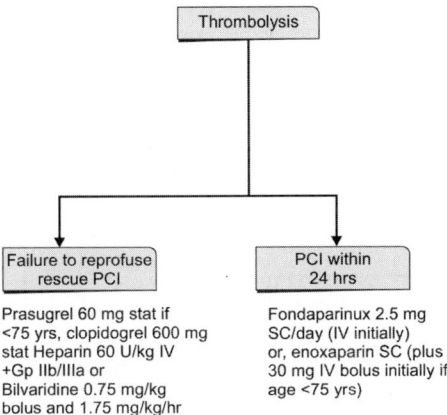

Risk Factors

High: Female, age >70 yrs, LVF, LBBB, STEMI, HR >150, SBP >150, raised troponin, renal failure, prolonged prehospital delay, diabetes mellitus (DM), cerebrovascular disease, peripheral vascular disease, anemia.

Causes of ST segment elevation: STEMI, LBBB, pericarditis, LVH, hyperkalemia, Brugada syndrome.

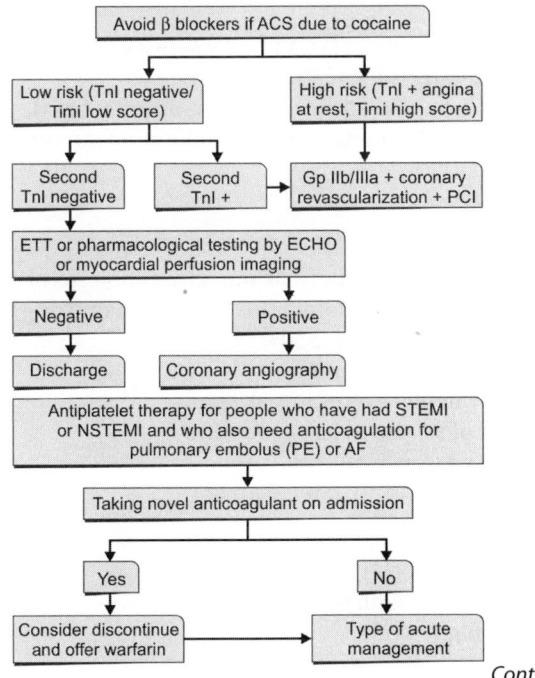

Contd...

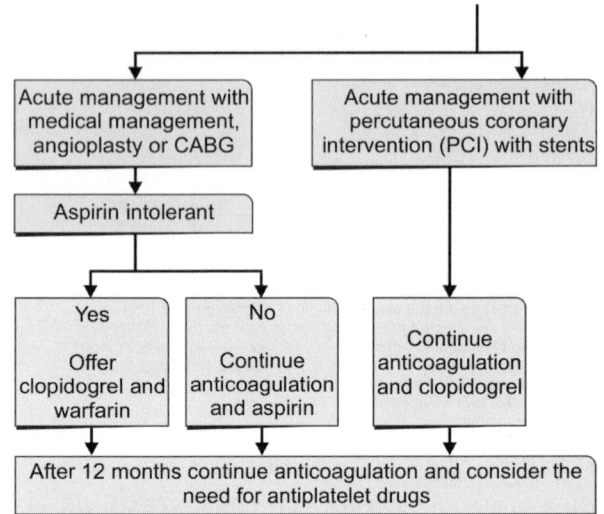

- Anteroseptal infarct left anterior descending (LAD) raised ST V1-V4 or new LBBB.
- Inferior infarct R coronary artery (RCA) raised ST segment in lead II, III, AVF.
- Lateral infarct left circumflex (LCX) raised ST I, AVL, V5, V6.
- Posterior infarct (LCX) ↑ST V7-V9 ↓V1-V3.
- RV infarct (RCA) ↑ST V4R-V6R.
- Door–needle-30 minutes (for thrombolysis), pain to needle 60 minutes, door to balloon-90 minutes (PCI).

Timi Risk Score

- >65 yr age
- 3 risk factors (hypertension, raised cholesterol, familial hypercholesterolemia (FH) diabetes, smoking)
- Coronary stenosis >50%
- ST changes >0.5 mm
- Two angina events in last 24 hrs
- Use of aspirin in last 24 hrs and
- Raised trop T.

Risk

- 0–2, low
- 3–4, intermediate
- >5, high

- If risk score >3 then early angiography within 24–48 hrs as in NSTEMI.

STEMI: Ischemic pain of >20 minutes and <12 hr (within 24 hrs if chest pain and ST elevation 2 mm still present in two chest leads and or 1 mm in limb leads or new LBBB on 12 lead ECG will benefit from PCI or thrombolysis.

ST segment depression >2 mm in precordial leads V1-V3 (acute posterior) do not benefit from thrombolysis. Consider posterior MI if ST segment depression in V1, V2 with large R wave, at V7, V8.

Most cases of STEMI are due to atherosclerotic plaque rupture and thrombotic occlusion. Other causes are stent thrombosis, spontaneous coronary artery dissection, coronary spasm, coronary embolism, recreational drugs (cocaine), thrombophilia, trauma and Kawasaki disease.

TROPONINS

Troponins are released from cardiac myocytes by toxins, inflammation and necrosis.
- Trop T (0.03 ng/mL), Trop I (0.5–1.5 ng/mL) is raised in STEMI.
- Tn is best negative predictive value after 12 hrs.
- Patients with troponin rise and NSTEMI needs aggressive management.
- Positive troponin indicates a need for antithrombotic (Fondaparinux 2.5 mg SC unless eGFR <20 or LMWH enoxaparin 1 mg/kg unless eGFR <30 or heparin or bivalirudin if patient going for angiography.
- Anti-platelet therapy aspirin 300 mg stat and 75 mg/day, clopidogrel 300 mg stat then 75 mg/day, glycoprotein IIb/IIIa (abciximab IV) before angiography and anti ischemic therapy β-blockers, nitrates or CCB.
- Raised troponin indicates need for early revascularization.
- In troponin normal patients, ETT may help to decide further invasive testing.
- Troponin levels do not rise significantly until at least 6 hr after the onset of pain.
- Peak level of Tn (troponin) is in 12–48 hrs and remains elevated for 2 wks.

Troponin are also raised in sepsis, TIA's, stroke, heart failure, renal failure, pulmonary embolism, tachyarrhythmia, hypo or hypertension, aortic dissection, hypothyroidism, scleroderma, hemochromatosis, severe asthma, pheochromocytoma, critically ill patient, marathon exercise, scorpion bite, snake venom, primary pulmonary hypertension, SVT, cardiac surgery, chest wall trauma, cardiac amyloidosis, sarcoidosis, cardioversion, dilated cardiomyopathy, postviral, aortic stenosis or regurgitation or dissection, eclampsia and gestational hypertension.

Pharmacological Management of ACS

- The GTN spray or tablet (0.3–1 mg SL) repeat after 5 min × 3 if required. O_2 should be given if patient has severe pain, is breathless or SaO_2 <96%.
- Opioids if pain not relieved by 3 doses of GTN spray. Correct major arrhythmia or hypotension and relieve severe pain with diamorphine 2.5–5 mg plus metoclopramide 10 mg IV or cyclizine 50 mg IV.
- Aspirin oral or P/R, 300 mg stat and 75 mg daily.
- Clopidogrel 300 mg stat and 75 mg/day for 12/12 (or prasugral 10 mg/day for 12 months if age <75 yrs and weight >60 kg). Consider clopidogrel 600 mg stat if patient is having invasive strategy within 24 hrs.

  Aspirin + clopidogrel for 4/52 in ST elevation ACS and for 12 months for non ST elevation ACS and 12/12 after PCI or stent.

  Prasugral 60 mg loading prior and then 10 mg/day for 12/12 in diabetic patients having PCI after ACS or stent thrombosis with clopidogrel treatment.
- *Anticoagulants*: Fondaparinux 2.5 mg SC daily for 2 days, unless invasive strategy is planned within 24 hrs or serum creatinine >265 micro mu/L.

  Enoxaprin 1 mg/kg SC twice daily is alternative to fondaparinux but increased bleeding rates.

  Unfractionated heparin 100 U/kg/hr IV with dose adjustment depending on APTT if patient is for angiography within 24 hrs or creatinine >265 mu/L.
- *Anti-ischemic therapy*: β-blockers oral within 24 hrs (no role for IV β-blockers),

  ACE inhibitors/ARB oral within 24 hrs, statins (Atorvastatin 80 mg/day if already not on statin).

  CCB (Amlodipine), long acting nitrates.

  Omacor 1 gm/day for 4 yrs (if not having 7 gm of omega 3 fatty acids/wk through diet alone).

Eplerenone if LV EF < 40% with heart failure or DM.

Intravenous Gp IIb/IIIa at presentation in high risk (waiting angiography) cases with diabetes, until after PCI.

Glycoprotein IIb/IIIa inhibitor not recommended with thrombolytic therapy but use only if PCI performed.

Device Therapy

Implantable cardioverter defibrillator therapy (ICD): Post STEMI (4 wks), EF <35% and spontaneous nonsustained VT or sustained monomorphic VT by electrophysiological testing.

Cardiac resynchronizations therapy (CRT): EF <35% with heart failure in spite of maximum therapy, LV dilatation and QRS duration >120 msec.

Call to balloon (C2B): Rescue PCI performed within 12 hrs of thrombolysis for recurrent infarction or incomplete resolution of ST segment (<70%) in 60–90 minutes after thrombolysis.

Routine angiography within 24 hours after thrombolysis should be considered.

History is important in differentiating these patients. Reproduction of pain on exercise or radiation of pain to the jaw, shoulders and arms increases the likelihood of pain being due to MI. Unfortunately 10% of patients with MI describe the pain as burning, 10% as stabbing, and in 8% of patients it can be reproduced by palpation.

Consider atypical presentation in females, diabetics and elderly.

Consider potentially lethal causes in all patients with chest pain: acute coronary syndrome (STEMI, NSTEMI and unstable angina), pulmonary embolism and aortic dissection.

- Check pulse, BP and listen over lungs, attach an ECG monitor and record an ECG. Take a preliminary history of chest pain (instantaneous, dissection), peaking over many seconds (MI) while recording ECG; is it consistent with MI or are there features suggestive of aortic dissection (instantaneous onset, associated neurological symptoms even minor transient blurring of vision, pain radiating to back and unequal BP in

both arms >15 mm Hg difference and presence of asymmetry of major pulses).
- Look at previous ECGs if available. ST elevation convex upwards (concave upwards in pericarditis in both chest and limb leads) >1 mm in 2 or more limb leads and >2 mm in 2 or more chest leads or new LBBB and chest pain consistent with myocardial ischemia lasting >20 minutes, working diagnosis is myocardial infarction (MI) and PCI or thrombolysis should be given. Normal ECG is unhelpful in excluding MI. Additional right and posterior leads and serial ECGs can increase the number of patients eligible for thrombolysis or PCI.
- If clinical picture and ECG are not diagnostic of MI then full history, examination, chest X-ray, blood test for troponin T or I, CRP, BNP (B type natriuretic peptide), glucose, FBC and U and E should be done. Enquire about previous history of exertional angina or MI.

  On chest X-ray particularly look for PE (focal infiltrate, segmental collapse, raised diaphragm or pleural effusion).

  Aortic dissection (widening or double lumen to aortic knuckle, irregular aortic contour, discrepancy in diameter of ascending and descending thoracic aorta, pleural effusion, mediastinal widening and displacement of calcified intima).
- If JVP is raised, consider PE or pericardial effusion. If there is early diastolic murmur of aortic regurgitation then aortic dissection must be excluded.

  Other risk factors for aortic dissection are Marfan syndrome, dilated aortic root or bicuspid aortic valve or pregnancy.

  Chest X-ray and pulses are normal in 50% of patients with aortic dissection.

  If you suspect esophageal rupture, put the patient nil by mouth and start antibiotics co-amoxiclav and metronidazole and discuss with gastroenterologist.

  In esophageal rupture there may be mediastinal and subcutaneous emphysema, paraspinal mass, pleural effusion and pneumothorax.

  Did the pain follow after esophageal instrumentation (perforation) or after insertion of central line (pneumothorax) or after vomiting (suspect esophageal rupture)? Here pain comes after vomiting while in MI pain comes before vomiting.

Exacerbating or relieving factors: Ask about pain on swallowing (esophageal motility disorders), pain on deep breathing (pleurisy or pericarditis) and movement of trunk and arms (musculoskeletal).

Remember myocardial ischemic pain and esophageal pain (due to acid reflux or spasm) may be indistinguishable. Both radiate to back or arms, may be burning or gripping in quality and both may be relieved by belching.

- Angina may occur after meals but usually during exercise after meals.
- Normal ECG does not exclude unstable angina and presence of ST segment depression or T-wave inversion favors acute coronary syndrome rather than esophageal pain.
- Hyper acute peaking of T-wave may be 1st sign of MI, if present give aspirin, nitrate and repeat ECG after 30 minutes.
- If history is compatible with myocardial ischemia or patient is at moderate or high risk of IHD, repeat ECG after 1 hr and 6 hr and wait for troponin levels.
- If ECG is normal thrombolysis should not be given even if history is suggestive of MI and T-wave inversion is not an indication for thrombolysis.

THROMBOLYTICS

Tissue Plasminogen Activator (TPA)

- This is preferred when BP <90 mm Hg and PCI not possible.
- Anterior MI <55 yr presenting <4 hr of onset of chest pain.
- Caution in frail elderly with inferior MI, risk: benefit ratio is marginal.
- Tissue plasminogen activator is given 15 mg IV over 2 minutes followed by 50 mg (0.75 mg/kg maximum 50 mg) over 30 minutes and then 35 mg (0.5 mg/kg max 35 mg) over 60 minutes.
- Door to needle time usually no more than 20 minutes.
- Concurrent heparin via separate venflow 4000 unit's bolus and 900 units/hr for 48 hrs should be given. APTT estimation should take place at 6 hr and dose adjusted to maintain ratio of 2.0 (range 1.8–2.5). Poor control increases the risk of hemorrhagic stroke.

- *Other TPA's*: Reteplase (bolus repeated after 30 minutes), tenecteplase.
- 20–30 lives saved/1000 patients (<12 hrs).

Has Reperfusion Occurred?

- 70% reduction of ST elevation 90 minutes after initiation of thrombolysis.
- Relief of symptoms, hemodynamic and electrical stability. Seek cardiology opinion and consider repeat thrombolysis with TPA or urgent cardiac angiography if persistent symptoms or persistent raised ST elevation.

Failure to Reperfusion

- <50% reduction in raised ST segment after 90 minutes of thrombolysis.
- On-going persistent pain, arrhythmia or hemodynamic instability.

Management

Rescue PCI and coronary angiography. Do not repeat thrombolysis.

Contraindications to Thrombolytic Therapy

Absolute

- Active internal bleeding or proven active peptic ulcer.
- Suspected aortic dissection or pericarditis.
- Intracranial neoplasm, history of hemorrhagic stroke, CVA in past 6 months.
- BP >180/110 mm Hg after pain relief and nitrates.
- Pregnancy.
- Recent surgery.

Relative

- Recent trauma or traumatic resuscitation or major surgery including dental (within 6 wk).
- Chronic severe hypertension with or without therapy.
- Symptoms suggestive of active gastric ulcer (GU).
- Known bleeding diathesis or current use of anticoagulants.

- Significant liver dysfunction or esophageal varices.
- Lactation/peripartum.
- Severe renal disease.
- Acute pancreatitis.
- Bacterial endocarditis.

Management of Hypertension before Thrombolysis or in Aortic Dissection

- *Pain relief*: Morphine 10 mg (or diamorphine 5 mg) in 10 mL of water for injection and give 2 mg/min slowly IV until pain relief along with cyclizine 50 mg or metoclopramide 10 mg. Assess for bradycardia HR <60/min, heart block, cardiac failure, asthma, COPD and critical limb ischemia.
- Buccal or IV GTN 0.6 mg/hr and increase by 0.3 mg/hr every 5 minutes until BP controlled or ISMN 2–10 mg/hr IV, and continue to monitor closely. Sodium nitroprusside might be considered as an alternative vasodilator.
- If hypertension is resistant to GTN and HR >100, IV beta blockade should be considered if there is no contra indications. Metoprolol IV 1–2 mg/min up to 5 mg with continuous ECG monitoring. Repeat after 5 minutes if required and maximum dose 10–15 mg. Commence thrombolysis when BP <180/110.

In aortic dissection with hypertension atenolol orally or IV labetalol plus GTN should be used and GTN IV single therapy should be avoided.

Angioplasty (PCI)

- Consider this in all patients with NSTEMI or STEMI.
- BP <100 mm Hg or HR >100 in a patient over 70 with anterior MI.
- Early presentation <6 hr of onset of pain.
- Expected time to angioplasty <90 min.
- Salvage procedure after failed thrombolytic therapy.

Complications in 1st 24 hrs after STEMI

- VF or VT 35% (in 4 hrs).
- AF 10–15%.
- *Heart blocks*: 20% in inferior MI (1% permanent pacing), 1% in anterior MI (usually large), cardiogenic shock.
- Severe MR, VSD, angina.

Stable Angina

Optimal drug treatment
- One or two antianginal drugs
- Beta-blocker
- Calcium channel blocker (Amlodipine or diltiazem)
- Short acting nitrate
- Aspirin and statin for secondary prevention of cardiovascular disease.

If calcium channel blocker or beta-blocker contraindicated or not tolerated then add
- Long acting nitrate or
- Ivabradine or
- Nicorandil or
- Ranolazine
- Consider adding 3rd antianginal drug only when two anti-angina drugs do not control symptoms
- Patient is waiting for coronary revascularization or revascularization is not appropriate or acceptable.

Unstable Angina

- Angina occurring at rest or on minimal exertion.
- New or recent onset of cardiac chest pain.
- Increased frequency and/or severity of exertional chest pain inpatients with known IHD.

Investigations

- ECG on admission and during pain if possible, repeating 5–10 minutes after sublingual GTN and after 12–24 hrs of admission.
- ECG may be normal, unchanged from previous ECG, ST segment depression (usually only present during chest pain), T-wave inversion (non-specific).
- *Blood*: Check FBC, U and E, glucose, cholesterol, Tn, and repeat troponin 12–24 hrs after admission.
- *High risk patients (TIMI risk >3)*: Patients with ACS (unstable angina or NSTEMI) who present with ST segment depression have similar mortality rate at 1 month as those with STEMI and increased mortality rate at 3 months (15% annual death rate/MI).

- If TIMI risk 6-7 in an unstable angina patient then consider IV Gp IIb/IIIa (Tirofiban) and angiography <48 hrs.

	Thrombolysis	Primary angioplasty (PCI)
Availability	+++	Limited
Applicability	60–70%	>90%
Early reocclusion	10%	5%
Late occlusion	20–30%	5%
Stroke	1%	0.1%

PCI with stent (reduces reocclusion and restenosis within 6 months) should be considered in high risk groups including shock, elderly, RV involvement, late presenters and those ineligible for fibinolysis. 1/3 pts with anterior MI are late arrival or have non-diagnostic ECG or are of advanced age.

Adjunctive Pharmacology during Percutaneous Intervention (PCI)

- *Aspirin*: For all clinical settings. Aspirin given before percutaneous intervention reduces the abrupt arterial closure by 50–75%. It is a mild antiplatelet agent and in 10% of patients it has no apparent effect.
- *Clopidogrel*: For stenting, unstable angina or NSTEMI. It irreversibly inhibits adenosine diphosphate (ADP) during platelet activation. The combination of aspirin and clopidogrel has become standard treatment during stenting. Dose is 300 mg stat at stenting or 75 mg/day before and continued for 1 yr after stenting.
- *Unfractioned heparin*: For all clinical settings. For patients already on LMWH who require urgent revascularization are switched to unfractionated heparin. LMWH is longer acting and only partially reversible with protamine. Direct thrombin inhibitors (Hirudina, bivalirudin, pepperdine and argatroban) at present are used in patients with heparin induced thrombocytopenia.
- *Glycoprotein IIb/IIIa receptor inhibitors*: They are potent antiplatelet inhibitors and are used with aspirin, clopidogrel and unfractioned heparin in elective PCI in chronic stable angina; unstable angina, NSTEMI

and STEMI. Gp IIb/IIIa are only indicated in patients at high risk (TIMI score) of ischemic complications. Gp IIb/IIIa in primary PCI reduces sub-acute thrombosis, recurrent ischemia and repeat revascularization during 1st month.

- *Abciximab*: Platelet inhibition 24–48 hrs; (12 hrs infusion), causes in 1% of patient's severe thrombocytopenia reversible with platelet transfusion. This is the only drug to demonstrate benefit in post MI PCI.
- *Eptifibatide*: Platelet inhibition 4–6 hrs; (18 hrs infusion). Large trials have shown that use of abciximab or eptifibatide during stenting for elective and urgent percutaneous procedures reduces the risk of MI during procedure and the need for urgent repeat percutaneous interventions by 35–50% and reduces mortality from 2.4% to 1% in 1 yr.
- *Tirofiban*: Platelet inhibition 4–8 hrs; (18 hrs infusion).

Low Risk Patients (TIMI Risk 1–2)

- Patients with ischemic chest pain and few TIMI risk factor (1–2) and normal ECG should be observed for 6–12 hrs with serial ECGs and troponin levels. If negative, patient then undergoes ETT before discharge.
- They should receive LMWH, aspirin 300 mg, clopidogrel, beta blockers and nitrates while awaiting blood results. Clopidogrel should be continued for 12 months.
- Patients with recurrent episode of chest pain despite appropriate treatment, new ST or T-wave changes on ECG have high risk of future cardiac events despite normal Tn levels, should be referred to cardiology for angiogram.

Exercise Stress Testing

Majority of late death occurs in 1st 3 months after discharge, so exercise ECG should be done prior to or early after discharge for intermediate or high risk patients with negative biochemical markers of myocardial injury.

Exercise ECG should not be done on patients with positive troponin or patient unfit for revascularization.

High risk features are ST depression >2 mm or chest pain before 6 minutes of Bruce protocol.

Indications for Myocardial Perfusion Scan

- Patient unable to exercise.
- LBBB
- Equivocal exercise ECG results.

Mortality: In hospital—11% STEMI, 33% LBBB. 1 year mortality 20% in STEMI and 55% in LBBB.

Recurrent Pain

- ECG should be recorded during pain if possible. Additional opioid, buccal GTN and optimal beta blockade (heart rate <70/min) should be considered.
- Recurrent pain with new or increased ST elevation, which is not due to pericarditis should be treated with further thrombolytic therapy or angiography and should be discussed with cardiologist.

Implantable Cardioverter Defibrillator and Pacing

Implantable cardioverter defibrillators (ICD) should be routinely considered as secondary prevention for the following (in the absence of treatable causes):
- Cardiac arrest due to either VT or VF
- Spontaneous sustained VT causing syncope or significant hemodynamic.

Compromise
- Sustained VT without syncope/cardiac arrest, and who have an associated reduction in ejection fraction (<35%) but are no worse than NYHA III

Implantable cardioverter defibrillators should be routinely considered as primary prevention for the following (in the absence of treatable causes):
- A history of previous MI and all of the following:
  - Non-sustained VT on Holter (24-hour ECG) monitoring
  - Inducible VT on electrophysiological testing

– Left ventricular dysfunction with an ejection fraction less than 35% and no worse than NYHA III.
- A familial cardiac condition with a high risk of sudden death, including long QT syndrome, hypertrophic cardiomyopathy, Brugada syndrome, arrhythmogenic right ventricular dysplasia and following repair of tetralogy of Fallot.

Indication for Pacing after MI

Emergency

- Asystole.
- Symptomatic sinus bradycardia with hypotension and first or 2nd degree A-V block with hypotension not responding to atropine.
- Bilateral bundle branch block (BBB or RBBB with alternating LAHB (L axis -30 +qR in I and AVL and rS in II, III AVF).
- New bifascicular block with 1st degree A-V block.
- Mobitz type II second degree block.
- Bradycardia not associated with MI
- On 24 hrs Holter monitor, asystole (3s may be, 4s definitely) or heart rate <40 when awake.
- IInd or 3rd degree A-V block with hemodynamic compromise (systolic BP <100) or syncope at rest.
- Trifascicular block (prolonged PR interval and LBBB).
- Ventricular tachyarrhythmia secondary to bradycardia.
- Elective
- General anesthesia with IInd or IIIrd degree AV block, intermittent AV block, 1st degree AV block with LBBB or bifascicular block.
- *Cardiac surgery*: Aortic surgery, tricuspid surgery, VSD closure and ostium primum repair.
- Over drive suppression of tachyarrhythmia.

Drug Therapy at Discharge after MI

- Aspirin (75–300 mg/day), clopidogrel 75 mg/day.
- Beta-blockers (if there is no contraindication).
- Lipid lowering therapy.
- ACE inhibitors in all patients with confirmed coronary heart disease with or without LV dysfunction. All patients should be given GTN spray and advice about smoking cessation, diet, exercise and alcohol intake.

- Nicotine replacement therapy (NRT) is safe in stable angina and should be avoided in unstable angina or 1st 2 wks of post MI. If patient is struggling then NRT as inhaler or micro tab preferable to patches. All MI patients should have angiography for revascularization or exercise test 4–6 wks after discharge.

Pericarditis

This occurs in 20% of patients after MI and causes pain, which is similar to initial MI pain. It is sudden in onset, substernal or left precordial radiating to trapezius ridges and less often to jaw, arms, neck, shoulder, back. It is worse on inspiration, recumbence and improves on sitting and leaning forward.

Most common causes are RA, Lupus, MI, viral, idiopathic, trauma and neoplasm.

Pericardial rub may be heard along the left sternal edge and tends to come and go over hours.

ECG shows ST (J point) elevation with PR segment depression (TP segment base line) in most leads and reverse in aVR, V1.

Treatment is with aspirin, ibuprofen 800 mg tds plus colchicine 0.6 mg bd. (Ibuprofen as NSAID also causes increased coronary blood flow, colchicine prevents recurrence).

Right Ventricular Infarction / ↑JVP Clear Lungs, Breathlessness

Right ventricular failure (RVF): Raised JVP in the absence of clinical/radiological evidence of pulmonary congestion suggests the possibility of right ventricular infarction, or PE or pericardial effusion or aortic dissection with AR. V3R and V4R will show raised ST segment in RV infarction.

The ECHO or pulmonary artery catheter will confirm showing low pulmonary artery wedge (PAW) pressure with elevated RA and RV pressures (>10 mm Hg).

Patient with hypotension without pulmonary edema has two possibilities, normal JVP (hypovolemia due to sweating, vomiting, previous diuretic therapy) and raised

JVP (RV infarction). For both initial treatment is IV fluids, give colloid 500 mL IV over 30 minutes followed by further 500 mL over 60 minutes if systolic BP remains <100 mm Hg and there are no signs of pulmonary edema. If hypotension persists then start dobutamine infusion, diuretics and vasodilators should be avoided.

Mild Pulmonary Edema without Hypotension

- Give furosemide 40–80 mg IV.
- Nitrates by IV infusion (isosorbide dinitrate 2 mg/hr increasing by 2 mg/hr every 30 minutes till breathlessness is relieved or BP <100 mm Hg or maximum of 10 mg/hr), buccal administration (GTN 5 mg).
- Start ACE (Ramipril 1.25 mg bd).

Cardiogenic Shock

Consider this if there is hypotension, tachycardia, poor peripheral perfusion and oliguria.

- Give O_2 60% humidified (in severe COPD 24–28%) maintaining SaO_2 >92%.
- Treat any arrhythmia appropriately where ever possible (beware negative inotropic effects).
- Check electrolytes and ABG.
- Put a urinary catheter, target >30 mL/hr.
- Immediate ECHO should be performed to exclude cardiac tamponade, acute mitral reflux and VSD.
- Consider invasive monitoring (pulmonary artery catheter).
- Start inotropic/vasopressor therapy (BP <90 mm Hg dobutamine, 80–90 mm Hg dopamine, <80 mm Hg noradrenaline). When BP >100 then nitrate infusion (isosorbide dinitrate 2 mg/hr). Consider PCI and seek cardiologist help.

Hypokalemia

Supplement potassium if <4.0 mmol/L or any arrhythmia with low normal potassium.

Diabetic Control

DIGAMI protocol: All patients with acute MI within preceding 24 hrs who are known diabetics or have random blood sugar >11 mmol/L should be started on IV insulin/dextrose for 24–48 hrs. Start a drip infusion of 5% dextrose running at rate of 500 mL/12 hrs.

Use 50 IU of actrapid or Humulin S in 50 mL of 0.9% saline equivalent to 1 IU/mL. Blood sugar 0–4 (no insulin), 4.1–6.9 (1 IU/hr), 7.0–10.9 (2 IU/hr), 11–15 (3 IU/hr), >15 (6 IU/hr).

All known or suspected diabetics should have HBA1c.

TACHYARRHYTHMIA

- For patients with arrhythmia, plasma K should be kept at 4–5 mmol/L. Regular broad complex tachycardia (>120/min) after infarction is almost always VT rather than SVT with aberrant conduction.
- If in doubt treat as VT with lidocaine or synchronized DC shock.
- In AF high risk (HR >150, on-going chest pain, critical perfusion) or intermediate risk (HR 100–150, breathlessness, poor perfusion) patients treatment is heparin and synchronized DC shock.

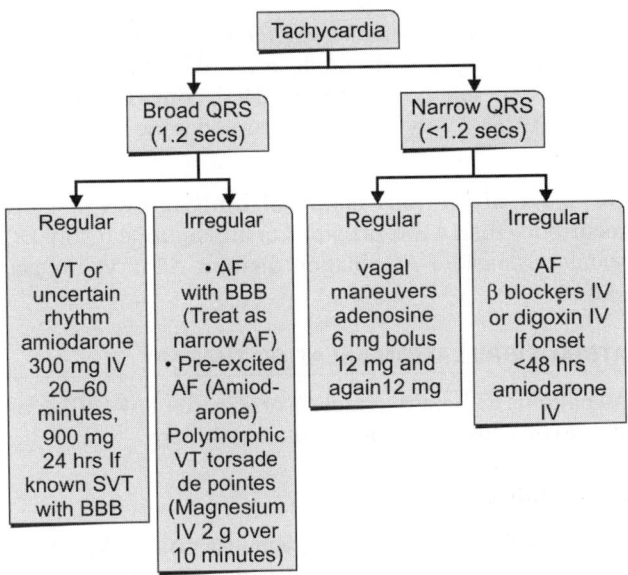

Atrial Fibrillation and Paroxysmal Atrial Fibrillation

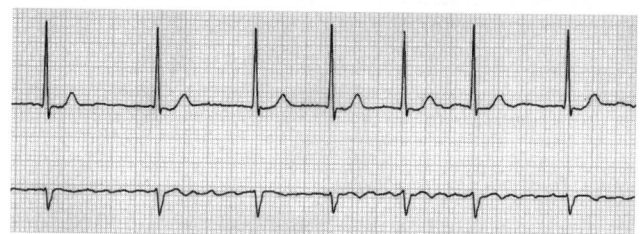

Paroxysmal atrial fibrillation (AF): Lasting <7 days (often <24 hrs).
Persistent AF: Lasting >7 days.
Permanent AF: Lasting >1 yr.

ECHO should be considered if for rhythm control or cardioversion or young patient.

Cardioversion: If AF <24–48 hrs, pharmacological or DC shock, after 48 hrs DC shock should be preferred.

Pharmacological cardioversion for persistent AF (lasting more than 7 days): IV flecanide or propafenone if no heart disease ischemic heart disease (IHD), congestive cardiac failure (CCF), LV dysfunction or amiodarone if any heart disease.

DC shock: If previous failure of cardioversion or early recurrence then 4 wks of sotalol or amiodarone before DC shock or consider AF ablation therapy. AF in young age <60 yrs.

ATRIAL FIBRILLATION ABLATION THERAPY

All patients with paroxysmal AF or persistent AF (AF <1 yr) should be considered for AF ablation therapy.

Contraindication to DC

Atrial fibrillation >12 months, age >65 yrs, marked atrial dilatation on ECHO, left ventricular hypertrophy, low left ventricular ejection fraction, high BMI and history of symptomatic heart failure are adverse features for maintenance of sinus rhythm after DC shock cardioversion or ablation therapy.

Treatment

- Beta-blockers, calcium antagonist (Verapamil, diltiazem), digoxin, warfarin if AF >24–48 hrs (heparin till INR >1.8), TOE before DC shock and warfarin for 1/12 after restoration of SR.
- Amiodarone
- Sotalol (avoid if severe LV dysfunction).
- Flecainide and procainamide (if no IHD, hypertension or structural heart disease).
- Atrial flutter treated as AF.

Wolff-Parkinson-White Syndrome

Initially adenosine to confirm, once confirmed amiodarone and procainamide 15 mg/kg over 20–30 minutes.

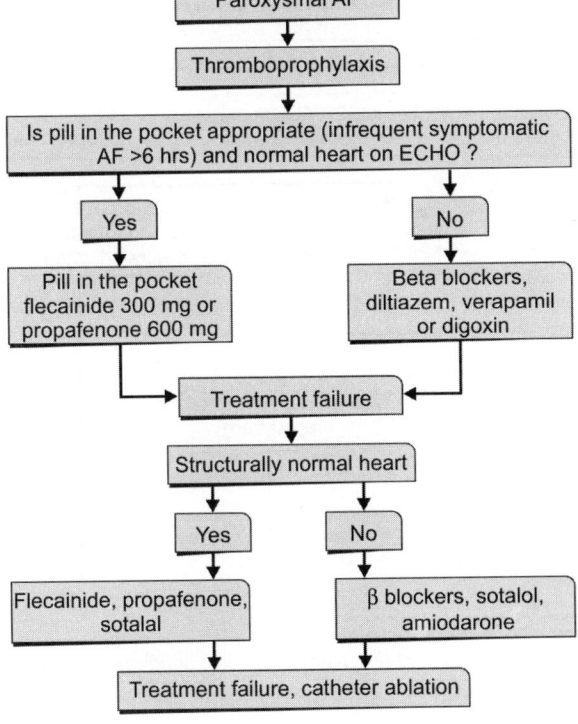

- Patient suspected of paroxysmal AF should have 24 hrs ECG if standard ECG is normal and the patient is having asymptomatic episodes or symptomatic

episodes <24 hrs apart. If symptomatic episodes are >24 hrs apart then 7 day ECG or event recorder ECG.
- Patients with infrequent paroxysm with few symptoms or with known precipitants (caffeine, alcohol) with low stroke risk (<65 yrs, CHA2DS-VASC = 0 should be offered pill in the pocket).
- Patients with symptomatic paroxysms with or with heart disease should be offered beta blockers.

Antithrombotics

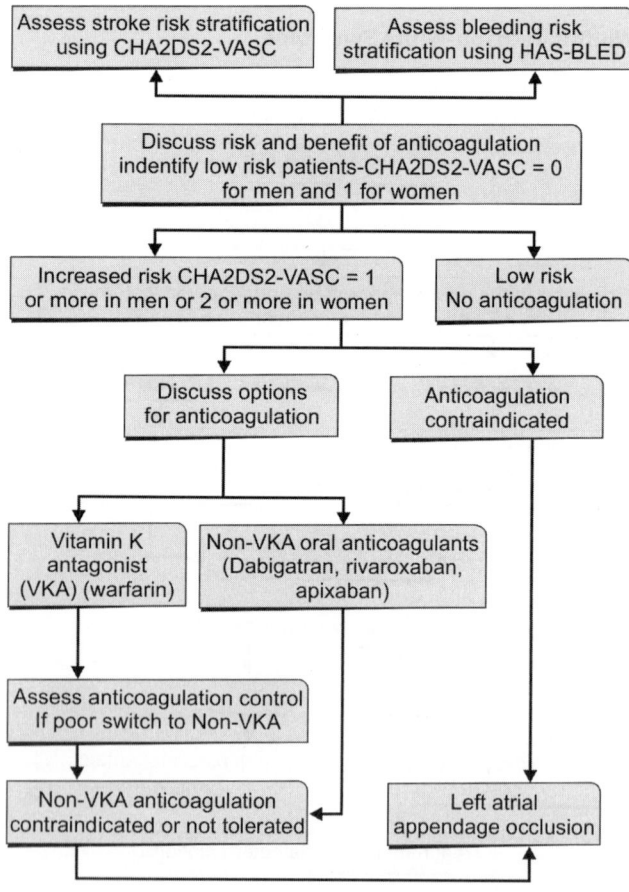

CHA2DS2-VASC	score	HAS-BLED bleeding risk	score
Congestive heart failure or LVF	1	Hypertension	1
Hypertension	1	Abnormal renal or liver function	1
Age >75 yrs	2	Stroke	1
Diabetes	1	Bleeding	1
Stroke or TIA	2	Labile INR	1
Vascular disease	1	Elderly age >65 yrs	1
Age 65 yrs to 75 yrs	1	Drugs like aspirin or NSAIDs or alcohol	1
Female sex	1	Maximum score	1

All patients with non-valvular AF with CHA2DS2-VASC >0 should be considered for long-term warfarin or new direct oral anticoagulants (Non-VTA) dabigatrin (renal excretion 85%) 150 mg twice daily or 110 mg bid in patients 75–80 yrs, rivaroxaban (renal excretion 33%) 20 mg/day with evening meal, reduce to 15 mg/day if eGFR15–50 mL/min or apixaban (renal excretion) (25%) 5 mg bid reduced to 2.5 mg bid if eGFR 15-30 mL/min can be used.

Dabigatran (primarily renal excretion) should not be used in renal impairment and over the age of 80 yrs while Apixaban is safe over 80 yrs.

Non-VTA anticoagulant should not be used if eGFR is <15 mL/min.

Rivaroxaban only has licence for the treatment of pulmonary embolus (PE) or deep venous thrombosis (DVT) and apixaban should be considered if there is history of gastric bleed in the past.

Reversal of Non-VTA

- Anticoagulants in severe bleeding as there is no specific antidote.
- *For minor bleed*: Discontinue the drug.
- For moderate to severe bleed
- Oral activated charcoal is helpful if non-VTA ingested in previous 2–3 hrs.
- If dabigatran is the drug then hemodialysis may be helpful as it is primarily renally excreted. Fresh frozen plasma (FFP) is not helpful.

- Activated prothrombin complex concentrate (PCC) is useful.
- Red cell transfusion and antifibrolytics such as tranexamic acid are useful.

Acute Atrial Fibrillation Complicating Intercurrent Illness or Surgery

- Rate control with digoxin plus calcium antagonist or beta blockers is needed if ventricular rate >120/min. Aim is resting HR <90/min and on exercise <110/min.
- Anticoagulation by SC heparin (LMWH) and if AF is still present after 2 days then anticoagulate with warfarin.
- Cardioversion should be considered if still in AF after 4–6 wks, unless there is thyrotoxicosis in which case defer cardioversion until euthyroid for 6 wks.
- Warfarin for 4 wks is essential before and after elective cardioversion.

Atrial Fibrillation (<48 hrs), No Intercurrent Illness

- Consider modifying current therapy if known paroxysmal.
- Requests ECHO looking for structural heart disease (LVH, LV dysfunction, large left atrium or mitral valve thickening).
- IF structurally heart is normal or hypertension without LVH then treatment options are chemical cardio version with flecainide or propafenone or sotalol or DC synchronised cardio version without anticoagulation.
- If there is structural heart disease then options is trans esophageal ECHO (TOE) to exclude thrombus and DC cardio version or amiodarone or sotalol can be used to restore sinus rhythm and maintain it.
- Digoxin is useful for rate control only, usually with beta blockers (Bisoprolol) or diltiazem or amiodarone but will not restore sinus rhythm.
- Never combine verapamil and beta blocker as risk of asystole.
- For oral anticoagulation and outpatient review in 3–4 wks to consider DC cardio version.

Atrial Fibrillation Longer than 2 days or Uncertain Duration

- Start anticoagulation unless contraindicated (active bleeding, tendency to fall, high and variable alcohol intake).

- Elderly with recurrent falls or patients with lone AF with low risk CHA2Ds2-VASc score 0 in men and 1 in female (young people <60 yrs with favorable ECHO) should receive aspirin instead of warfarin.
- Rate control or amiodarone and planned DC cardioversion if chemical cardioversion has not occurred and chances of maintaining sinus rhythm are high (no significant structural abnormality, duration <3 months).
- Annual stroke rate in untreated rheumatic AF is 15-20% (untreated), 12-15% (treated with aspirin), 5-10% (treated with warfarin), and while in non-rheumatic is 5-6% (untreated), 2-3% (treated with aspirin) and 1-2% (treated with warfarin).
- The incidence of annual stroke rate with lone AF is 1% (untreated), <1% (treated with aspirin or warfarin).
- There is no advantage of anti-arrhythmic drugs over rate control in AF.
- No distinction should be made between paroxysmal, persistent and permanent AF.
- If AF rate control is not achieved by drugs then catheter ablation of AV node with permanent pacemaker should be considered (ablate and pace policy).

Rate Control

- Digoxin loading dose IV (0.75-1.0 mg in 50 mL of 5% dextrose or normal saline over 2 hrs) or oral (0.5 mg bd for 2 days). Maintenance dose 0.625-0.25 mg/day taking in account of age, renal functions and drugs interactions.
- Diltiazem slow release 90 mg twice daily increasing to 120 mg twice daily or verapamil IV 5 mg over 2 minutes, if no response after 5 minutes give further doses of 5 mg every 5 minutes to a total dose of 20 mg (10 mg in patients with IHD or >60); orally 40-120 mg tds.
- *Beta blockers*: Atenolol IV 5-10 mg slowly or sotalol 20-60 mg IV slowly, orally bisoprolol 2.5-5 mg/day or sotalol 80-160 mg bd.
- Amiodarone loading dose IV (300 mg in dextrose 5% by infusion over 20-120 minutes (5 mg/kg), followed by 900 mg over 24 hrs. Orally 200 mg tds for 1 wk (started concurrently with IV loading) followed by 200 mg bid for 1 wk. Maintenance dose orally 100-200 mg/daily.

5. Flecainide IV 2 mg/kg (maximum 150 mg) over 10–30 minutes. Then if necessary 1.5 mg/kg over 1 hr and then if necessary 100–250 µg/kg over 24 hrs maximum dose in 24 hrs 600 mg). Orally 50 mg bid initially, increasing to 100 mg bid. Flecainide should be avoided in the presence of IHD and impaired LV functions.

Atrial Flutter

- Rapid regular or irregular narrow complex tachycardia of 150 bpm with a saw tooth baseline appearance.
- Carotid massage or vagal maneuvers (caution if possible digoxin toxicity, acute ischemia or presence of carotid bruit) may slow the ventricular response revealing flutter waves.
- Adenosine may help by slowing AV conduction and revealing flutter waves.
- Rapid IV bolus of 6 mg followed by saline flush, up to 12 mg IV a total of 3 times at 1–2 minutes interval may be if tolerated. Half-life of adenosine is 10 sec and clinical effects lasts 2 minutes and warn the patient about chest tightness and flushing.
- Do not use in asthmatics, or those taking dipyridamole, carbamazepine and 2nd or 3rd degree heart block.
- Atrial flutter tends to be sustained and does not respond readily to AV node blocking drugs, so every patient with sustained atrial flutter should be considered for cardio version.
- Immediate management is same as for AF with IV amiodarone, beta blockers and calcium antagonists.

Supraventricular Tachycardia

Referral to Electrophysiologist

- Wide QRS tachycardia.
- SVT with syncopy or severe symptoms. Patient with drug resistance or intolerance or patient who prefers to be free of drugs.
- Pre-excitation syndrome with or without supraventricular tachycardia (SVT).
- *Brugada syndrome*: RBBB with raised ST segment in V1-V3. This predisposition to fatal arrhythmia in young people, some times presenting as syncope and treated by ICD.

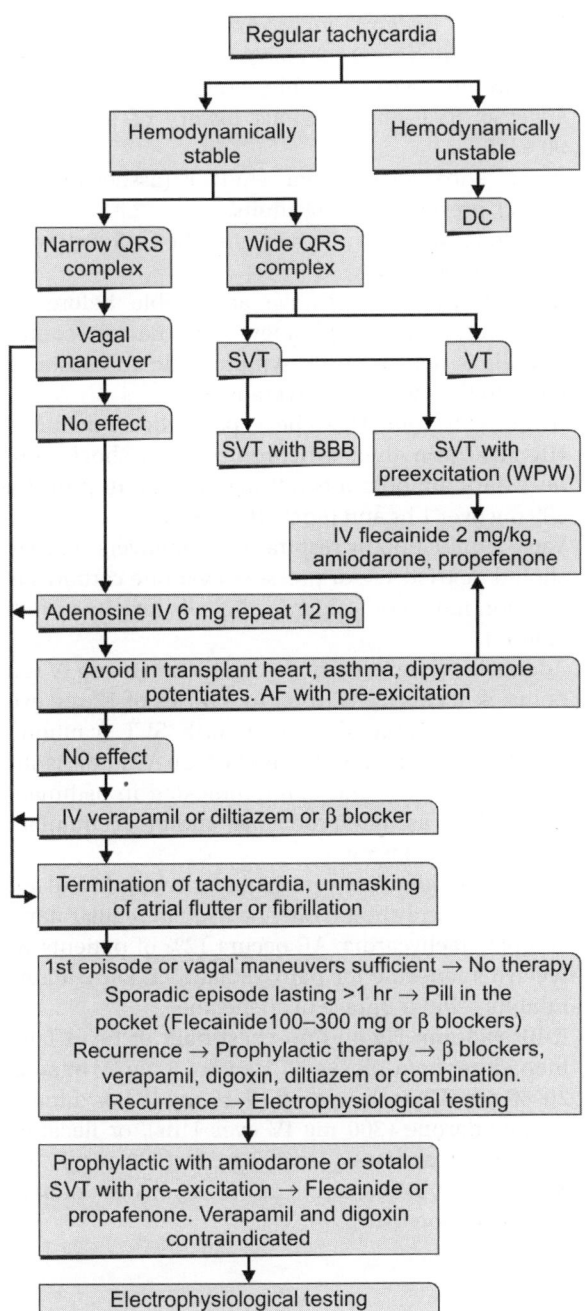

- *AV node re-entry tachycardia (AVNRT)*: Usually presents in young persons, common in females. Usually no P-waves visible. Previous history of SVT suggests SVT and previous history of MI suggests 90% VT.
- AV re-entry tachycardia (AVRT) (associated with WPW), present in young adults.

  Inverted P-wave may be seen after the QRS and pseudo RBBB pattern in V1.

  Atrial tachycardia, P-wave are visible before QRS but with abnormal morphology. Most narrow complex tachycardia is benign and if symptomatic and sustained, responds to Beta blockers or verapamil.
- If BP <90 mm Hg, chest pain, heart failure or HR >200/min then synchronized DC shock and if necessary amiodarone 150 mg IV over 10 min, then 300 mg over 1 hr and repeat the shock.
- Vagal stimulation by respiratory maneuvers (Valsalva) should be tried 1st, or pressure over one carotid sinus (caution in recent ischemia, digitalis toxicity or in the elderly).
- Adenosine (blocks AV node conduction) 6 mg IV rapid bolus, if necessary with up to 3 doses of 12 mg every 1–2 minutes may slow or abolish SVT (caution in known WPW patients). It has effect on AV node, is short lived (10–15 sec) and contraindicated in asthmatics. Doses given are often too small and no accumulation with multiple dosing.
- Adenosine can cause ventricular arrhythmia and atrial fibrillation and should only be used in regular narrow complex tachycardia. AF occurs 12% of patients who receive adenosine for paroxysmal SVT. Dipyridamole inhibits cellular uptake of adenosine.
- If BP >90 mm Hg and no chest pain or heart failure then either beta-blockers (Atenolol 5 mg IV or sotalol 20–60 mg IV) or verapamil (5–10 mg IV) or diltiazem or amiodarone (300 mg IV over 1 hr), or flecainide, repeated if necessary and digoxin (500 mg IV over 30 minutes). Diltiazem is as efficacious as verapamil but less hypotensive.

Cardiovascular 227

Broad Complex Tachycardia

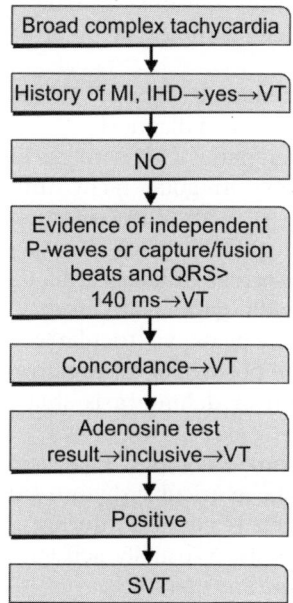

- All broad complex regular tachycardia treat as VT unless proved otherwise.
- All irregular broad complex tachycardia consider W-P-W and avoid digoxin, beta blockers, verapamil and adenosine. Low thresh hold for DC cardioversion.
- VT (monomorphic) nonsustained lasting less than 30 sec and sustained lasting more than 30 sec. Polymorphic VT is Torsade-de-pointes which has a distinct pattern.

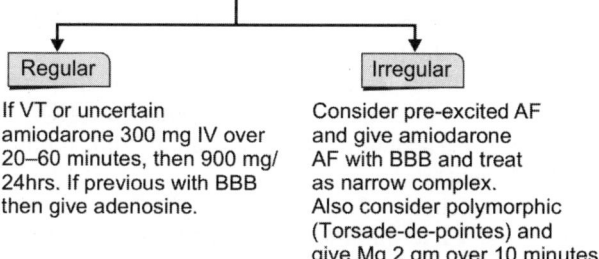

DIAGNOSIS

- In a patient with previous MI, IHD, cardiomyopathy, age >60, broad complex tachycardia is always due to VT.
- In young patients <40 suspect WPW or BBB, adenosine may be used to assist diagnosis.
- Do not use verapamil if VT is not excluded.
- Broad complex irregular tachycardia is due to AF with LBBB, AF with WPW or torsade's-de-pointes tachycardia.
- Broad complex regular tachycardia is due to VT when associated with QRS >140 msec, AV dissociation, capture/fusion beats, ventricular concordance (QRS complexes all positive or all negative) or extreme left axis deviation or definite axis shift as compared to previous ECG.
    - Regular broad complex tachycardia <120 bpm is due to idioventricular rhythm (>120 bpm due to VT), which is common during reperfusion after thrombolysis, is usually self-terminating and do not require any therapy.

    VT which looks like RBBB, in VT the 1st deflection is larger than 2nd while other way round in RBBB.
- Presence of frequent ventricular ectopic (VE) with significant left ventricular impairment (EF <35%), consider 24 hrs cardiac monitor to exclude non sustained VT.
- QRS amplitude alternans suggests SVT and essential to rule out pericardial effusion by ECHO.

    VT and sudden cardiac death in people with low EF <30%.

Management VT

- If cardiac arrest or severely compromised hemodynamic state (pulse less VT): DC shock.
- If the patient is hemodynamically stable, correct electrolyte abnormalities keeping potassium (K) >4.0 mmol/L, Ca (calcium), Mg(magnesium) >0.7 mmol/L, O_2 (Oxygen).

    Thump chest

    Drugs VT termination: Lidocaine (19%), procainamide (36%), flecainide (60%), amiodarone (12%), sotalol (56%), quinidine (24%), disopyramide (31%).

Give lidocaine 100 mg (5 mL of 2% solution) IV over 30s (After MI maintenance IV infusion of lidocaine 4 mg/min for 30 minutes, 2 mg/min for 2 hrs, and 1 mg/min for 12–24 hrs). If this fails to restore sinus rhythm, give procainamide 200 mg IV over 1 minute or amiodarone or sotalol. If VT persists, give synchronized DC shock.

- After correction of VT, establish the cause.
- Correct hypokalemia (keep K between 4–5 mmol/L), hypomagnesemia, long QT interval, hypoxia and cardiac ischemia.
- For VT suppression load with amiodarone (1st 24 hrs) and after that with phenytoin.
- Suggest chest X-ray, ECG and ECHO to exclude MI, pulmonary edema and LV dysfunction.
- The etiology of VT will determine long-term strategy.
- Coronary intervention (PCI).
- Electrophysiological intervention.
- Drug therapy.
- Implantable cardioverter-defibrillator (ICD). Do not hesitate to ask cardiology opinion.

RVOT Tachycardia (RV Outlet Tachycardia)

- VT associated with normal heart.
- Usually in young people.
- Frequently nonsustained and exercise induced.
- LBBB with R axis.
- Responds to beta blockers and good prognosis.

Fascicular Tachycardia

- VT associated with normal heart.
- Young people.
- LAD with RBBB.
- Terminated with verapamil.
- Good prognosis.

Sudden Cardiac Death

Initial evaluation (all 1st degree relatives of patients with inherited cardiac disease or victims of sudden arrhythmic death syndrome).

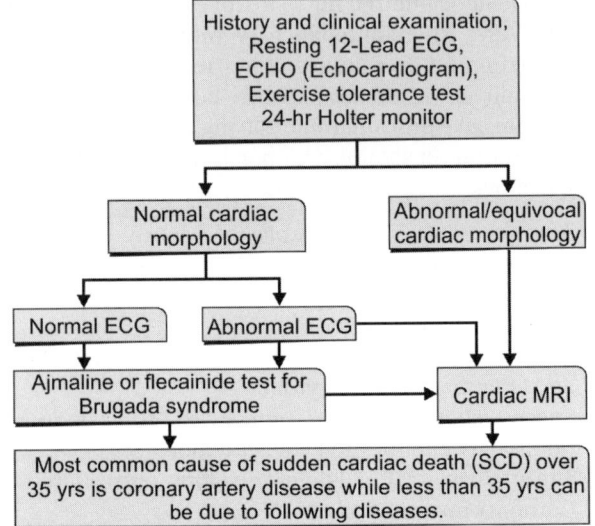

Hypertrophic cardiomyopathy (HCM), arrythmogenic right ventricular cardiomyopathy (ARVC), Brugada syndrome, long QT syndrome, short QT syndrome, Wolff-Parkinson-White syndrome (WPW) and catecholaminergic polymorphic ventricular tachycardia.

HYPERTROPHIC CARDIOMYOPATHY

- Left ventricular hypertrophy (LVH) in absence of hypertension or valvular heart disease.
- Presents with angina or breathlessness, unheralded syncope, ventricular tachycardia (VT).
- LVH >30 mm and (FH) of premature sudden cardiac death <40.
- There is asymmetric sepal hypertrophy and dynamic LV obstruction on ECHO and flat BP response (Systolic BP rise <25 mm Hg rise with exercise).
- HCM is the most common cause of SCD in young athletes.

Treatment

- Beta blockers or diltiazem or verapamil.
- Implantable cardiac defibrillator (ICD).
- Screen 1st degree relatives.

ARRHYTHMOGENIC RIGHT VENTRICULAR CARDIOMYOPATHY (ARVC)

- Presents with palpitation, syncope, sudden cardiac death (SCD), congestive cardiac failure (CCF), ventricular tachycardia (VT), thromboembolic event at young age on exercise.
- ECG shows T-wave inversion V1-V4 and ventricular ectopic of left bundle branch block (LBBB) pattern in V1-V4 indicating right ventricular origin.

Treatment

Avoid strenuous exercise, beta blockers, ICD and screen 1st degree relatives.

BRUGADA SYNDROME

- Partial right bundle branch block (RBBB) with coved raised ST segment >2 mm with inverted T-wave in V1-V2 on ECG.
- Presents as syncope or seizure.

Treatment

Implantable cardioverter-defibrillator (ICD) therapy.

LONG QT SYNDROME (A DISEASE OF THE YOUNG, UNUSUAL AFTER 40)

Long QT syndrome is associated with sudden death in young fit healthy persons due to VF or syncope due to polymorphic VT (Torsa-De-Pointes Tachycardia) precipitated by physical stress or emotional stress or loud noises (LQT2), diving, swimming (LQT2), sleep or rest (LQT3).

The risk of death or syncope is decreased in pregnancy but increased in postpartum period. Three genes LQT1 (most common), LQT2 and LQT3 are recognized.

Presents as palpitation or syncope or SCD. QTc is >440 msec in males and >460 msec in females (risk 20% for QTC >446 msec and 70% for QTc >498 msec).

Causes

Hypocalcemia, hypothyroidism, antiarrhythmic drugs (Sotalol), haloperidol, methadone and pentamidine can also cause long QT syndrome.

Therapy

- Avoid competitive sports.
- Beta blockers (long acting atenolol or nadolol) and ICDs for QTc >460 msec in women and >440 msec in men.
- ICD for survivors of cardiac arrest or having syncope while on Beta-blockers or patients with QTc >500 msec.
- Avoid all class 1 drugs.
- Screen 1st degree relatives. L cardiac sympathetic denervation (L stellate ganglionectomy) if recurrent syncope in spite of beta-blockers.

TORSADES-DE-POINTES TACHYCARDIA

- Characterized by rapid broad QRS polymorphic VT and can be mistaken for VF.
- Consider torsade when polymorphic VT with long QT interval and changing axis.

Causes

- Bradycardia.
- Electrolyte disturbance (Hypokalemia/hypocalcemia/severe hypomagnesemia). Tricyclic antidepressants.
- Thioridazine.
- IV erythromycin.
- Antihistamines (terfenadine).
- Anti-arrhythmic (Sotalol, amiodarone, disopyramide, procainamide).
- Myocardial ischemia, subarachnoid hemorrhage (SAH).
- Congenital long QT syndrome or base line prolonged QT >500 msec.
- Recent conversion of AF by QT prolonging drugs.

Management

- Withdraw any drug likely to prolong QT interval.
- Give magnesium sulfate 8 mmol IV over 10–15 minutes, repeated if necessary. Correct calcium and potassium.
- Consider beta blockers atenolol or nadolol.
- Consider temporary atrial or ventricular pacing.
  LQT3 is due to defect in sodium channels rather than K channels and is treated with flecainide.

Hereditary short QT syndrome—rare, QT is <300 msec. Sudden cardiac death due to VF and AF can occur. Quinidine is effective in prolonging the QT interval and preventing arrhythmia, but ICD implantation is desirable.

BRADYCARDIA AND PACEMAKER

Sinus or junctional-rate < 60 bpm, P-wave inverted or buried within or after QRS in junctional rhythm. Common after inferior MI, also consider hypothyroidism, drugs (Beta blockers overdose, glucagon 5 mg IM or IV to reverse it), hypothermia and raised intracranial pressure.

Treatment

- Indicated, if BP <90 mm Hg, HR <40 bpm, ventricular arrhythmia, or heart failure.
- Give atropine 0.6 mg IV, repeated at 5 minutes interval if the HR remains <60 to a total dose of 3 mg.
- If unrelated to MI, then it usually is due to effect of beta-blockers or sick sinus syndrome.
- If due to beta-blockade causing pulmonary edema then give atropine and isoprenaline 0.5–10 µg/min till the HR >60.
- If BP remains low then start dobutamine infusion 10 µg/kg/min. Glucagon 50–150 µg/kg with 5% glucose IV can be combined with isoprenaline or dobutamine.
- No action is necessary if patient is asymptomatic and HR is >40 bpm, if symptomatic (syncope or presyncope) or HR <40 bpm, stop any drugs that may be contributing and put in a temporary pacing wire.

FIRST DEGREE HEART BLOCK

Regular sinus rhythm with PR interval >0.2 sec, not uncommon after acute inferior MI and needs temporary pacing if associated with bifasicular block (RBBB with LAD >−30 or RAD >+90 degree axis) or complete LBBB. It may also indicate septal abscess formation in aortic valve endocarditis indicating the need for transesophageal ECHO and referral to cardiologist.

- Left axis deviation (LAD).
- Right axis deviation (RAD).

SECOND DEGREE HEART BLOCK

- 2nd degree block—Mobitz type 1 (Wenckebach)—Progressive lengthening of PR interval followed by a dropped beat.
- In inferior MI, if there is hypotension unresponsive to atropine then needs pacing.
- If unrelated to MI exclude digoxin toxicity, beta-blockers.
- If there are symptoms of syncope or presyncope then arrange temporary pacing and permanent pacing later.
- If asymptomatic, record 24 hrs ECG and discuss with the cardiologist whether permanent pacing is indicated.
- Mobitz type 2 Block (usually 2 : 1) Characterized by constant PR interval and the sudden failure of conduction through AV node. This occurs in a cyclic pattern.

THIRD DEGREE ATRIOVENTRICULAR BLOCK

- Complete AV dissociation with all atrial impulses blocked within the conducting system.
- In anterior MI development of 2nd or 3rd degree heart block needs temporary pacing wire initially and permanent pacing before discharge.
- Even in asymptomatic patient without MI, this carries a risk of sudden death, put in temporary pacing wire if there is syncope or presyncope or HR <40/min and arrange permanent pacing later.

TRANSVENOUS TEMPORARY PACING

Indication

- Any bradycardia unresponsive to atropine associated with syncope or symptomatic hypotension (BP <100 mm Hg), CCF or ventricular arrhythmia or asystole >3 sec night time and >2 sec day time may be for pacing, and if >4s then definite for pacing on 24 hrs tape.
- Bifasicular (RBBB with LAD >-30 or RAD >+90) or trifasicular block (bifasicular or LBBB with 1st degree heart block).
- 2nd or 3rd degree heart block in MI with hypotension. If thrombolysis has been given in the preceding 36 hrs or patient is on anticoagulants then peripheral or femoral veins should be used and not the central vein.

Pacing threshold usually should not exceed 1 volt and over the succeeding days it should not rise above 2–2.5 volts without repositioning. Pacing threshold should be checked twice daily and sudden increase in threshold usually indicates need for repositioning. Pacing should be at 2–2.5 times of pacing threshold and not above 3.5 volts and should always be in demand mode.

Chest X-ray should always be done to check electrode position and assess for pneumothorax.

Need for pacing wire should be reviewed daily and catheter removed at the earliest opportunity and if infection is suspected then swab from wound and tip of the needle should be sent for culture.

RISK OF PACEMAKER

One percent pneumothorax, 1% risk of bleeding and 1%/year of infections.

SUSPECTED MALFUNCTION OF PERMANENT PACEMAKER

- Check details (single or dual chamber and what is the pacing mode), contact hospital where the system was implanted.
- Obtain 12 lead ECG and penetrated chest X-ray to see position of leads.
- If there are no spikes then consider normal sensing, spikes buried in QRS, malfunction of pulse generator and electromagnetic interference.
- Spikes without capture or failure to capture (high threshold, lead displacement, myocardial fibrosis, myocardial perforation, lead not properly connected to pulse generator, depletion of battery of pulse generator or spike in ventricular refractory period.
- Spikes without sensing or failure to sense, lead displacement, and low intrinsic QRS current should be considered.

Heart Failure (Mild/Moderate) in Acute Coronary Syndrome

- Raised JVP, mild breathlessness at rest or on minimal exertion, basal crepitation, and upper lobe diversion on chest X-ray and persistent tachycardia.

- B type natriuretic peptide (BNP) is secreted by myocytes in response to myocardial strain and it causes natriuresis, diuresis and vasodilatation.
- BNP <100 pg/mL nearly rules out CCF.
- BNP > 400 likely CCF (ECHO within 2 wks) and BNP >1000 (urgent ECHO) specific for CCF.
- Isolated raised JVP reflects right ventricular MI; diuretics in this situation may be harmful.
- BNP is decreased in obesity. Treat with ACE or ARB or Beta blockers or diuretics or aldosterone antagonist.
- BNP is raised in CCF, diabetes mellitus (DM), sepsis, age >70, LVH, IHD, tachycardia, RV overload, hypoxia, cirrhosis, GFR <60.

Management of CCF with Normal or Reduced Ejection Fraction

- O_2 and monitor SaO_2 keeping >95%.
- Consider stopping or reducing beta-blockers temporarily.
- Ensure the patient is on ACE inhibitors/AII receptor antagonist and spironolactone unless contraindicated.
- In African descent patient intolerant to ACE and ARB consider hydralazine and nitrates.
- Consider oral diuretics and assess their need daily.
- Diuretics are useful in the management of mild chronic LVF or acute exacerbation of chronic LVF.
- In resistant heart failure consider edematous GI tract, excessive oral salt intake, low albumin (secretion to nephron is predominantly bound drug), oral cimetidine (competes for secretion in nephrone) and blunting of initial naturetic response (distal part of tubule will increase reabsorption of Na because of increased delivery of Na) so increase the frequency of furosemide as it lasts only 6 hrs.
- Consider the need for IV nitrates.
- Assess LV function by ECHO before discharge.
- Consider starting beta-blockers once the patient is stable with no signs of fluid retention.
- Avoid NSAID, rate-limiting calcium antagonists (Diltiazem and verapamil), tricyclic antidepressants.
- Life style modification (stopping smoking, excessive alcohol, losing excess weight, taking regular exercise and avoiding salt rich foods).

- Annual immunization for influenza and *pneumococcus* is recommended.

Cardiac resynchronization therapy (CRT): CCF (NYHA class II, III or IV) with EF <35% and evidence of dyssynchrony (QRS >150 ms LBBB). This is achieved by pacing right atrium, right ventricle like DDD pacemaker but also pacing left ventricle (coronary sinus).

Implantable Cardiac Defibrillator (ICD)

- Primary prevention.
- MI >1 month ago, EF <30% QRS >120 ms.
- MI >1 month ago. EF <35% and nonsustained VT.
- Secondary prevention survivors of VT or VF causing syncope or severe hemodynamic compromise.
- If LV ejection fraction is <35% then consider ICD and CRT.

SEVERE HEART FAILURE

- Patient breathless at rest, tachypneic, sinus tachycardia or rapid AF, gallop rhythm, wide spread crepitation and chest X-ray showing pulmonary edema.
- Chronic heart failure made worse by anemia, sepsis and intense vasoconstriction.

Management

Identify and treat separately those few (5–10%) with low filling pressures.

Fluid Resuscitation

Relieve the intense vasoconstriction
- Give high concentration of O_2 to achieve SaO_2 >92%.
- GTN 2 Puffs sublingual.
- Give morphine 2–10 mg or diamorphine (reduces anxiety causes some vasodilatation) 2.5–5 mg IV preceded by metoclopramide 10 mg IV
- IV nitrate is treatment of choice in LVF complicating MI. Give GTN 0.3–0.6 mg/hr. Vasodilators are the drugs of 1st choice in acute LVF except tight aortic stenosis.
- Consider CPAP and IV diuretics (Furosemide 50–100 mg IV).

- Inotropes if BP is low: Dobutamine 5–20 µg/kg/min and adjusting by 2.5 µg/kg/min increments or epinephrine 0.05 µg/kg/min and adjusting by 0.02 µg/kg/min.
- Nebulized salbutamol 2.5–5 mg if there is bronchospasm.
- Monitor urine output and SaO_2.

Exclude VSD, mitral regurgitation, cardiac tamponade and left ventricular aneurysm by ECHO.

Treat tachy/bradyarrhythmias.

If patient becomes drowsy, consider opiate antagonist.

Also consider ICU referral and pulmonary artery catheter and consider inotropes if BP is low. Digitalis IV may be used as inotropes.

DIGOXIN TOXICITY

Often associated with bradycardia, ventricular bigeminy, paroxysmal atrial tachycardia with variable AV block and accelerated idioventricular rhythm. But almost any arrhythmia can occur. Nausea, vomiting, anorexia and visual disturbance are also common.

Treatment

- Discontinue digoxin and check blood levels and U and Es.
- Correct any fluid and electrolyte imbalance especially hypokalemia.
- If hypokalemia is present then assume the presence of hypomagnesemia and correct it.
- Treat SVT and VT as discussed before and avoid DC cardioversion for danger of precipitating VF. Temporary pacing wire can be inserted in profound bradycardia.
- Consider digibind.

Hypertensive Emergencies and Resistant Hypertension

Causes

- *Malignant hypertension:* Most cases have secondary pathology, 80% renal disease (glomerulonephritis, tubulo interstitial nephritis, pyelonephritis and renovascular disease).

- *Endocrine*: Pheochromocytoma 1%, Conn's 10% (family history of stroke, young patient with refractory hypertension needing 3 drugs) and Cushing's disease.
- Drugs (Cocaine, MAOI's).
- Aortic dissection/coarctation and pre-eclampsia.
- Essential 20%.

  Hypertensive encephalopathy (headache, focal CNS signs, seizures and coma), heart failure, eclampsia and dissecting aneurysm are indications for rapid controlled reduction in BP. Hypertension after stroke is not treated for 2/52 unless systolic BP > 220 and diastolic >140.

Clinical Presentation

- Headache, epistaxis, faintness, chest pain, dyspnea, neurological deficit, pulmonary edema, encephalopathy, cerebral hemorrhage and psychomotor retardation.
- Control should be achieved in 2–3 hrs in hypertensive encephalopathy, 6–12 hrs in subarachnoid hemorrhage (SAH) and after 2 wks in stroke.

Endocrine Hypertension

- K <3.5 mmol/L, consider hyperaldosteronism with familial hyperaldosteronism (FH) of stroke, young patient with resistant hypertension requiring >3 drugs. Blood aldosterone level >450 pmols/L.
- Or loss of fall <140 pmols after 2 L of normal saline IV over 4 hrs.
- *Diagnosed by aldosterone*: Renin ration in the blood.
- Ratio is increased by beta blockers, calcium antagonist and decreased by ACE, diuretics. So when testing for aldosterone rennin ratio beta blockers, diuretics, ACE and calcium antagonists should be stopped and patient put on alpha blockers before testing. If bilateral hyper aldosteronism then treated with spironolactone or eplerenone.

Treatment

Relieve pain and anxiety. Most of these patients are dehydrated.

Drugs to Avoid

- Nifedipine, hydralazine and minoxidil.
- Nifedipine may cause precipitate drop in BP and has variable sublingual absorption.
- Hydralazine (10–20 mg IV bolus than 20–40 mg 6 hrly) is safe and proven in pregnancy, but may cause precipitate drop in BP, so start with a small dose and built up.
- Nitroprusside IV (0.3 µg/kg/min titrated upto 6 µg/kg/min, e.g. 50 mg in 1 L 5% dextrose and expect to give 100–200 mL/hr for few hours only to avoid cyanide risk). It is the drug of choice but should be monitored closely.
- *High renin and high aldosterone*: Renal artery stenosis.
- *Low rennin and low aldosterone*: Pheochromocytoma, Cushing, cocaine, renal, amphetamine.
- If with LVF
  - IV nitrate (GTN), furosemide. 2nd choice nitroprusside
- If with ACS
  - GTN infusion + Beta blocker 2nd choice nitroprusside
- Aortic dissection
  - Nitroprusside + Beta blockers 2nd choice IV labetalol 50 mg IV/1 min repeated every 5 minutes max dose 200 mg.
- Pheochromocytoma
  - IV fluids (as most of patients are dehydrated) + IV Phentolamine + oral phenoxybenzamine. Avoid beta blockers until fully alpha blocked.
  - 2nd choice nitroprusside + GTN.
- SAH
  - Nimodipine, nipride
- Intracerebral hemorrhage (ICH)
  - Labetalol 50 mg bd, 2nd choice nitroprusside.
- Pregnancy
  - Methyldopa 250 mg tds to 500 mg tds, labetalol, prazosin and amlodipine.
  - Avoid sublingual (SL) nifedipine and diuretics. ACE contraindicated as teratogenic.
- Acute kidney injury (AKI)
  - Labetalol, 1 and 2nd choice nitroprusside reduced dose

- *Eclampsia/pre-eclampsia*: Hypertension, oliguria, proteinuria, edema and fits.
- Correct hypovolemia.
- $MgSO_4$ 40–60 mg/kg, 2–4 g/hr infusion and maintaining serum Mg >1.5–2 mmol/L + hydralazine
- Deliver the child.

RESISTANT HYPERTENSION

- Resting BP >140/90 and ambulatory BP >135/85 in spite of being on 3 anti-hypertensive drugs.
- Initially angiotensin converting enzyme inhibitors (ACE) or angiotensin receptor blocker (ARB) plus calcium channel blocker (CCB) plus thiazide diuretics (A + C + D), if resting BP still >140/90 mm Hg or ambulatory BP >135/85 mm Hg then add spironolactone 25 mg/day initially later increasing to 50 mg/day keeping serum potassium <4.5 mmol/L. If spironolactone produces side effects (gynecomastia, breast tenderness) then consider amiloride or eplirinone.
- If the BP still remains poorly controlled there is option of adding alpha or beta blockers or centralling acting alpha agonist (methyldopa or clonidine) or vasodilators (hydralazine or minoxidil).

Characteristic of Patient with Resistant Hypertension

- Old age >75 yrs.
- High base line blood pressure and chronicity of uncontrolled hypertension.
- Target organ damage (left ventricular hypertrophy, chronic kidney disease.
- Diabetes, obesity, ethnicity (black), sex (female), excessive and dietary sodium.

Contributing Factors

- *Life style factors*: Obesity, high alcohol intake (>21 units/wk for men and >14 units/wk for women), excessive dietary sodium >6 gm/day, cocaine and amphetamine use.
- *Drugs related*: NSAID (nonsteroidal anti-inflammatory drugs), contraceptive hormones (but not postmeno-

pausal hormone replacement therapy), steroid hormones (Cushing's syndrome), sympathomimetic agents (nasal decongestants, diet pills), erythropoietin, cyclosporine, tacrolimus and liquorice.
- *Volume overload*: Progressive renal insufficiency, high salt intake and inadequate diuretic therapy.
- *Secondary causes*:
  - *Primary hyperaldosteronism*: Hypokalemia, fatigue, low renin levels inspite of being on 3 antihypertensive drugs A + C + E (which slightly raise renin levels).
  - *Renal artery stenosis*: Carotid or abdominal or femoral bruits, history of flash pulmonary edema. Young female (fibromuscular dysplasia), history of atherosclerotic disease.
  - *Renal parenchyma disease*: Albuminuria or microscopic hematuria, nocturia, edema and biochemical disturbances
  - *Obstructive sleep apnea*: Obesity, short neck, day time somnolence, snoring, frequent night time awakenings and witnessed apnea.
  - *Pheochromocytoma*: Episodic palpitations, headaches, sweating.
  - *Thyroid disease*: Eye signs, weight loss/gain, heat/cold intolerance, heart failure, tachycardia, bradycardia, anxiety or fatigue, hypo or hyperthyroidism.
  - *Coarctation of aorta*: Radioradial or radiofemoral delay, diminished femoral pulses and rib notching on chest X-ray.

Acute Aortic Dissection

Risk factors are hypertension and Marfans syndrome (autosomal dominant, tall stature, long limbs, lower segment >upper segment, arachnodactyly, joint laxity, aortic root dilatation, lens dislocation and striae in skin).

Peak incidence 6–7th decade, if presenting <40 yrs then the cause is pregnancy or Marfan syndrome. It occurs 65% in ascending aorta, 20% in descending aorta, 10% aortic arch and 5% in abdominal aorta.

Increased susceptibility in hypertension, Marfans syndrome, aortic root dilatation, bicuspid aortic valve and pregnancy.

Presenting Features

- Very severe instantaneous anterior chest pain (like hammer-blow or tearing in quality).
- Severe back pain.
- Syncope and hypotension.
- Ischemic coronary, cerebral, upper limb, renal and lower limb symptom (focal neurological deficit, stroke).
- Cardiac tamponade.
- Acute aortic regurgitation.
- Asymmetry of pulses, difference in systolic BP in both arms (normal <15 mm Hg).
  Chest X-ray may be normal (50%) or may show mediastinal widening, widening or double lumen of aortic knuckle, irregular aortic contour or pleural effusion.

Management

- High index of clinical suspicion.
- High flow O_2 by face mask.
- Diamorphine 2.5–5 mg IV preceded by IV 10 mg metoclopramide or cyclizine 50 mg.
- Chest X-ray, FBC, U and E, LFT, troponin, group and save, cross match and clotting screen.
- Spiral CT with contrast has high diagnostic accuracy. If aortic dissection involves ascending aorta then urgent cardiothoracic surgical opinion but if dissection limited to arch or descending aorta then conservative management.
- Arrange urgent transthoracic ECHO/TOE looking for an intimal flap (50% of proximal dissections), dilatation of ascending aorta to 5 cm or more, aortic regurgitation and pericardial fluid. If ascending aorta appears normal or not well seen then TOE should be performed.
- ECG to exclude MI (rarely dissection can involve right coronary artery causing inferior MI).
- Transfer the patient to CCU and aggressive BP control (systolic 100–120 mm Hg) with labetalol (1 mg/min) or esmolol (50–200 microgram/kg/min).
- Put a bladder catheter to monitor urine output.
- Early mortality in acute aortic dissection is 10% per hour. Surgery can be life-saving and should not be

delayed and never transfer a patient for surgery without adequate BP control with IV therapy as described above.

Infective Endocarditis

Infective endocarditis (IE) should be suspected in ill patient with known cardiac disease or new cardiac murmurs (especially after dental, invasive diagnostic or surgical treatment) or signs of new embolic or vasculitic complications.

Micro or macro ulcers on the valvular endocardium, contact with the blood forms coagulum, pathogens in bacteremia bind avidly to the coagulum, attract and activate monocytes to produce cytokines resulting in enlargement of infected vegetation.

Clinical Features

Pyrexia >38°C, remitting, rigors, weight loss, fatigue and arthralgia, new or worsening regurgitant cardiac murmurs or development of cardiac failure are salient features. Emboli from valve vegetation can go in any major vessels or signs of vasculitis, i.e. splinter hemorrhages, Osler's nodes (small tender subcutaneous nodules palpable in pulp of finger lasting hours to days), Jane way lesions (small erythematous or hemorrhagic non tender macular lesions in palm and soles), Roth's spots (oval retinal hemorrhage with pale center), conjunctival petechiae, glomerulonephritis, emboli to brain, lung and spleen. Fever may be absent in the elderly and immune suppressed patients.

Strep viridans (50-70%), *Staph aureus* (25%) and enterococci (10%) are the organism responsible in native valve IE and late prosthetic valve endocarditis (PVE). In early PVE staph epidermidis and staph aureous are the most common organism.

HIGH RISK PATIENTS

Previous IE, prosthetic heart valve, mitral valve prolapse with regurgitation or thickened valve leaflets or congenital heart disease.

MODERATE RISK PATIENTS

Rheumatic heart disease, hypertrophic obstructive cardiomyopathy, atrial septal defect (ASD), PDA, VSD and coarctation.

Diagnosis

Three blood cultures 1 hr apart, peaks of temperature not essential as constant bacteremia; if culture negative (14%) then serology for legionella, Q fever and PCR for other pathogens and fungus infections should be done.

- ECHO (transthoracic) if negative and low risk: IE less likely.
- Transesophageal ECHO (TOE) if high risk and transthoracic ECHO negative.

Five variables: Absence of prosthetic valve, IV drug use, positive blood cultures, central venous access or signs of embolic phenomena makes likelihood of IE zero.

Duke Criteria

Major criteria
- Positive blood culture and identification of microorganism from at least two blood culture bottles drawn 12 hrs apart or all three blood culture bottles +. If the patient is ill with high suspicion of IE then take 3 sets of blood cultures >1 hr apart; if not acutely ill then 6 sets of blood cultures within 24–48 hrs.
- Evidence of endocardial involvement, e.g. ECHO showing vegetation on intracardiac valve.
- Clinical evidence of new valvular regurgitation.
- Positive serology in culture negative for Q fever, *Bartonella and Chlamydia psittaci*.

Minor criteria
- Predisposing heart condition or IV drug abuse.
- Fever >38 °C.
- *Vascular phenomena*: Major arterial emboli, septic pulmonary infarct, mycotic aneurysm, intracranial hemorrhage, conjunctival hemorrhage, Jane way lesions, new clubbing, splinter hemorrhages and splenomegaly.
- *Immunological phenomena*: Glomerulonephritis, Osler's nodes, Roth spots, positive rheumatoid factor, high ESR, high CRP >100 mg/L.

- Positive blood culture but not meeting major criteria as defined above.

Infective endocarditis diagnosed 2 major criteria or 1 major + 3 minor criteria or 5 minor.

Treatment

In sick patient antibiotic treatment should be commenced immediately after taking blood cultures.

- If IE due to penicillin sensitive *Strep viridans* or *Streptococcus bovis*
  Benzyl penicillin 7.2–12 g IV/24 hr in 4–6 doses 4–6 wks + gentamycin 3–5 mg/kg (max 240 mg/day) IV/day in 2–3 doses for 2 wks.

  For patients allergic to penicillin vancomycin 30 mg/kg/day in 2 doses for 4 wks + gentamycin as above.

- Infective endocarditis due to *Staphylococcus* on native valve
  Penicillin sensitive (non beta-lactamase producers)
  Benzyl penicillin 12–14 g IV/day in 4–6 doses for 6 wks + gentamycin 3–5 mg/kg/day IV in 2–3 doses for 3–5 days.

- Methicillin sensitive staph (Beta-lactamase producer)
  Flucloxacillin 8–12 g/day IV in 4 doses for 6 wks + Gentamycin for 3–5 days in the same doses as above.

- Infective endocarditis due to methicillin-resistant *Staphylococcus aureus* (MRSA)
  Vancomycin 30 mg/kg/day IV (over 2 hrs) in 2 doses for 6 wks + gentamycin 3–5 days on the same doses.

- Infective endocarditis due to enterococci
  Benzyl penicillin 10–12 g IV/24 hrs in 4–6 doses for 4–6 wks or ampicillin or amoxicillin 12 g IV/24 hrs in 4–6 doses for 4–6 wks + gentamycin for 4–6 wks in the same doses as above.

Selected patients with streptococcal IE may be suitable for once daily ceftriaxone as outpatient treatment.

Surgery is indicated in severe valvular regurgitation, annular or aortic abscess, large mobile vegetation, prosthetic valve endocarditis (PVE), infection resistant to antibiotics and fungal IE.

Surgery should be considered in hemodynamically unstable patients, persistent fever despite appropriate antibiotics, development of fistula or abscess, prosthetic valve IE, highly resistant organisms and large vegetations (>10 mm).

Prophylaxis

- Patients at risk are valvular heart disease with stenosis or regurgitation.
- Valve replacement.
- Previous infective endocarditis.
- Hypertrophic cardiomyopathy and congenital heart disease excluding isolated ventricular septal defect (VSD), fully repaired ventricular septal defect (VSD) and patent ductus arteriosus (PDA).
- Amoxicillin 3 g oral 1 hr pre-procedure or 2 g IV <30 minutes pre-procedure.
- If allergic to penicillin then clindamycin 600 mg oral 1 hr pre-procedure or 300 mg IV <30 minutes pre-procedure or IV clindamycin 150 mg 6 hrs later.

Patients with Previous IE

- Amoxicillin 2 g IV <30 minutes + gentamycin 1.5 mg/kg IV <30 minutes pre-procedure and 1 g IV or orally 6 hrs postprocedure.
- If allergic to penicillin then vancomycin 1 g IV over 2 hrs 1-2 hrs preprocedure + gentamycin as above.

No Prophylaxis

- For dental procedures, upper and lower GI procedures (OGD, sigmoidoscopy or colonoscopy), urological, gynecological, child birth, upper and lower respiratory tract (ENT and bronchoscopy).
- Maintain good oral health.
- Outline the symptoms of infective endocarditis and when to seek medical help.
- Explain the potential risk of body piercing and tattooing.
- Promptly investigate and treat any infection to reduce the risk of subsequently developing infective endocarditis.
- If a person at risk is having antibiotics because they are having GI or GU procedures at a site where there is suspected infection then individual should receive antibiotics that cover infective endocarditis.

Aortic Stenosis

Small volume, slow rising pulse, Jugular venous pressure (JVP) not raised (unless CCF), apex position normal or slightly displaced, forceful sustained heaving, systolic thrill palpable over aortic area, over carotids and some times over apex. There is harsh ejection systolic murmur over aortic area radiating to neck, A2 is soft or absent. BP is usually low with low pulse pressure.

If carotid pulse is normal (not slow rising), apical impulse not displaced, no thrills, ejection systolic murmur is not harsh or loud, audible only in the aortic area, faintly in the neck. A2 is well heard or presence of physiologically normal split S2, and BP is normal or hypertensive, suggests aortic sclerosis or minimal aortic stenosis.

Other causes of short systolic murmur are mitral valve prolapse or trivial mitral regurgitation (MR) in HCM.

Risk factors are hypertension, age, male gender, diabetes, hyperlipidemia and smoking.

Causes of Aortic Stenosis

Rheumatic heart disease (RHD) is common in developing countries and usually associated with mitral lesions.

Congenital bicuspid (unicuspid usually fatal before the age of 1), common in males 50–60 yrs, while tricuspid 70–80 yrs, (calcification at the free margins of the cusps).

Bicuspid aortic valve becomes regurgitant only after antecedent infection (IE).

Degenerative calcification (calcification at the base) in elderly and stenosis is usually mild). The murmur of mitral stenosis should be particularly sought in female patient.

Symptoms

- Onset of symptoms is associated with ominous prognosis (50% mortality in 2 yrs).
- Gradual decrease in exercise tolerance, dyspnea, angina and syncope are main symptoms.
- ECHO for assessment of severity, anatomy of the valves, LV systolic and diastolic function.

Mild	Moderate	Severe
Velocity 2.5–3.0 m/sec	3–4 m/sec	>4 m/sec
Valve area of >1.5 cm^2	1–1.5 cm^2	<1 cm^2
Gradient <25 mm Hg	25–40 mm Hg	>40 mm Hg

Severity: Early peaking murmur (mild), late peaking murmur (severe) and disappearance of 2nd heart sound

(severe). Murmur is muffled in CCF, obesity, chronic obstructive pulmonary disease (COPD) and left ventricular (LV) dysfunctions.
- ACE is safe and can be used cautiously in mild aortic stenosis only.
- The average rate of decrease of valve area is 0.1 cm^2/yr with average increase in aortic velocity is 0.3 m/sec/yr.
- Consider endocarditis prophylaxis in all patients.
- Average survival after onset of symptoms is 2–3 yrs.
- High resolution computed tomography (HRCT) is routinely done before aortic valve surgery to assess coronary artery disease as 50% have significant coronary artery disease.
- All patients are advised about avoiding competitive sports, IE prophylaxis.
- Co-existing hypertension should be very gradually treated, as there is risk of excessive hypotension, as cardiac output cannot increase in response to peripheral vasodilatation.
- Medical therapy directed at symptoms relief is ineffective and hazardous.

Indication for Surgery

- *Symptoms*: Syncope, angina, dyspnea.
- Systolic pressure gradient >50–60 mm Hg or aortic orifice <1 cm^2.
- Patients with mild to moderate aortic stenosis having coronary artery bypass grafting (CABG) surgery.
- Asymptomatic severe stenosis with pressure gradient >60 mm Hg, valve area <1 cm^2 and jet velocity >5 m/sec and operative mortality <1% are for surgery.

In children and young adults, valvotomy rather than valve replacement as operative risk is less.

Sinus rhythm (SR), slow rising pulse (may be bisferien), JVP normal, apex is forceful sustained heaving, palpable systolic thrill over aortic and carotid area, harsh ejection systolic murmur over aortic area radiating to the neck, A2 soft, an early diastolic murmur down the left sternal edge when patient sitting forward in expiration.

This patient has mixed aortic valve disease with predominant aortic stenosis because of slow rising pulse, systolic thrill, forceful heaving apex and A2 is soft.

Large volume collapsing pulse, thrusting apex beat in anterior axillary line 6th intercostal space, wide pulse pressure, absence of thrill, will favor predominant lesion as acute aortic regurgitation due to endocarditis or dissection and treatment is surgery and IV nitroprusside.

Aortic Regurgitation

Large volume pulse is collapsing, JVP not raised but arterial pulses can be seen in the neck. Apex beat is thrusting, in anterior axillary line in 6th intercostal space, early diastolic murmur heard best left sternal edge and aortic area when patient sitting up leaning forward in expiratory phase and wide pulse pressure.

There is often accompanying systolic murmur in aortic area (flow murmur and not AS). If there is mid diastolic murmur at the apex (Austin-Flint murmur, vibration of anterior mitral cusp due to AR) can be distinguished from mitral valve disease by absence of opening snap and loud 1st heart sound.

Ventricular dilatation maintains normal ventricular diastolic pressure in aortic regurgitation (AR) while in AS there is ventricular hypertrophy but no dilatation.

There is rise in diastolic pressure in acute AR and sudden rise in LV diastolic pressure results in pulmonary edema.

Severity of AR can be judged by pulse volume and diastolic pressure which in severe cases is <60 mm Hg.

Causes

- *Chronic leaflet abnormality*: Rheumatic heart disease (RHD), bicuspid valve.
- Dilatation of aortic root
  - Hypertension, Marfan syndrome (tall with long extremities, arachnodactyly, and high arched palate). Syphilitic aortitis (AR pupil, aneurysm of ascending aorta), seronagative arthropathies (ankylosing spondylitis, psoriatic arthropathy, Reiter syndrome) and RA.

Acute: Infective endocarditis and dissection of aorta.
- In acute AR peripheral signs of aortic regurgitation (wide pulse pressure) may be absent, patients are in cardiogenic shock and only to and fro noise is heard on left sternal border.

- Increase in intensity in early diastolic murmur implies increased severity in AR while decrease in intensity in ejection systolic murmur implies fall in cardiac output in AS.
- Asymptomatic initially, till decreased exercise tolerance and CCF indicate LV dysfunction.
- ECHO to assess severity.
- After load reduction therapy with ACE or nifedipine prevents dilatation and delays surgery. Endocarditis prophylaxis is routine.

Indication for Surgery

- Ejection fraction <50%.
- LV end diastolic dimension >75 mm, LV end systolic dimension >55 mm.
- Early LV dysfunction.
- Infective endocarditis (emergency).

Mitral Regurgitation

Causes

Degenerative, ischemic, papillary muscle dysfunction, cardiomyopathy, mitral valve prolapse, IE, rupture of chordae tendinae (acute severe MI), connective tissue disorders (SLE, RA, ankylosing spondylitis), congenital anomalies Marfan syndrome, Ehler's-Danlos syndrome (hyper extensible skin and joints, thin scars) pseudo-xanthoma elasticum (loose skin or chicken skin appearance in antecubital fossa, inguinal region and neck), and rheumatic heart disease (RHD).

Symptoms

- Acute severe MR presents as pulmonary edema while chronic severe MR as gradual onset of breathlessness and any infection or AF leads to acute cardiac failure.
- Usually SR, JVP not raised, apex beat thrusting in the 6th intercostal space in anterior axillary line, systolic thrill, left parasternal heave, 1st sound is soft and loud pan systolic murmur radiating to axilla (it may be quiet in ischemic MR).

- In mitral valve prolapse murmur may commence in mid systole preceded by a click.
- Left parasternal heave suggests pulmonary hypertension.
- Pansystolic murmur of TR can be heard over apex and left sternal edge. In this systolic venous pulsation in the neck, increase in murmur on inspiration and lack of transmission to axilla differentiates it from MR.
- ECHO assesses the severity.
- *Nonischemic mitral regurgitation*: A symptomatic patient with moderate or severe MR should be followed 6–12/12 with ECHO. Vasodilators have no role in slowing ventricular dilatation.
- Aim for surgery before severe symptoms or LV dysfunctions develop.
- Most patients with cardiomyopathy with MR are managed as CCF and a few with severe MR will benefit from repair.

Indication for Surgery

- Moderately breathless patient with normal house hold activity despite medical treatment.
- Left ventricular systolic dimensions >45 mm.
- Left ventricular progressive dysfunction EF declining <60%.
- Repair reconstruction (annuloplasty) in young patients and valve replacement in IE and rupture chordae tendinae.
- No LV dysfunction and no AF or PH → yearly review.
- Surgery contraindicated if EF <30%.

Mixed Mitral Valve Disease

- Malar flush, AF, JVP not raised, apex beat tapping and not displaced, left parasternal heave, loud 1st heart sound, a pan systolic murmur radiating to axilla, loud P2, an opening snap and mid diastolic murmur localized to apex.
- This patient has mixed mitral valve disease with predominant mitral stenosis because of tapping cardiac impulse, loud 1st sound and not displaced cardiac apex.

- However, if cardiac impulse was thrusting, displaced and 1st heard sound was soft then it will be mixed mitral valve disease with mitral incompetence as predominant lesion.
- Innocent systolic murmurs (soft <2/6, upper sternal edge, normal splitting of 2nd sound and normal pulses).

Mitral Stenosis

Rheumatic heart disease (RHD) Rheumatic fever group A B hemolytic streptococci.

Clinical Features

- Short of breath, fatigue, AF, RHF (right sided heart failure), systemic thromboembolism.
- Malar flush, pulse AF or SR low volume, JVP not raised, no ankle or sacral edema.
- Apex is tapping (palpable 1st heart sound) and left parasternal heave.
- 1st heart sound loud (pliable valve), P2 loud (if pulmonary pressure raised), opening snap (OS) after S2 followed by rumbling mid diastolic murmur with presystolic accentuation (if SR) localized to the apex when patient in left lateral position.
- Longer the murmur tighter is the stenosis.
- Systolic murmur is with accompanying MR or TR.
- In tight mitral stenosis opening snap soon after 2nd sound (mean left atrial pressure >20 mm Hg), if longer after 2nd sound (L atrial pressure <15 mm Hg).
- OS after S2 absent if mitral valve calcified (1st heart sound soft), tighter the stenosis the closer the OS to S2

Echocardiography (ECHO)

- Mitral valve area severe (<1 cm^2), moderate (1–1.5 cm^2) and mild 1.5–2.2 cm^2).
- Advise antibiotic prophylaxis.
- Anticoagulation if atrial fibrillation (AF) or SR if left atrial size >5 cm or history of thromboembolism.
- Beta blockers or rate limiting and calcium antagonists for AF rate control.
- Diuretics for RHF.

Surgery Indicated

- If significant symptoms limiting normal activity.
- Pulmonary edema without precipitating causes.
- Recurrent emboli.
- Hemoptysis
- Atrial fibrillation (AF) causing clinical deterioration and not responding to medical treatment.

Criteria for balloon valvuloplasty: Mobile valve (1st sound, opening snap, absence of calcium on X-ray screening) and absence of MR.

Grades of Intensity of Murmurs

- Heard by an expert in optimum conditions.
- Heard by a non-expert in optimum conditions.
- Easily heard, no thrill
- Loud murmur with a thrill
- Very loud, often heard over a wide area with a thrill
- Extremely loud, heard without stethoscope.

PROSTHETIC MITRAL AND AORTIC VALVES

Bileaflet mechanical valves are used in young 50–70 yrs (longevity 20–30 yrs but require anticoagulation INR 3–4) while biological xenograft valve (from porcine aortic valve or bovine pericardium) are used in elderly >75 (less durable 5–15 yrs, no anticoagulants). In patients <50 either auto graft or homograft's are used as they are more durable than xenografts and avoids anticoagulation.

Contraindications to anticoagulation (avoid mechanical valve): Liver failure, previous hemorrhagic stroke, GI bleed or other bleeding diathesis, alcoholisms or recurrent falls, women considering pregnancy and poor compliance.

Implant of choice for mitral valve is mechanical valve. In this patient has midline sternotomy scar, click with the 1st heart sound (closure of mitral prosthesis), opening click in diastole with a mid-diastolic murmur (flow murmur) or pan systolic murmur (suggest leakage from mitral prosthesis).

In aortic prosthesis, midline sternotomy scar, 1st heart sound is normal (unless mitral stenosis), ejection click (opening of prosthesis) with ejection systolic murmur and click at the 2nd heart sound (closure of prosthesis). If there is early diastolic murmur with collapsing pulse and wide pulse pressure suggests leakage of the valve.

Consider infective endocarditis when leakage develops.

Thromboembolic disease (anticoagulants and antiplatelet drugs reduce but do not abolish these complications).

DEXTROCARDIA

- Apex beat is not palpable on the left side, and may have difficulty in listening the heart sounds. But as one moves the stethoscope to the right side the heart sounds get louder and apex beat is palpable in the 5th intercostal space in the mid clavicular line on the right side.
- ECG show P-wave and QRS complex negative in lead 1 and upright in aVR and R-wave progressively become smaller as one moves from V1 to V6.
- Patient has dextrocardia.
- Pulse and JVP are normal and usually has sign of bronchiectasis in the chest.
- If situs inversus is present, patient is usually otherwise normal. Liver is palpable on the left side. Dextrocardia without situs inversus is usually associated with cardiac malformation.
- *Kartagener's syndrome*: Dextrocardia, bronchiectasis, situs inversus, infertility, dysplasia of frontal sinuses, sinusitis, and otitis media. These patients have ciliary immobility.

Dilated Cardiomyopathy

Causes

- Post viral infections, alcohol, myocarditis, Fe overload, uremia, pheochromocytoma, deficiency states (Beriberi, selenium deficiency), sarcoid, dermatomyositis and idiopathic.
- Mostly middle aged men, progressive right and left heart failure and dilation of annulus of mitral and tricuspid with MR and TR and reduced ejection fraction <40%.
- Prognosis poor and 70% dying within 10 yrs of diagnosis.

Hypertrophic Cardiomyopathy

- There is myocardium hypertrophy, asymmetrical septal hypertrophy, and dynamic obstruction of left ventricular cavity and systolic anterior movement of the anterior leaflet of the mitral valve.
- This results in mid-late sub aortic obstruction.
- It is caused by autosomal dominant gene (1/500–1/1000) with variable penetrance and a family history is common. Hypertrophic cardiomyopathy (HCM) is the most common cause of sudden cardiac death in young adults.

Clinical

- Syncope with exertion, dyspnea due to impaired filling of left ventricle, raised left atrial pressure and pulmonary veins pressure.
- Angina due to inadequate perfusion of the hypertrophied myocardium, cardiac arrhythmia and sudden death.

Signs

Sharp carotid pulse (compared to AS slow rising pulse), forceful apex beat (may be double), 4th heart sound, systolic murmur caused by mitral regurgitation or out flow obstruction and loudness of the murmur increases with Valsalva maneuver (which increases the out flow obstruction).

Investigations

- *ECG*: LVH, deep Q-waves and conduction defects. 24 hrs holter monitoring required.
- *ECHO*: Hypertrophied non dilated left ventricle.

Risk factors and for prophylactic cardiac defibrillator:
- Family history of sudden death if 2 or more than prophylactic cardioverter defibrillator fitted, if one than risk explained.
- Extreme thickness of left ventricular wall >30 mm in young patients.
- Unexplained syncope (not neurotriggered) in young patients.
- Nonsustained VT <30, even 3–4 beats, if frequent.

- If hypotensive response to exercise or on standing then for prophylactic cardioverter defibs.

Treatment

Heart Failure

- Beta blockers and small doses of diuretics. ACE should be avoided as they increase outflow obstruction by decreasing after load. Verapamil can be used if angina.
- Anti-arrhythmic drugs like amiodarone long-term improve the prognosis.
- Beta blockers for angina.
- Dual chamber pacing and implantable cardiac defibrillator (ICD).
- Patients with outflow obstruction gradient >50 mm Hg and severe symptoms (NY 3 or 4), should be considered for surgical myomectomy and therapeutic septal MI.
- *AF*: Amiodarone or beta blockers or verapamil.
- Prophylaxis for infective endocarditis if outflow obstruction at rest.
- Clinical screening of 1st degree relatives every 2 yrs in young and 5 yrs in adults.

PULMONARY EMBOLISM, DEEP VEIN THROMBOSIS

Pulmonary Embolism in Pregnancy

Risk Factors

- Hyperemesis, surgery for ectopic, pre-eclampsia, nephrotic syndrome, multiparity, obesity.
- Risk of PE higher in pregnancy (X5) and postpartum period (X15).
- D-dimer not helpful,
- Ultrasound lower limbs (L) as isolated iliac vein thrombosis is more common in pregnancy.
- Chest X-ray as standard (lead apron) if normal then VQ (ventilation/perfusion) scan half dose (perfusion only), if abnormal and high suspicion then CTPA.
- Echocardiography for right ventricular dysfunction.
- CTPA delivers lower radiation dose to fetus than VQ scan (lead apron) but gives increased radiation to the breast. So instead of CTPA half dose VQ scan or VQ SPECT scan or MRI should be considered in pregnancy.

- Treat with low molecular weight heparin (LMWH) and use unfractionated heparin (UFH) during peri-delivery. Avoid warfarin (teratogenic) and for thrombolysis if hemodynamic unstable BP <90 mm Hg, monitor platelets and anti-factor Xa every month.

Radiation dose	Mother (msv)	Life time risk of cancer	Fetal (mGy)	Cancer risk to age 15
VQ	0.7	1/24000	0.15	1/220,000
CTPA	5.8	1/2900	0.02	1/6.5 millions

- If PE on pill then thromboprophylaxis when pregnant.
- Pregnant patient with pneumonia or pyelonephritis require thrombo prophylaxis.
- If initial event pregnancy related needs prophylaxis in next pregnancy.
- 50% silent PE in DVT and 80% PE have DVT.
  In nonpregnant patient is:

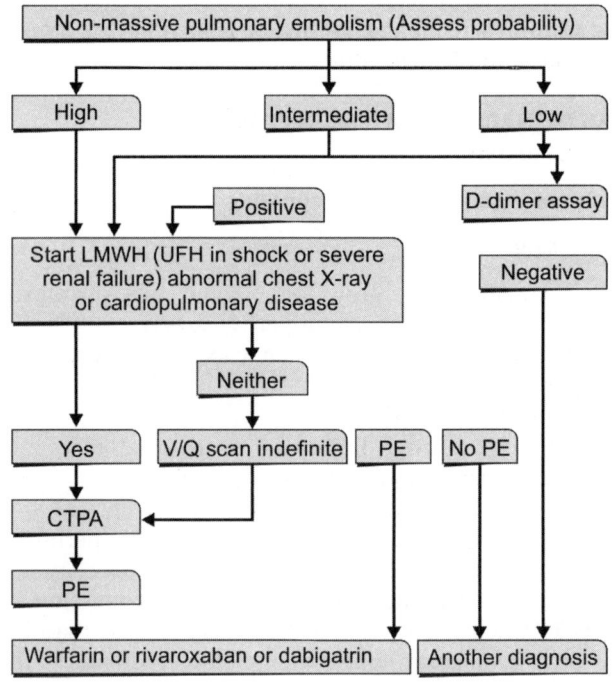

- Consider PE in any patient with acute breathlessness (respiratory rate >20) with hypoxia (but arterial O_2 saturation may be normal).
- Pulmonary embolism should be suspected if unexplained tachycardia, normal chest X-ray, worsening of chronic breathlessness (COPD, heart failure) or syncope or leg pain, warm and swelling of the leg >3 cm than other side or prominent collateral superficial veins are present.
- Pulmonary embolism is unlikely if RR <20 and no hypoxia and HR <100.

Symptoms

Pleuritic chest pain, dyspnea, cough or hemoptysis and syncope.

Signs

- Tachypnea, crackles, tachycardia, 4th heart sound and accentuated P2, pleural rub and hypoxia.
- One or more risk factors for DVT are present in 80–90% of patients with PE.

Risk Factors

Risk increases with age >40 yrs. Annual incidence <40 yrs—1/10,000; 60–69 yrs—1/1000 and >80 yrs—1/100.

Major

- Deep vein thrombosis (DVT) or pulmonary embolism (PE) in the past, major abdominal, pelvic, hip or knee surgery, malignant disease (adenocarcinomas of hepatobiliary, ovary, lung, colon, Hodgkin's and non-Hodgkin's, lymphomas), immobility, pregnancy or puerperium, fracture, polycythemia and thrombocytosis.
- Thrombophilia screening considered if strong family history of unprovoked VTE in a young patient, warfarin induced necrosis, cerebral venous thrombosis, splanchnic vessel thrombosis, thrombosis at unusual site, recurrent VTE and recurrent miscarriage.
- Test for deficiency of antithrombin 3, protein C or S, presence of factor 5 Leiden, raised homocysteine, lupus anticoagulant and anticardiolipin antibody.

- Testing for thrombophilia should be considered in <50 yrs and those with a strong family history.

Minor

- Oral contraceptive, HRT, antiphospholipid syndrome, nephrotic syndrome, Behçet syndrome, obesity, hyperhomocysteinemia, travel (>5–6 hrs) and COPD/CVS/CNS disease.
- Look for DVT (swelling of calf, warm, dilated superficial veins, tender, positive Homan's sign (pain in the calf muscle on sudden flexion at the ankle when knee is flexed at 90 degree).
- Look for signs of RV strain (raised JVP, parasternal heave, loud P2, S3).

Investigations

- ECG and chest X-ray, FBC, U and E, LFT, Tn (troponin), D-dimer and ABG.
- ECG may show sinus tachycardia, non-specific ST/T wave changes.
- In ECG look for T-wave inversion in V1/V2. RBBB, right axis deviation (RAD), S1Q3T3 are uncommon and may be seen with major pulmonary embolism.
- Chest X-ray is often normal or may show non-specific abnormalities such as raised hemidiaphragm, pleural effusions, infiltrates, atelectasis and wedge infarct.
- If clinical suspicion is high, start therapeutic LMWH pending the results of investigation.
- D-dimers (degradation product of cross-linked fibrin) are detectable at levels >500 ng/mL of fibrinogen equivalent units.
- A negative D-dimer with low clinical probability (e.g. alternative diagnosis with no risk factors) may be useful exclusion test, but with high or intermediate probability objective testing is needed such as VQ scan or CTPA.
- D-dimer also may be useful in non-diagnostic lung scans.
- VQ scanning is used for small or intermediate PE. VQ is often done when CTPA is contraindicated because of renal failure).
- If high probability of PE then continue heparin and consider CTPA (ideally within 24 hrs and preferably within 4 days) and ECHO looking for dilated RV, RV

hypokinesia, tricuspid regurgitation and rarely visible free clot.
- CTPA is preferred if high probability of PE in the presence of abnormal chest X-ray or chronic cardiac or lung disease or previous PE. CTPA use should be minimized in females under 40 yrs because of associated risk of breast cancer.
- Normal chest X-ray and normal VQ scan excludes PE.
- Normal D-dimer excludes thrombosis in low or medium risk patients, although raised value is not specific for this.

When not to do D-Dimer

- Pregnancy, cancer, sepsis, liver disease, renal disease, DIC, when diagnosis other than PE is highly likely, anticoagulated, and postsurgical inpatient.
- Negative predictive value is unpredictable if symptoms present for more than 2 wks.
- Left leg ultrasound is 1st line investigation in pregnancy.

Wells Scoring System for PE

- Clinical signs/symptoms of DVT (minimum of leg swelling and pain with palpation of deep veins of the leg). 3
- No alternate diagnosis likely or more likely than PE 3
- Heart rate >100/min 1.5
- Immobilization or surgery in last 4 wks 1.5
- Previous history of DVT or PE 1.5
- Hemoptasis 1
- Cancer actively treated within last 6 months 1

Risk: Low 0–1, moderate 2–6, and high >6.

Management

- If SaO_2 <90% then give high concentration O_2 (60%).
- Intravenous access and heparinize (LMWH does not need monitoring). Raised Tn or BNP is poor prognosis.
- Monitor ECG, SaO_2 and BP.

Massive PE

- Systolic BP <90 mm Hg, hypoxia refractory to 60% O_2, raised JVP, right ventricular gallop. AF or atrial flutter on ECG should be treated with IV digoxin 0.5–1 mg over 2 hrs.

- Start infusion of colloid gelofusine 10 mL/kg until systolic BP >90 mm Hg.
- Get cardiology advice and immediate ECHO showing dilated right ventricle and raised PA pressure.
- Heparin 10,000 units IV.
- If after gelofusin BP <90 mm Hg, start dobutamine 10 µg/kg/min increase it as needed to 40 µg/kg/min until systolic BP >90 mm Hg.
- If systolic BP still remains <90 mm Hg, dopamine or noradrenaline should be used.
- If the BP <90 mm Hg at 30–60 min and there is clinically definite PE then thrombolysis should be considered. Most deaths from major PE occur within 1 hr.
- Thrombolysis should not be delayed beyond 30–60 minutes.
- If cardiac arrest due to PE—Resuscitate (CPR), 50 mg IV alteplase and reassess in 30 minutes.
- If deteriorating due to PE—contact consultant, 50 mg IV alteplase and urgent ECHO or CTPA.
- If stable heparin 10,000 units IV.

Reversal of Anticoagulation

- *Heparin (unfractioned)*: Stop heparin, give protamine by slow IV injection (1 mg neutralizes 100 units). Give less dose if longer time has elapsed (heparin is rapidly excreted) and max dose of protamine is 50 mg. Excess protamine is anticoagulant. FFP is not helpful, as it has no heparin neutralizing activity.
- LMWH Stop heparin, IV protamine as above (less neutralizing effect on LMWH than heparin). FFP is not helpful as above.
- Warfarin—(Immediate reversal):
    - Stop warfarin, vitamin K 1 mg IV, FFP 2–4 units IV;
    - *Delayed reversal*: If INR <8, stop warfarin, recheck in 3 days. If INR >8, stop warfarin, give vitamin K 5–10 mg PO and recheck in 24 hrs.

Pulmonary embolism with hypotension or cardiogenic shock should be considered for thrombolysis with Alteplase (T-PA). T-PA is most commonly used as in MI

- *Alteplase*: Regime is 10 mg bolus over 1–2 minutes then 90 mg by IV infusion over 2 hrs.
- Warfarin should be started during heparin therapy, overlapping 3–4 days.

- Heparin can be stopped after 5 days provided INR is >2.0.
- Warfarin or rivaroxaban or dabigatran (Rivaroxaban or dabigatran do not require monitoring) is usually given 3 months for 1st PE (target INR 2–3 with warfarin use).
- In unprovoked PE 10% recurrence in 1 year and 30% at 5 yrs. Pulmonary hypertension 10% and post-thrombotic syndrome 30–50% after DVT.
- There is lower risk of recurrence if normal D-dimer level a month after stopping the anticoagulant therapy.
- *1st proximal DVT*: Full length TEDS for 2 yrs + oral anticoagulant for 6/12.
- Indefinite treatment may be indicated for patient with massive PE or 2nd unprovoked PE/DVT and presence of active cancer.

Placement of Vena Caval Filter

- Contraindication to anticoagulation.
- Major bleeding complication during anticoagulation.
- Recurrent embolism while on adequate anticoagulant therapy.

Filters are effective in preventing pulmonary embolism but they increase the incidence of DVT and do not prolong survival. Usually filters are retrieved after one year.

Upper Limb DVT

- Catheter associated (repetitive micro trauma to subclavian vein), cancer associated 38%, usually in women.
- Catheter removal not usually recommended unless there is infection associated with it or malfunctions of the catheter or no longer required.
- Strenuous exercise of upper arms (painting, car repair, playing baseball, badminton, weight lifting, rowing) in men.

Complication	Upper limb DVT	Lower limb DVT
PE	6%	15–32%
Post-thrombotic syndrome	5%	56%

- Presents with swelling, discoloration, edema and visible venous collaterals of the arm.

Superior Vena Cava Syndrome

- Facial swelling, headache, nausea and dyspnea.
- Diagnosed by ultrasonography when undeterminant then CTA or MRA.

Treatment

- Low-molecular-weight heparin (LMWH) for 6 months if cancer associated otherwise.
  LMWH followed by warfarin for 3–6 months.
- Unfractionated heparin (UFH) if severe renal failure.
- Thrombolysis if extensive swelling and functional impairment of the arm and symptoms duration <10 days.
- Mechanical catheter interventions (aspiration, fragmentation, thrombectomy, balloon angioplasty) only if there are severe symptoms after adequate anticoagulation.
- SVC filter if contraindication to warfarin or progression of thrombus or PE in spite of adequate anticoagulation.

Pulmonary Hypertension

Pulmonary artery pressure >25 mm Hg or above at rest and 30 mm Hg or above on exercise.

Causes

- *Idiopathic pulmonary hypertension*: Slowly progressive disease, 1–2 cases/million/year, three times common in females and without targeted therapy median survival 2–3 years.

  Incidence in associated conditions is systemic sclerosis (10–20%), sickle cell disease (20%), HIV infection (0.5–2%), portal hypertension (1–2%), drugs and toxins.
- Pulmonary chronic thromboembolic disease (CTEP).
- Chronic interstitial lung disease, COPD
- Congenital heart disease ASD, VSD, PDA.
- LVF, mitral valve disease, left atrial tumor or thrombus.

Signs and Symptoms

- Breathlessness, chest pain and syncope on exertion.

- Signs of right heart failure (RHF), tachycardia, raised JVP, right ventricular heave, loud P2 with systolic murmur, hepatomegaly with abdominal distension, ascites, ankle swelling and general fatigue.

Investigations

- FBC, U and E, thrombophilia screen and autoimmune screen and arterial blood gases (ABG).
- HIV testing if indicated.
- ECG.
- ECHO—systolic pulmonary artery pressure (sPAP) <30 + RA and DLCO >50%—Low probability, if SOB then further investigation.
- ECHO sPAP 30–40 + RA—intermediate probability—if DLCO >50% and SOB or DLCO <50% then refer specialist center.
- ECHO sPAP >40 + RA—high probability—refer.
- Chest X-ray
- VQ scan or CTPA.
- High resolution CT and MRI angiography if indicated.
- Lung function tests.
- Patients at risk of PH can be identified after the diagnosis of massive or submassive PE by ECHO sPAP >50 mm Hg on admission or ECHO sPAP >40 mm Hg at 6 wks, on-going dyspnea following PE or new onset of dyspnea with previous history of DVT or PE.

Treatment

Family members of idiopathic pulmonary hypertension (IPH) are at risk of developing IPH with autosomal dominant inheritance and 10–20% penetrance can be identified by genetic screening or exercise testing but should be approached sensitively.

Disease locus PPH1 has been identified on long arm of chromosome 2.

- Supportive treatment is warfarin, diuretics, digoxin and O_2 therapy.
- IV Iloprost given via Hickman line as continuous infusion or nebulizer 6–9 times/day because of short half-life. With continuous infusion life threatening infection is the side effect.
- Calcium channel blockers are advocated but their efficacy is limited to a small minority of patients with

a vasodilator response (fall in PAP of 20% after NO or epoprostinol).
- Endothelan receptor antagonist bosentan improves the symptoms and physiological markers of the disease.
- Sildenafil is going phase 3 study and results eagerly awaited.

Surgery

- Pulmonary endartertectomy in thromboembolic PH in patients with PAP >50 mm Hg.
- Heart-lung or lung transplantation for patients not responding to medical therapy.
- Atrial septostomy is effective way off loading right ventricle.

General Surgery and Cardiac Patient

Clinical Predictors of Increased Perioperative Risk (MI, CCF, Death)

Major

Unstable ACS (acute or recent MI), decompensated CCF, significant arrhythmia (A-V block, VT, SVT with uncontrolled HR), severe valvular disease.

Intermediate

Mild angina, previous MI by history or Q-waves, compensated CCF, IDDM, and renal failure.

Minor

Advanced age, ECG (LVH, LBBB), AF, history of stroke and uncontrolled hypertension.

Surgery Specific Risk

Major (>5%): Emergency operation in the elderly, aortic and other major vascular surgery, peripheral vascular surgery, anticipated prolonged vascular procedure.

Intermediate (<5%): Carotid endarterectomy, head and neck surgery, intraperitoneal and intrathoracic surgery, orthopedic and prostate surgery.

Low (<1%): Endoscopic procedure, superficial procedure, cataract surgery and breast surgery.
- Beta blockers (Bisprolol oral/IV 5 mg) reduce perioperative ischemia, ideally started 1 wk before to achieve HR 50-60 and continued for 1 wk. CABG before elective vascular surgery does not alter outcome.
- Exclude severe aortic stenosis (AS), left ventricular ejection fraction (LVEF) <20%.
- In diastolic heart failures with dilated left atrium avoid vasodilators.

7

Gastrointestinal

ABDOMINAL PAIN

Consider medical mimics of surgical abdomen (basal pneumonia, myocardial infarction (MI), diabetic ketoacidosis and porphyria).

- Always look at the hernia orifices.
- Constant severe generalized pain exacerbated with slightest movement—peritonitis.
- Abdominal pain and patient writhes around—visceral pain, colicky pain.
- Pain early hours of the morning or nightly bouts of pain, relief with food—DU.
- *Pain worse with food*: Esophagitis, gastritis, obstruction.
- *Epigastric pain*: Esophagus, duodenal ulcer, Pancreatitis (discomfort in the back).
- Para umbilical—small bowel.
- Para umbilical bruising (Cullen' sign) and bruising in the flank (Grey Turner's sign) of pancreatitis.
- Colonic—local over the area.
- Right upper quadrant (RUQ)—biliary.
- Diffuse abdominal pain 2 minutes to 1 hr after meal in arteriopath—abdominal angina.
- Amylase raised in DU, cholecystitis but X5 in pancreatitis.
- Investigations.
- Full blood count (FBC), U and E, LFT, amylase, CRP, blood glucose, erect and supine abdominal X-ray, CT abdomen if suspicion of peritonitis and abdominal US if biliary disease suspected.
- *Irritable bowel syndrome*: Treated with soluble fiber (Ispaghula), antispasmodics (Hyoscine) and peppermint oil.

Acute Upper Gastrointestinal Hemorrhage

Most common cause peptic ulcer, *Helicobacter pylori*, NSAID and liver disease.

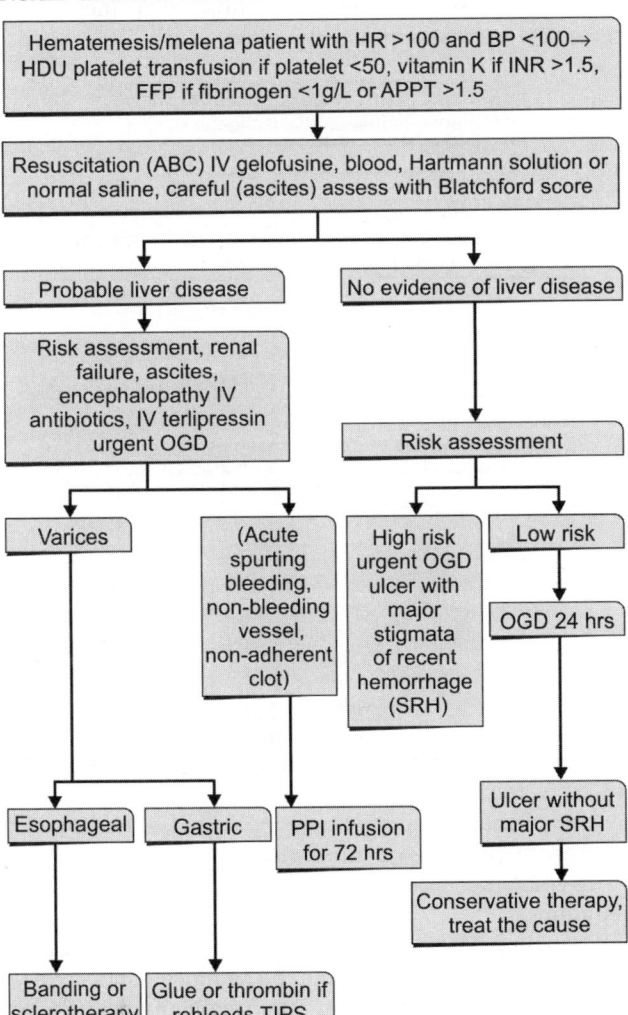

Terlipressin 72 hrs infusion (beware coronary artery spasm, abdominal colic, limb ischemia).

Blatchford score (Hb >12.9 gm, BP >109 mm Hg, pulse <100/min, urea <6.5 mmol/L. No melena or syncope, liver disease or heart failure, no admission required and treated as outpatient.

Any patient with iron deficiency anemia (ferritin <50) should have OGD (men Hb <11 and women Hb <10 g/L), beware thalassemia.

Gastrointestinal bleed and antiplatelet therapy in recent MI or stent or prosthetic valve:

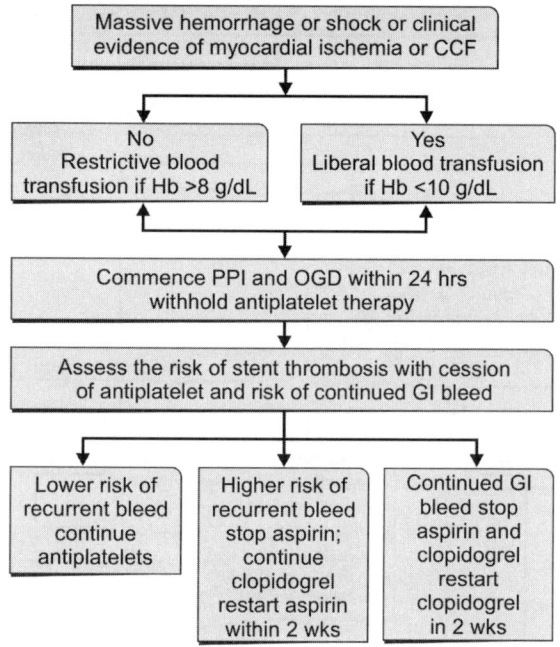

Risk of stent thrombosis—4% off warfarin, 2.2% on aspirin, 1% on warfarin.

PPI decrease the effect of clopidogrel. Effect smaller with esomeprazole or pantoprazole.

Hematemesis or melena (suggests source proximal to jejunum).

Bleeding PR, do not assume colonic unless bright red and no hemodynamic compromise, shock, syncope, dizziness, weakness, unexplained hypotension (BP <100 mm Hg, HR >100) or hepatic encephalopathy.

Note any previous history of GI bleed, DU or GU, NSAID, aspirin and other antiplatelet agents use, warfarin, usual and recent alcohol intake, evidence of liver disease (splenomegaly, spider naevi, abdominal veins, ascites) and whether vomiting preceded hematemesis (suggestive of Mallory-Weiss tear).

Ten percent of PR bleeds from upper GIT, 10% of melena from lower GIT with variable loss of blood.

Etiology

- DU or GU (secondary to *H. pylori* or NSAID) 50%.
- Esophageal varices (secondary to chronic liver disease) 5-10%.
- Esophagitis (secondary to acid reflux or drugs) 10%.
- Mallory-Weiss tear 5% and vascular malformation 5%.

Resuscitation

Class

- 0.75 L   10–15% loss   No clinical signs
- 1.5 L   15–30% loss   Postural hypotension, vasoconstriction, urine output <20–30 mL/hr.
- 2 L   30–40%   Hypotension, HR >120, tachypnea RR >20, confused, urine <20 mL/hr.
- 3 L   >40%   Marked hypotension, tachycardia, tachypnea, comatose, no urine output.

Risk of Rebleeding and Mortality (Rockall Score)

Risk of rebleeding is greatest in 1st 48 hours and can be predicted by age, severity of shock (systolic BP <100 and HR>100) and comorbidity.

Score	0	1	2	3
Age	<60 years	60–79 years	>80 years	
Shock	SBP >100 mm Hg	SBP >100 + tachy	SBP <100 mm Hg	
Pulse	Pulse <100/min	Pulse >100		
Comorbidity	None		CCF, IHD, diabetes, CVA	Renal and Liver failure
Total score	0	2	4	6
Mortality	0.2%	5%	24%	49%

Consider no admission or early discharge if pre-endoscopy Rockall score 0, age <60, no hemodynamic compromise and no significant comorbidity.

Management

- O_2, high concentration at least 60% in a shocked patient.
- IV access (if peripheral veins are not accessible even in antecubital fossa in a shutdown patient then consider inserting femoral venous (vein medial to artery) catheter and do not attempt subclavian or internal jugular). IV fluids 0.9% saline or colloid, avoid saline in liver disease.
- Blood for cross match, FBC, U and E, LFT, PT/clotting.
- ECG if age >40.
- Estimate the blood loss.
  Major bleed >1500 mL (pulse >120, tachypnea RR >20, systolic BP <120 mm Hg, cool and cold extremities, agitation, confusion, reduced conscious level).
  Minor bleed <750 mL (pulse <100, systolic BP >120 mm Hg, normal RR, normal profusion of extremities and normal mental state.
- Give IV fluids 0.9% Hartmann solution or gelofusin 10–20 mL/kg (500–1000 mL). If major bleed or signs of intravascular volume depletion (postural hypotension sitting versus lying), give 1 L fluids (colloid or 0.9% saline as fast as possible and repeat examination and if still has signs of intravascular depletion, give further 500 mL as fast as possible. Use blood instead of colloid as soon as possible.
- Inform gastroenterologist.
- Use O negative blood if patients BP is <100 mm Hg and 1 L colloid has been given and cross matched blood is not available.
- A urinary catheter should be inserted in major bleeds to measure exact urinary output.
- Nasogastric intubation is not necessary.
- Use blood warmer if large volumes are to be given.
- Coagulopathy should be corrected. If prothrombin time (PT) is >1.5 × control then give vitamin K 1 mg IV (not IM) and 2 units of fresh frozen plasma. If platelet count is <50,000 give platelet concentrate.

- Early endoscopy (within 24 hrs) should be performed after resuscitation for all major bleeds and suspected varices.

Endoscopy provides definitive diagnosis and opportunity for treatment.

Adrenaline injection and heater probe are effective in 85–90% of patients with bleeding DU or GU (*H. pylori* checked and successfully eradicated lowers the risk of long-term recurrence). Patients who continue to bleed need 2nd attempt at endoscopic treatment before surgery.

Risk of Rebleeding after Endoscopy

- Spurting artery (80–90%), oozing (50–70%), Non bleeding visible vessel (50–60%), adherent
- Clot (25–35%), black spot in ulcer base (0–8%), clean ulcer base (0–12%).
- Consider IV pantoprazole or omeprazole 80 mg stat slowly, then 8 mg/hr infusion for 3 days in bleeding peptic ulcers or oral omeprazole 40 mg 12 hrly for 3 days.
- *In vitro* studies platelet aggregation and blood coagulation are impaired when the gastric pH is below 6.8. Low pH activates pepsin which lyses the clot and inactivates platelets.
- Therefore hemostasis may improve by suppressing acid secretion. So PPI should be used when there is increased risk of rebleeding (adherent clot, visible vessel) or delayed endoscopy in major bleed.
- Tranexamic acid use further reduces mortality (30–40%). Dose 3–6 gm/daily IV 2–3 days than orally 3–5 days.

High-risk Patient for Emergency Endoscopy (next 4 hrs)

- Hypotensive (systolic BP <100) after initial resuscitation (500–1000 mL of 0.9% saline or gelofusine) or failure to stabilise after 4 units of blood.
  Hb <100 g/L, high rockall score >4.
- Vericeal bleeds likely (known cirrhosis, jaundice, splenomegaly, ascites, low platelets, high MCV, raised PT, low albumin, urea and Na.
- Obvious signs of chronic liver disease or deranged clotting.

- Continuing hematemesis, melena or rebleed.
- Next day endoscopy.
- No history of collapse, Hb >100 g/L.
- Rockall score <4.

Endoscopy Risk Score

Mallory-Weiss tear, or no lesion and no stigmata of recent hemorrhage	0
Clot, spot and free blood	2
Suspected upper GI malignancy	2
All other diagnosis	1

Postendoscopic Management

- If postendoscopy risks score 0–2 discharge home
- If score > or = 3—then observe for rebleed.
- Further hematemesis or melena with fall in Hb 2.0 g/L over 24 hrs or hypotension/tachycardia, rescope if <60, else surgery.
- If peptic ulcer injected confirmed then omeprazole 80 mg IV stat and 8 mg/hr IV for 3 days or oral lansoprazole 60 mg bid for 3 days then 60 mg/day for 2/52 then 30 mg/day.
- Re-bleeding risk reduced from 22.5 to 6.7%.
- Consider surgery if rebleeding or persistent hemodynamic instability, transfusion required 8 units of colloids/blood (4 units if >60).

Negative Endoscopy, Continued Bleeding (OGIB) Occult Gastrointestinal Bleed

- Consider repeat endoscopy, colonoscopy.
- CT angiography, angiography, capsule endoscopy and balloon enteroscopy.
- 5% of all GI bleeds are occult (OGIB). Midgut investigations like capsule endoscopy should be considered if transfusion dependent.

HEYDE'S SYNDROME

Acquired Von Willebrand disease in aortic stenosis and GI bleeding and bleeding will not stop till aortic stenosis is corrected by valve replacement. Diagnosed by raised Von Willebrand multimers in the blood and AS by ECHO.

Eosinophilic Esophagitis

Young patient, atypical dysphagia, history of atopy, PPI resistant reflux.

Treatment

- Six elimination diet (soya, cow milk protein, wheat, egg, sea food and peanut).
- Elemental diet, steroids (fluticasone inhaler).
- Systemic steroids/azathioprine.
- Endoscopic dilatation.

Variceal Bleeding

- Known cirrhosis, portal vein thrombosis or portal hypertension, jaundice, splenomegaly, ascites and stigmata of chronic liver disease.
- Mortality from variceal bleeding is 25-30% with 1st bleed, therefore all cirrhotic patients should have screening endoscopy.
- Large bore peripheral IV access.
- *Bloods*: FBC/clotting screen × match 6 units, fibrinogen. U and E, LFT, glucose, amylase and bicarbonate. Blood and urine culture, chest X-ray.
- Urgent endoscopy is required to define the source of bleeding.
- Terlipressin given prior to endoscopy if variceal bleed suspected, 2 mg stat over 3-5 minutes and then 1-2 mg 4-6 hrly for 72 hrs or till bleeding stops but not in patients with IHD/ischemia.
- ECG prior to injection.
- Intravenous octreotide/somatostatin are alternative for those where terlipressin is contraindicated.

Antibiotics tazocin IV or (Cefotaxime 1 g BD + metronidazole 500 mg TDS) before endoscopy has proven benefit even in the absence of clear sepsis as bacterial infection produces endothelin causing contraction of stellate cells which increases intrahepatic portal pressure, variceal pressure and variceal bleeding.

- Emergency therapeutic (sclerotherapy or banding of varices) endoscopy is required if major bleed (pulse >100, systolic BP <100 mm Hg and Hb <100 g/L) or

likely variceal (stigmata of liver disease, abnormal LFT and clotting).
- Elective endoscopy (pulse <100, systolic BP >100 mm Hg and Hb >100 gm/L.
- Resuscitate and correct clotting abnormality, avoid saline and use colloids or blood. Platelet transfusion if baseline count <50,000. Two units of FFP every 4 units of blood if PT >20 secs. Vitamin K 10 mg IV three times. Cryoprecipitate if fibrinogen <0.2 g/L. After sending blood culture, tazocin 4.5 gm IV or cefotaxime 1 gm IV bid + metronidazole 500 mg tid even in absence of infection.
- Give terlipressin as a bridge to endoscopy (causes less myocardial ischemia than vasopressin, more effective than octreotide) 2 mg IV stat followed by 1–2 mg 4–6 hrly for 72 hrs or until bleeding is controlled. ECG prior to treatment. It reduces in hospital mortality by 28%. However, as it is associated with cardiac complication it is usually given with nitrates. Somatostatin and octreotide are also effective at inducing hemostasis and have fewer side effects but have never been shown to have any effect on survival.
- Infection is a common complication of bleeding (up to 66%) and may contribute to poor prognosis. Prophylactic antibiotics, such as ciprofloxacin or cefotaxime for one week increases survival by 9.1%.
- Omeprazole 40 mg IV or oral daily to prevent stress ulcers.
- Lactulose 30 mL 3 hrly to prevent encephalopathy.
Endoscopic variceal ligation now seems superior to sclerotherapy with ethanolamine or cyanoacrylate or human thrombin (equal efficacy but fewer complications). Perform within 6 hrs but after resuscitation. Anesthetist present as high risk of aspiration if bleeding, sedated or encephalopathic.
- If bleeding continues uncontrolled postendoscopy, insert Sangstaken-Blakemore (Minnesota) tube through mouth. It should be placed by the GI team. The gastric balloon inflated with 300 mL air and tube held in place by two tongue depressors taped together and padded. Aim to remove S-B tube <24 hrs.
- Transjugular intrahepatic portosystemic shunting (TIPS) is a useful rescue procedure for refractory bleeding (30% risk of encephalopathy, predicted

by severe liver disease). However, it does not influence survival. Surgery such as portal shunting, devascularization or transection has a mortality of 80% and only should be offered in selected patients.

- *Contraindication of (transjugular intrahepatic Porto-systemic shunt) TIPS*: Right heart disease, severe liver disease. Polycystic liver disease and hepatobiliary sepsis.
- *Complications*: Encephalopathy 25%.
- Worsening hemodynamic state. After the acute episode, Beta-blockers perhaps with nitrates appear to reduce rebleeding and improve survival both as secondary and primary prevention.

Surveillance and Primary Prophylaxis for Varices

On endoscopy
- *No varices*: Re-endoscope 3-4 yrs
- *Grade 1 varices*: Re-endoscope 1 yr
- *Grade 2-3 varices*: Propranolol 80-160 mg/day—intolerant—variceal band ligation.

Severity of Cirrhosis

	1	2	3
Encephalopathy	0	I/II	III/IV
Ascites	Absent	Mild/moderate	Severe
Bilirubin (micromol/L)	<34	34–51	>51
Albumin	>35 g/L	28–35	<28 g/L
INR	<1.3	1.3–1.5	>1.5

Score of 6 or less — Child-Pugh class A
Score of 7–9 — Child-Pugh class B
Score of 10 or more — Child-Pugh class C

PREVENTIVE STRATEGIES IN CIRRHOSIS OR MANAGEMENT OF PORTAL HYPERTENSION

Ultrasound (US) to ensure patency of portal vein and exclusion of hepatocellular carcinoma (HCC).

Stable cirrhosis is a procoagulant state and there is risk of portal vein thrombosis without warfarin or heparin

- Nonselective beta blockers (Propranolol 80 mg bid) reduce bacterial translocation. If propranolol is not tolerated then consider carvedilol or ACE.

- Statin (Simvastatin 40 mg/day) improves hepatic function, perfusion and prevents hepatic cell carcinoma.
- Nonabsorbable antibiotics (Norfloxacin 400 mg/day).
- Anticoagulants (Warfarin or heparin).
- Isosorbide mononitrate (ISMN) reduces intrahepatic resistance.

Lower Gastrointestinal Bleeding

Altered red blood per rectum usually localizes the source to the left colon, while dark red blood per rectum (PR) usually arises from more proximal colon and bright red from anorectum.

Hematemesis and fresh rectal bleed suggests massive hemorrhage with a poor prognosis.

HISTORY

- Anorexia, weight loss, recent alteration in bowel habit (consider malignancy), abdominal pain if long standing and intermittent (diverticular disease), if severe (mesenteric ischemia).
- Drugs that predispose to hemorrhage (Aspirin, NSAID, anti-coagulants).
- Presence of chronic liver disease (rectal varices).
- Family history of colonic polyp/neoplasia or hereditary hemorrhagic telangiectasia.

EXAMINATION

- Pulse, BP, temperature of peripheries, JVP, posture BP (sitting verses lying).
- Looking for jaundice, lymphadenopathy, mucus membrane for chronic anemia, abdominal masses or localized tenderness, telangiectasia on skin or mucus membrane.
- Rectal examination for piles, blood or masses.

Causes

Diverticular bleeding 24%, infective colitis 10%, inflammatory bowel disease 10%, colorectal carcinoma 10%, vascular lesions, colonic polyps, ischemia colitis and hemorrhoids.

Investigations

- FBC, U and E, LFT, coagulation screen, inflammatory markers.
- Sigmoidoscopy.
- Colonoscopy is successful at making a diagnosis in 80% of significant bleeds although mucosal visualization is impaired by the presence of blood. Colonoscopy is less frequently therapeutic. If there is no definite diagnosis and the patient rebleeds, upper endoscopy or CTA or mesenteric angiography with embolization or Tech99 MRBC scan should be considered.
- Capsule endoscopy if bleeding suspected from jejunum to terminal ileum.
- Enteroscopy if available is more useful in the 3–5% of patients with significant small gut bleeds.
- Resuscitation and management of GI bleed as described above.
- If portal hypertension present then consider terlipressin.
- *Poor outcome*: If low BP, on-going bleeding, raised PT, erratic mental state and comorbidities.

Acute or Chronic Liver Failure

FULMINANT LIVER FAILURE

Rapid development (<8 wks) of liver failure with impaired synthetic functions (INR/PT, alb) + encephalopathy in a previously normal or well compensated LFT or within 2 wks of developing jaundice. Cerebral edema is common, mostly due to paracetamol.

SUBFULMINANT

Rapid deterioration of LFT with encephalopathy <6 months, renal failure and portal hypertension are common, caused by alcohol, viral, cryptogenic, biliary cirrhosis, hemochromatosis and Wilsons disease.

In hepatic encephalopathy (HE) with hepatocellur failure, portosystemic shunting tends to be present. It is due to failure of detoxification of gut derived toxins normally cleared by liver. Causation is due to intrahepatic and extrahepatic shunting which occurs with liver failure. Abnormal blood-brain barrier also occurs.

Ammonia is one of the gut derived toxins and in the brain it is detoxified in the astrocytes and eliminated by amidation of glutamate. Glutamate, an excitatory neurotransmitter, after reacting with postsynaptic receptor is converted to glutamine in the astrocytes.

So in HE cerebral glutamine levels are increased and glutamate levels are decreased, glutamate reuptake mechanism are abnormal and glutamate binding sites on post synaptic neurons is down regulated.

Increased glutamine in the astrocytes causes osmotic stress, cellular swelling and cellular damage, called Alzheimer type 2 astrocytosis. Peripheral benzodiazepine receptor sites are also increased.

Abrupt onset of confusion, fetor hepaticus (exhalation of unmetabolized mercaptans) may progress within a few hours from mild confusion to deep coma.

Precipitating Factors

- GI bleed, ingestion of large protein meal, constipation, renal failure, electrolyte disturbance (hypokalemia), dehydration, paracentesis, infections and sedatives.
- States of circulation
  - Vital signs are normal in early stages.
  - Tachycardia and hypotension occurs late and bradycardia and hypertension occur very late. Liver is usually tender but normal size or slightly enlarged.
- If significantly enlarged then to consider hepatic venous obstruction (Budd-Chiari syndrome) or malignant infiltration or chronic liver disease.
- Ascites if significant consider Budd-Chiari syndrome.
- There is risk of hypoglycemia and raised intracranial pressure (ICP).
- Signs of chronic liver disease are absent, and nutrition is good.
- Focal neurological signs are absent, if present consider cerebral lesion (hemorrhage).
- Alcohol abuse, starvation, phenytoin and INH worsen liver damage.
- For liver unit if pH <7.3 or prothrombin time (PT) >50 sec, creatinine >300 micromol/L and encephalopathy grade 3.
- <10% will get cirrhosis.

- Sub clinical encephalopathy may affect visuospatial and psychomotor abilities (clock face or five pointed star).

Guidelines for referral for liver transplant	
Paracetamol overdose	*Non-paracetamol*
Arterial pH <7.30 or HCO$_3$ < 18	pH < 7.30 or or HCO$_3$ <18
INR >3.0 day 2 or >4.0 thereafter	INR >1.8
Oliguria and/or elevated creatinine	Age <10 years or >40 years oliguria/renal failure
Altered conscious level	Encephalopathy, hypoglycemia
Hypoglycemia	Shrinking liver size (<1000 mL need OLT) Na <130 mmol/L, Bilirubin >300 µmol/L

Necrosis of hepatocytes due to paracetamol is due to apoptosis (shrinkage of nucleus but no rupture of cell membrane) and no secondary inflammation but in non paracetamol acute liver failure there is secondary inflammation resulting in multiple organ failure.

Signs of Chronic Liver Disease

Patient is icteric, pigmented, clubbing, palmar erythema, leukonychia (white nails, other causes of white nails are injury to the base of the nail and diet low in potassium), Dupuytren's contracture and several spider naevi.

Flapping tremor of hands (Portosystemic encephalopathy), scratch marks, purpura, gynecomastia, scanty body hair and small testis, raised alkaline phosphatase and raised gamma glutamyl transpeptidase (γGT) or (gamma GT).

There may be hepatosplenomegaly, ascites, edema, distended abdominal veins with flow away from umbilicus. Diagnosis is cirrhosis with portal hypertension.

Causes

- Viral hepatitis (B, C), autoimmune hepatitis (smooth muscle antibody positive), primary biliary cirrhosis (PBC) positive antimitochondrial antibody,

hemochromatosis primary or secondary, sclerosing cholangitis (cryptogenic), hepatic vein obstruction, cardiac failure and constrictive pericarditis.
- Bilirubin, prothrombin time and albumin reflect synthetic functions.
- Hepatic encephalopathy (HE).
  - *Grade 0*: No abnormality.
  - *Grade 1*: Trivial lack of awareness, euphoria, anxiety, reduced attention span, impaired performance in addition or subtraction.
  - *Grade 2*: Lethargy, apathy, disorientation of time and place, personality change and inappropriate behavior.
  - *Grade 3*: Somnolence, semistupor, gross disorientation and confusion.
  - *Grade 4*: Coma.
- Most common cause of acute liver failure are paracetamol poisoning (50–75%), viral hepatitis A or B (8–40%), autoimmune liver disease [primary biliary cirrhosis (PBC), chronic active hepatitis (CAH), primary sclerosing cholangitis (PSC)], Wilson's disease, ischemia, Non A-E hepatitis, acute fatty liver of pregnancy, idiosyncratic drug reactions and Budd-Chiari syndrome.
- *Increased ALT*: Viral or autoimmune liver disease.
- *Increased ALP and gamma GT*: Obstructive jaundice, PBC, metastasis in liver, drugs (antibiotics).
- Precipitating factors for acute liver failure
  - Sepsis
- Low SBP.
- *Avoid*: Renal failure, CNS active drugs, electrolyte abnormalities, fluid restriction if hyponatremia, diuretics over use and gastrointestinal bleeding

Treatment

- For N acetylcysteine in acute liver failure due to paracetamol or nonparacetamol cause.
- General supportive measures, consider Wernicke's encephalopathy (opthalmoplegia nystagmus horizontal or vertical, failure of conjugate movement or eye abduction, confusion, ataxia) if alcohol related or poor nutrition give IV pabrinex or thiamine before giving IV dextrose and supplement with oral

thiamine 300 mg/day and vitamin B complex strong 2 tablets tid.
- Hydration even in a patient with ascites, colloids if BP <100 or hypervolemia.
- Removal of precipitants.
- Vitamin K orally or IV.
- Full septic screen.
- H2RA or PPI for stress ulcers.
- Short-term protein restriction (60–40 g/day).
- Lactulose 30 mL bid or tid or metronidazole if comatose.
- Nutrition (enteral feed) + steroids + pentoxiphiline are core management.
- ITU should be considered for fulminant failure.
- All patients with HE should be considered for liver transplantation.
- *Treatment for hepatorenal syndrome (HRS)*: Terlipressin + human albumin 40 g/day.

Hepatorenal Syndrome

Characterized by renal failure due to severe renal vasoconstriction in a patient with cirrhosis and ascites due to extreme under filing of arterial circulation and mesenteric vasodilatation.

Its incidence is 10%. There is progressive oliguria and rise in creatinine.

Often it is precipitated by spontaneous bacterial peritonitis.

Criteria for Diagnosis

- Raised serum creatinine >140 µmol/L and creatinine clearance <40 mL/min.
- Absence of shock, fluid loss, on-going bacterial infection and no current treatment with nephrotoxic drugs.
- Absence of sustained renal improvement (decrease in serum creatinine) after stopping diuretics and a trial of plasma expansion with 1.5 L saline.
- Absence of proteinuria (<500 mg/day) and hematuria (<50 RBC/high power field).
- Urinary Na <10 mmol/L, urinary volume <500 mL/day, urine osmolality >plasma osmolality and serum Na <130.

- Normal renal ultrasound (excludes obstructive uropathy or parenchymal disease).

Treatment

- Fluid support, volume expansion, broad spectrum antibiotics and terlipressin.
- Later permanent abstinence and liver transplantation.
- Dopamine and prostaglandins are ineffective.
- Administration of one of the following drugs or combination along with albumin 1 g/kg IV on day 1 followed by 20–40 g/day for 5–15 days and stopped when serum creatinin <132 mmol/L.
- Terlipressin 0.5–2 mg IV 4–12 hrly; or
- Norepinephrine 0.5–3 mg/hr IV or
- Midodrine 2.5–7.5 mg orally tds with octreotide 100–200 µg SC tds
  Duration of therapy 1–2 weeks.
  The transjugular intrahepatic Porto-systemic shunt (TIPS) can also be used for treatment of hepatorenal syndrome.
  Hemodialysis only used as a bridge to liver transplantation.

Viral Hepatitis (HBV, HCV)

- *Aspartate amino transferase (AST)*: Alanine amino transferase (ALT) >2—suggestive of alcoholic liver disease. They also have raised gamma GT and high MCV.
- *AST*: ALT <1 hepatic steatosis or viral hepatitis.
- High ALT >30 IU/mL in men and >19 IU/mL can be due to alcohol, type 2 diabetes mellitus (T2DM) and obesity, if persistently raised then consider US of liver and liver screen (blood test for hepatitis B, hepatitis C, ferritin, antinuclear antibody (ANA), anti-smooth muscle antibody, antimitochondrial antibody, copper, ceruplasmin, alpha 1 trypsin and transient elastography).

HEPATITIS A AND E

- *Hepatitis A virus (HAV)*: Spread by fecal/oral route, epidemics are water/food borne and shell fish is a potent source of transmission (because they may ingest sewage).

- Blood transmission is rare.
- *Incubation period*: 3–5 wks and virus is shed fecally till the jaundice stage.
- IgM antibodies indicate recent infection and IgG antibodies pastinfection.

Treatment

- Attention to hygiene, human immunoglobulin containing anti HAV can be given 2 IU/kg to people at risk (close contacts, controlling epidemic in institution and nonimmune people traveling to endemic area).
- It may have prolonged cholestatic phase.
- Monitor prothrombin time (PT) if prolonged by 20 secs transfer to liver unit.
- If jaundice and increased PT, suggests significant liver damage.
- Trial of steroid if antinuclear antibody (ANA) mildly positive autoimmune?
- Virus D and E cause acute hepatitis (except HCV).
- Flue like symptoms, anorexia, nausea and muscular pains, followed by dark urine, pale stools and jaundice. Symptoms resolve after 2–6 wks.
- Treatment is symptomatic and avoidance of fatty food.

Hepatitis B

- Sexual transmission, IV drugs or blood transfusion.
- Viruses HAV (RNA virus A), HBV (DNA virus B), HCV (RNA flavi virus C).
- *Hepatitis B*: Incubation 3–6 months, spreads parenterally by blood products (needles or sexually) or vertically (mother to baby) and rarely mouth to mouth, excreted by body fluids (saliva, serous exudates, semen, vaginal and menstrual discharge). Most cases of chronic infection are acquired through mother to child at birth or through exposure to the virus in early childhood.
- *Incidence*: 0.4% in UK, 0.5% in USA and 15% in Far East and Africa. Most chronic HBV patients acquire infection at a young age often as new born.

Testing for hepatitis B virus: (For presence of hepatitis B virus or immunity to the virus)
- People born in countries with high or intermediate prevalence, i.e. Asia, Africa, Central America and Eastern Europe.

- Infants born to women with chronic hepatitis B infection.
- Family, sexual or household contact of some one with hepatitis B infection.
- Adults at high risk of infection (IV drug users, multiple sexual partners, men who have sex with men and sex workers).
- Diagnosis of another infection with shared mode of acquisition (hepatitis C virus or HIV).
- People presenting with abnormal liver function test results or evidence of acute or chronic liver disease or hepatocellular carcinoma or mental handicap institutions.
- People having chemotherapy or immunosuppressive therapy (risk of reactivation of hepatitis B virus).
- Pregnant women (Routine antenatal screening test).

Hepatitis B surface antigen (HBsAg): A marker of current infection acute or chronic.

Hepatitis B surface antibody (anti-HBs): A marker of immunity through vaccination or previous exposure.

Hepatitis B core antibody (anti-HBc): A marker of previous exposure.

Anti-HBc IgM: Marker of recent infection.

Anti-HBc IgG: Marker of chronic infection.

HBs Ag negative and positive anti-HBc and anti-HBs, in this scenorio there is previous exposure to hepatitis B virus with resolution of infection by sero conversion. These people are at risk of reactivation or flare up of hepatitis in the setting of immunosuppression or rituximab therapy.

In response to vaccination only anti HBs antibody are present and titer >10 mIU/mL is considered to be protective. If all three markers HBs, anti-HBs and anti-HBc are negative patient has neither vaccination nor exposure to the virus. Vaccination should be offered if there is risk of infection.

Acute viral hepatitis HBV resolves in 80%. 20% become chronic carriers and 20% of these develop chronic hepatitis.

- *Anti-HBsAg*: Past history of infection or vaccination.
- *HBsAg present*: Current infection with HBV.
- *Anti-HBcAg*: Little viral replication and low level of viremia and infectivity.

- *HBcAg present*: Active viral replication and high level of viremia and infectivity.
- *IgG anti-HBc*: Evidence of infection in the past.
- *IgM anti-HBc*: Recent HBV infection.
- If HBsAg persists for >6/12, patient has chronic hepatitis.
- *Healthy carrier*: Absence of significant liver damage (ALT normal), HBeAg negative and HBV titer <10^4 IU/mL. These do not require treatment but require lifelong surveillance (3 monthly for 1st year and then yearly measuring HBV DNA and liver function tests to detect conversion from inactive to active disease) as serum titers may subsequently rise.

Stages of HBV Infection

- *Stage 1*: Incubation/active viral replication—asymptomatic, lasts a few weeks, HBsAg is positive as are HBV DNA (indicating active viral replication), HBeAg and anti-HBc IgM present. Transaminases are normal.
- *Stage 2*: Symptomatic with jaundice and hepatitis with raised ALT lasting few weeks. HBcAg present but HBV DNA falls as the infected cells decline. Stage 2 can last for years leading to cirrhosis. Seroconversion refers to HBcAg to anti-HBcAg.
- *Stage 3*: Immune response eliminates infected cells and HBcAg is negative and has anti-HBcAg. HBV DNA may be detectable with PCR and ALT is normal.
- *Stage 4*: Most patients will become HBsAg negative and develop anti-HBsAg antibodies. HBV DNA is undetectable by PCR and reactivation or re-infection is unlikely. Anti HBcAg and anti-HBc IgG are present.

Anti-HBc, IgG, anti HBcAg is present with past history of infection HBV and persist life long and anti-HBsAg antibodies present after infection or vaccination.

Clinical Course of Hepatitis B Infection

To determine the phase of the disease patients who are positive for HBsAG require testing for hepatitis Be antigen (HBeAg) a marker of wild type infection usually associated with high viral levels and anti-HBe (a marker of clearance of HBeAg).

Stage 1	Stage 2	Stage 3	Stage 4
Immune tolerance	Immune clearance	Immune control	Immune escape
Initial 15–30 yrs of infection	High HBV DNA	Low HBV DNA	High HBV DNA
High HBV DNA level	>20,000 IU/mL	<2000 IU/mL	>2000 IU/mL
Normal LFT	Abnormal LFT	Normal LFT	Abnormal LFT
HBeAg positive	HBeAg positive	HBeAg negative	HBeAg negative
Monitor 6–12 monthly	Risk of progression	Liver US 6–12 months.	Anti-HBe positive
HBeAg and anti-HBe	Cirrhosis and hepatic carcinoma		High risk of progression
Liver function test	Consider treatment		Cirrhosis, hepatic carcinoma Consider treatment

Following should be seen by liver specialist

Patients seropositive HBsAG (present more than 6 months) with chronic hepatitis with fluctuating ALT regardless of positive or negative HBeAg.

Any feature of advanced fibrosis or cirrhosis on US or splenomegaly or low platelet count.

Any woman found seropositive HBsAG during antenatal screening with high HBV DNA antiviral treatment in 3rd trimester and infant should have vaccination and hepatitis B immunoglobulin within 12 hrs of birth.

Treatment

- Life style modification and before starting treatment for hepatitis B, HIV test should be done.
- For transient elastography (US test for liver fibrosis) as initial test to assess severity of liver disease and need for treatment.
- All adults (except who are pregnant or receiving immune therapies) are offered following treatment.
- Peginterferon-alfa-2a for 48 wks as 1st line.

- Consider changing treatment after 24 weeks if HBV DNA level decreased by less than 100-fold or HBsAg level is >20,000 IU/mL and offer 2nd line treatment with tenofovir or entecavir.
- Offer tenofovir or entecavir who do not undergo HBeAg seroconversion or who revert to being HBeAg positive after seroconversion.
- Consider stopping 2nd line treatment after 12 months of HBeAg seroconversion in people without cirrhosis but continue indefinitely in people with cirrhosis.
    - Transient elastography score >11 kPa (HBeAg positive, compensated disease and LFT stable) offer antiviral treatment.
    - Patients >30 yrs with HBV DNA levels >20,000 IU/mL and abnormal ALT.
    - Patients <30 yrs with HBV DNA levels >20,000 IU/mL and abnormal ALT and transient elastography score >6 kPa.
    - Patients with HBV DNA >20,000 with abnormal ALT of any age needs treatment.
    - Patients with cirrhosis and any detectable HBV DNA regardless of HBeAG status, HBV DNA levels or ALT levels needs treatment.
    - Transient elastography score between 6 kPa and 10 kPa consider liver biopsy before treatment.
- If ALT is normal and HBV DNA <2000 IU/mL do not offer liver biopsy or antiviral treatment.
- Offer annual assessment of liver disease by transient elastography who are not on antiviral treatment.
- Offer 6 monthly surveillance for hepatocellular carcinoma by hepatic ultrasound and alpha fetoprotein testing in people with hepatic fibrosis or cirrhosis.
- Pegylated interferon 180 µg/wk SC.
- *Side effects*: Influenza like symptoms, cytopenia, depression, anxiety, irritability and autoimmune disorders.
- Tenofevir 300 mg/day, oral, well tolerated monitor renal functions.
- Entecavir 0.5 mg/day, oral, well tolerated.

Hepatitis C Virus (RNA Flavivirus)

- Intravenous drug users (IVDU) or inoculation with blood or blood products is the mode of transmission.

- Now screening of blood donors and heat treatment of coagulation factors should prevent infection for the future.
- Parenteral drug users, tattooing, circumcision, dental or medical treatment where infection control is poor, children of infected people, sexual partners of infected people, continue to be at risk of HCV. Sexual and vertical transmission may occur but less often.
- Patients with chronic infection are often asymptomatic or suffer from mild fatigue.
- Many patients eventually develop cirrhosis (20% after 20 yrs and 50% after 30 yrs) and 2–5% of cirrhotic patients progress to hepatic cell carcinoma (HCC) per year.
- *Risk factors*: Male, obese, hepatitis B virus, HIV, alcohol, diabetes, old age.
- Genotypes 1–4, type 1 most virulent, >40, male, severe fibrosis but acute hepatitis rare.
- It causes chronic hepatitis leading to cirrhosis.
- Type 2 and 3 best response.
- *Treatment for HCV*: Interferon-alpha plus oral ribavirin. Telaprevir and boceprevir are likely to be introduced.
- Pegylated interferon weekly SC plus oral ribavirin 6/12 for type 2 and 3 and 12/12 for type 1. Failure to achieve good response at 12 wks means non response.

Hepatitis C Virus (HCV)

- Major public health concern worldwide. Incidence in UK 0.5%, 85% carrier rate eventual progression to cirrhosis and 1–4% HCC.
- Hepatitis C virus is a single stranded RNA virus, spread by sharing needles in drug users and transfusion of blood or blood products (eliminated from UK since 1991), sharing tooth brushes, razors, tattooing, body piercing, electrolysis, acupuncture. Sexual transmission and vertical maternal transmission rate is low.
- Hepatitis C virus needle stick injury 1:30.
- Hepatitis C virus antibody test is positive after 6/12 of exposure but HCV virus can be detected by PCR.
- Liver biopsy is the only way to assess severity as LFT fluctuates disproportionately.
- Investigations if only ALT is raised.

8

Nonalcoholic Fatty Liver Disease and Nonalcoholic Steatohepatitis

	NAFLD	Alcoholic liver disease
Body weight	Increased	Variable
HbA1c	Increased	Normal
ALT	Increased or normal	Increased or normal
AST	Normal	Increased
AST/ALT ratio	<0.8	>1.5
Gamma GT	Increased or normal	Considerably increased
Triglycerides	Increased	Variable may be considerably increased
HDL cholesterol	Low	Increased
Mean corpuscular volume	Normal	Increased

- If at any stage AST/ALT ratio >0.8, specialist referral
- Nonalcoholic steatohepatitis (NASH) = severe nonalcoholic fatty liver disease (NAFLD)
- NASH has double the risk of IHD.
- Risk is because of expanded and inflamed visceral adipose tissue.
- Normal liver (obesity) → insulin resistance ↑ leptin → steatosis ↑ SNS tone (sympathetic nervous system) → hypertension and fibrosis → adipocytokines and reactive O_2 species (ROS) → inflammation, and cirrhosis → hepatocellular carcinoma (HCC).
- Incidence 2–3%, hepatocellular steatosis (macrovesicular) is the hallmark.
- *Risk factors*: Obesity and metabolic syndrome (obesity, hypertension, dyslipidemia (raised triglycerides and

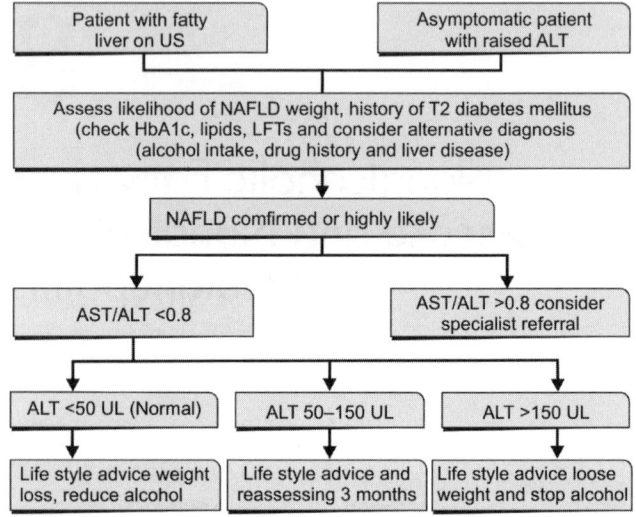

- low high density lipoprotein (HDL), insulin resistance, raised blood sugar and T2DM).
- Abnormal LFT (raised ALT × 3 the normal, raised gamma GT and cholestasis) with risk factors and ultrasound consistent with fatty liver (steatosis) are diagnostic after excluding other causes; alcohol, hepatotoxic drugs and liver screen for hepatitis B, C, auto antibodies, serum ferritin, ceruloplasmin and alpha 1 antitrypsin.
- This has good prognosis and the risk of developing cirrhosis is 1–2% after 15–20 yrs.
- Nonalcoholic fatty liver disease (NAFLD) patients with older age (45 yrs), increasing obesity (BMI >30), T2DM or raised fasting glucose, and AST/ALT >0.8 should be considered for liver biopsy for diagnosis of nonalcoholic steatohepatitis (NASH) which has increased propensity for fibrosis, cirrhosis and hepatocellular carcinoma (HCC) and needs long-term follow-up.
- Macrophages infiltration to adipocytes releasing cytokines which leads to extrahepatic insulin resistance with increased supply of free fatty acid (FFA) due to obesity causes the inflammation in the liver. Reduced production of adiponectin (anti-inflammatory cytokine) by adipocytes in obesity also contributes to liver inflammation and fibrosis.

- Natural history of NAFLD and NASH.
- Obese mothers may program their children to be obese and develop NAFLD and NASH.
- Steatosis in NAFLD leads to 47% fibrosis and 53% no change.
- NASH → 20% cirrhosis, 16% severe fibrosis, 32% no change and 32% improve.

Treatment of NAFLD is treatment of metabolic syndrome (Which is waist circumference in men >94 cm and in women >80 cm together with three of the following:
1. Hypertension >130/85 is treated with ACE.
2. Fasting glucose >5.6 or T2DM.
3. Hypertriglyceridemia >1.7 mmol/L or HDL <0.9 in men and <1.1 in women and treated with fibrates.

Treatment

- Stop smoking.
- Metformin in nondiabetic NAFLD normalizes ALT and decreases fibrosis.
- Pioglitazone increases insulin sensitivity and improve liver biochemistry and fibrosis.
- For hypertension ACE or A2RB or alpha blocker should be preferred.
- Weight loss, stopping smoking, increasing exercise, decreasing alcohol within limits of 21 U in men and 14 U in women.

Alcoholic Hepatitis

- Alcohol chronic liver disease (Binge drinking 5 pints of beer or 1 bottle of wine or 5 shots of spirits at single occasion).
- Recently cut down/stopped.
- AST, ALT almost always < 500 IU/L.
- Higher level ALT suggests viral, ischemic or drug hepatitis (e.g. paracetamol).
- Relatively lower ALT due to hepatic deficiency of pyridoxal-6-phosphate in alcoholics, a cofactor for ALT enzymatic activity.

Signs and Symptoms

Fever, hepatomegaly (tender), abdominal pain, jaundice, anorexia
- *Mild*: Asymptomatic

- *Severe*: Anorexia, malnutrition, weight loss, jaundice, malaise, pyrexia, and ascites may or may not be present with enlarged tender liver.
- Blood shows raised MCV, polymorph leukocytosis 20,000, raised gamma GT, raised bilirubin, raised PT, raised ALT usually <200, (markedly raised ALT indicates viral hepatitis or drug hepatotoxicity). Ferritin often is raised >1000 even in the absence of hemochromatosis.

Treatment

- Chlordiazepoxide 20 mg qid (day 1), 15 mg qid (day 2), 10 mg qid (day 3), 5 mg qid (day 4), 5 mg bd (day 5) or lorazepam for alcohol withdrawal.
- Use sedatives cautiously for risk of encephalopathy.

Low risk of encephalopathy	Thiamine 100 mg tds
Moderate risk	Pabrinex one daily for 3 days
Established	Pabrinex 2 pairs tds for 3 days

- IV pabrinex bd for 3 days and oral thiamine 100 mg tds/day for 14 days to prevent Wernicke's or Korsakoff if patient has confusion, ataxia or ophthalmoplegia at presentation.
- Pentoxifylline is helpful in alcoholic hepatitis.
- Hyponatremia is common in alcoholic hepatitis with ascites. Water restriction will worsen the condition (hepatorenal syndrome). Screen for infections.
- If patient presents with encephalopathy then rarely short course of steroids may be helpful (1-2 wks). Pentoxifylline 400 mg tds is also helpful for 4 wks. Lactulose is the mainstay treatment of encephalopathy.
- Consider terlipressin and moxifloxacin if variceal hemorrhage.
- Treat as spontaneous bacterial peritonitis (SBP) if ascites has neutrophils >250/cumm with 3rd generation cephalosporin.
  GAHS >9 will benefit from steroids.
  GAHS <9 mortality at 28 days 13% while GAHS >9 mortality is 54%.
- Steroids, Pentoxifylline—reduce mortality in selected cases.

Glasgow alcoholic hepatitis score (GAHS)			
	1	2	3
Age	<50 yrs	>50 yrs	
WCC	<15000	>15000	
Urea	<5 mmol/L	>5	
Bilirubin	<125 micromol/L	125–250	>250
PT	<1.5	1.5–2	>2.0

- Septic screen important.
- Discriminant function (Maddrey score) = (4.6 × [prothrombin time-control PT]) + (serum bilirubin).
- Score > 32 associated with a high short-term mortality.
- Used to decide treatment with prednisolone or pentoxifylline.

Detoxification

It is safe and humane withdrawal from a drug of dependence and can be done at home.

ALCOHOL WITHDRAWAL SYNDROME (DT)

- Early 3–12 hrs, peak 24–48 hrs and lasts 5–7 days (tremor, sweating, anorexia, nausea, anxiety, insomnia, tachycardia and systolic hypertension).
- Withdrawal seizures 10–60 hrs, peak 12–24 hrs, grandmal, usually self-limiting (predisposing factors low glucose, low K, low Mg and epilepsy).
- Delirium tremens (DT's): Incidence 5%, 48–72 hrs confusion, agitation, hallucination, paranoia, precipitated by febrile illness.
- Correct electrolyte abnormalities and dehydration.
- Treat infection if present.
- Thiamine 100 mg tds if absence of Wernicke's encephalopathy otherwise IV pabrinex.
- Chlordiazepoxide 20 mg qid (day 1), 15 mg qid (day 2), 10 mg qid (day 3), 5 mg qid (day 4), 5 mg bd (day 5) or lorazepam for alcohol withdrawal.
- Prophylactic phenytoin or carbamazepine if previous withdrawal fits.

Primary Biliary Cirrhosis

In primary biliary cirrhosis (PBC) there is granulomatous cholangitis and progressive destruction of intrahepatic small and medium size bile ducts. Antinuclear antibodies (ANA) are positive and antimitochondrial antibody (AMA) are also positive in 95%. In 10% AMA may be negative but other features of PBC like raised IgG, positive ANA, and raised liver enzymes like alanine aminotransferase (ALT) will help in diagnosis. AMA (gp210) is specific to PBC.

Clinical Features

- Xanthelasma, xanthomata, middle age women, tiredness, intense itching and isolated raised alkaline phosphatase. Later cholestatic jaundice, pigmentation around the face, hepatosplenomegaly and variceal bleeding may be present.
- May also have steatorrhea and malabsorption leading to osteomalacia.
- Drug hepatitis due to phenothiazine's and non-steroidal anti-inflammatory drugs (NSAIDs) should be excluded.

Treatment

- Ursodeoxycholic acid 10–15 mg/kg daily as single or divided doses.
- Cholestyramine 4–28 g/day or rifampicin 300 mg/day or naltrexone (opioid antagonist) 25 mg/day or sertraline 50 mg/day help the itching.
- Liver transplant is considered for advanced disease.
- *Associated diseases*: Rheumatoid arthritis, thyroid disease, Sjögren's syndrome, Addison's disease, fibrosing alveolitis and Raynaud's disease should also be considered.

Hemochromatosis

Hemochromatosis (HHC) is due to iron deposition in skin, pancreas, liver, heart and anterior pituitary.

Clinical

- Incidence is 0.4%. Thin male (presentation earlier in male and later in females, 40–60 yrs) patient has slate-gray pigmentation, decreased body hair, gynecomastia; testicular atrophy, hepatomegaly, fatigue, arthralgia, diabetes, pseudogout and idiopathic cardiomyopathy. Other features may be spider naevi, palmar erythema, ascites and jaundice.
- Autosomal recessive, HLA-A3 short arm of chromosome 6, single base mutation (cytosine to tyrosine C282Y) in HFE gene is the reason.
- Carrier rate is 1/10 and homozygous rate is 1/200 to 1/600.
- Less than 5% with genetic abnormality develop iron overload.

Diagnosis

- Diagnosis is suggested by high ferritin >1000, high serum iron, iron saturation >75% and high transferring saturation >55%. Diagnosis is confirmed by liver biopsy and genetic testing.
- Treated with weekly phlebotomy keeping ferritin <10 and Hb <110 g/L.
- Increased risk of hepatocellular carcinoma 33% in cirrhotic patients.
- Risk is 200 times more than normal population.
- At present screening is done in relatives of patients with HHC or any diabetic with abnormal liver biochemistry or symptoms and signs suggestive of HHC.

Wilson's Disease

Wilson's disease should be considered in any young patients with cirrhosis or neurological problems with tremor, dysarthria and involuntary movements.

Clinical

Uncommon, presents in childhood or early adulthood with liver or neurological manifestations as chronic active hepatitis, hepatic failure or decline in mental functions, tremor, dysarthria or involuntary movements and Kayser-Fleischer rings (rusty brown deposit of copper in Descemet's membrane of cornea at 6 or 12 o'clock), sometime detectable only with slit lamp.

- Choreiform movements are due to deposition of copper in basal ganglia.
- Liver cells are unable to excrete copper in bile due to mutation in copper transporting ATPase. Autosomal recessive, chromosome 13.

Diagnosis

- Serum copper may be normal, high or low. Low ceruloplasmin (copper carrying protein) and high urinary copper is diagnostic.
- Liver biopsy is diagnostic.
- Treatment is with penicillamine.
- Monitor prothrombin time (PT), bilirubin, and albumin. Most cases will respond to therapy and normalize LFT in 6 months. If encephalopathic then liver transplant.
- Asymptomatic siblings should be screened.

10
Autoimmune Hepatitis

Mainly affects young females (45 yrs, ratio M:F 1:3), presents with fatigue, right upper quadrant pain, arthralgia, and abnormal LFTs or isolated raised alanine amino transferase (ALT).

In 20% other autoimmune conditions are present such as rheumatoid arthritis (RA), SLE, scleroderma and thyroid disease. Raised ALT × 10 times the normal or five times the normal plus raised gamma globulin selective IgG (double the normal) on presentation and in them there is risk of developing cirrhosis usually in 5 yrs.

Smooth muscle antibody (SMA) positive 87%, antinuclear antibody (ANA) positive 13% and liver, kidney and microsomal (LKM) antibody positive 4%. SLA/LP (soluble liver antigen/liver pancreas antibody) appear when SMA and ANA are negative.

- *Type 1 AIH*: Most common (80%), young females, has high titers of antinuclear antibodies (ANA), anti-smooth muscle antibodies directed at actin (anti-SMA) and raised gamma globulin.
- *Type 2a AIH*: 20% in children. It is not associated with ANA but with anti-LKM (liver, kidney, microsomal antibodies), rapidly progressive without treatment.
- *Type 2b AIH*: 2a and HCV infection.
- *Type 3*: 2a, rapidly progressive, no significant hyper gamma globulinemia, positive anti-SLA (soluble liver antigen) directed at cytokeratin.

Differential diagnosis: Primary biliary cirrhosis (PBC), viral hepatitis, primary sclerosing cholangitis (PSC), non-alcoholic steatotic hepatitis (NASH).

Treatment: Steroids for 1 yr + azathioprine starting dose 1 mg/kg/day and tapering once in remission and lasting 3 yrs.

Budd-Chiari Syndrome (Hepatic Vein Obstruction)

Clinical

Young female, right upper quadrant abdominal pain, recent abdominal swelling and jaundice, raised alanine amino transferase (ALT), prolonged prothrombin time (PT) and ascites.

Diagnosis

Ultrasound shows hepatomegaly and Doppler of hepatic vein confirms obstruction of hepatic vein.

Causes

Myeloproliferative disorders 50%, estrogen use/pregnancy 10%, tumors 10%, hypercoagulable state 5%, paroxysmal nocturnal hemoglobinuria 5% and idiopathic 20%.

Treatment

If no hepatic decompensation—Diuretics and warfarin, if significant liver impairment—TIPPS, portocaval shunt and if encephalopathic—Transplant.

Hepatotoxicity is increased by enzyme inducing drugs (Phenytoin, carbamazepine, and rifampicin), malnutrition, recent surgery (because of decreased glutathione) and chronic alcohol misuse.

Prothrombin time (PT) is the best marker of liver injury.

Hepatocellular—ALT >2 × upper limit normal (ULN) or ALT/AP >5.

Cholestatic—AP>2 × ULN or ALT/AP (alanine amino transferase/alkaline phosphatase) <2.

CHOLESTATIC HEPATITIS

- Rarely can occur with co-amoxiclav, amoxicillin and flucloxacillin.
- There is increased risk in elderly.
- Latent period is up to 6 wks after discontinuation and can persist up to 6 months.
- Increased dose and duration >2 wks is also a risk factor.

Acute on Chronic Liver Disease

Presentation: Jaundice, ascites, peripheral edema.

Causes

- Alcoholic hepatitis, infection, dehydration, upper gastrointestinal (GI) hemorrhage.
- Pentoxifylline in alcoholic hepatitis is helpful (decreases mortality 37%).

History

Drug history, alcohol consumption, previous jaundice, transfusion or drug use, viral hepatitis, FH (Hemochromatosis, Wilson's disease, alpha 1 antitrypsin deficiency), travel history, and sexual history.

Complication

Encephalopathy, ascites, spontaneous bacterial peritonitis, hepatorenal syndrome, coagulopathy and GI bleeding.

Consider acute liver failure in any patient with jaundice, elevated transaminases, prolonged INR (which is not corrected by vitamin K 10 mg IV).

Fulminant hepatic failure is acute liver failure with abnormal behavior or reduced conscious level and asterisks (liver flap) or hepatic fetor.

Jaundice is not always present in fulminant hepatic failure.

Diagnosis is usually obvious in patients with known chronic liver disease or stigmata of chronic liver disease who develop jaundice, ascites or encephalopathy. These three complications are the prime manifestations of hepatic failure.

Indications for Liver Transplant

FULMINANT HEPATIC FAILURE

- Alcohol induced cirrhosis (if patient can stop alcohol)
- Hepatitis B or C induced cirrhosis
- Primary biliary cirrhosis (PBC), hereditary hemochromatosis, Wilson's disease.

- Hepatocellular carcinoma (HCC) <5 cm and cholangio-carcinoma.

Chronic Liver Disease

Age <60
- Grade 3 encephalopathy with pH <7.3 after fluid resuscitation, prothrombin time (PT) >50 sec, creatinine >300.
- Bilirubin >50 micromol/L and INR >1.5
- Jaundice to encephalopathy >7 days.
- No significant co-morbidity.

Contraindications for Liver Transplant

- On-going alcohol abuse
- Extra hepatic malignancy
- Hepatocellular carcinoma >5 cm.

Chronic Hepatic Failure

Occurs when there is decompensation in a chronic liver disease, e.g. spontaneous bacterial peritonitis in a patient with alcoholic cirrhosis.
- Note the presence of ascites, spider naevi, pruritus, splenomegaly, bruising and rashes.
- Establish if there is a history of drug misuse, blood products transfusion, hepatotoxic drug ingestion, alcohol abuse or foreign travel.
- Causes of decompensation in chronic liver disease—
  GI bleed,
  Drugs (diuretics, hypnotic, sedatives and narcotic analgesics).
  Hypoglycemia, hypokalemia and hyponatremia.
  Intercurrent infections (chest, UTI or spontaneous bacterial peritonitis).
  Alcoholic binge, acute viral hepatitis, major surgery and anesthesia.

Constipation

Development of hepatocellular carcinoma.

Investigations

Full blood count (FBC), U and E, glucose, liver function test (LFT), prothrombin time (PT), alpha-feto protein (AFP), blood culture, MSU, paracetamol level, viral hepatitis screen, autoantibody profile, ascitic tap for bacteriology and culture, ferritin, plasma ceruloplasmin in patient <50 yrs.

Chest X-ray, liver ultrasound, rectal examination, plain abdominal film, endoscopy and daily fasting weight.

Management

- Check blood glucose, if <3.5 mmol/L, give 250 mL of 10% dextrose intravenous (IV).
- O_2 high flow keeping SaO_2 > 92%.
- Avoid hypotension and electrolyte abnormalities (including hypophosphatemia).
- For constipation and/or encephalopathy, lactulose 30 mL oral 8 hrly and titrate to produce 2–3 bowel movements daily. Give phosphate enemas.
- Metronidazole 400 mg 8 hrly.
- Identify and treat infection (no role for prophylactic but low threshold for treating suspected infection) or bleeding and stop precipitant drug.
  If asicitic tap shows >250 WBC/cmm, of which 75% are polymorph treat with cefuroxime, gentamicin and metronidazole.
  Start cefotaxime and gentamicin if there is fever in the absence of focal signs of infections, after taking blood culture.
- Thiamine 300 mg oral daily and vitamin B complex 2 tab tds.
- Sedation should be avoided.
- Exclude focal neurology, e.g. subdural hematoma.
- Monitor renal function closely.
- Give prophylactic omeprazole or ranitidine or sucralfate.
- No-added salt diet, give K supplements to maintain level >3.5 mmol/L. If IV fluid is needed, use albumin solution or dextrose 5% and avoid saline. Give vitamin K 10 mg IV and folic acid 15 mg PO daily.
- Patients with ascites need increasing doses of diuretics, usually beginning with spironolactone 50–600 mg daily along with furosemide 40–120 mg daily. If this provokes deterioration in renal function or hyponatremia, then diuretics must be stopped; fluid restriction is the next course of action along with terlipressin 2 mg 6 hrly.

Hyponatremia is common and is due to water excess and should be treated with fluid restriction and not by infusion of normal saline.

Consider paracentesis with albumin support (100 mL 20% albumin per 2–3 liters ascites).

Check serum cortisol and short Synacthen test to exclude hypoadrenal disease.

Acute/Imminent Wernicke's Encephalopathy or Korsakoff's Psychosis

Diagnosis

- *Ocular signs*: Nystagmus, bilateral lateral rectus palsy, conjugate gaze palsy, fixed pupils and rarely papilledema.
- *Ataxia*: Broad base ataxia with cerebellar signs in limbs.
- *Confusion*: Restlessness, amnesia, apathy, stupor and coma.
- Give IV pabrinex slowly over 10 minutes or IV infusion in 100 mL 5% dextrose over 30 minutes.

Major Complications in Acute Liver Failure

- *Hypotension*: Correct hypovolemia with blood or 4.5% albumin solution. Use adrenaline or noradrenaline infusion to maintain mean arterial pressure >60 mm Hg.
- *Renal failure*: Correct hypovolemia. Avoid high dose furosemide. Consider terlipressin 2 mg 6 hrly. Consider renal replacement therapy if anuric or oliguric with plasma creatinine >400 micromol/L.
- *Coagulopathy*: Give vitamin K 10 mg IV daily. Give platelet transfusion if count <50,000. Give fresh frozen plasma only if there is active bleeding.
- *Gastric stress ulceration*: Prophylaxis with omeprazole or ranitidine or sucralfate.
- *Hypoxemia*: Many causes (inhalation pneumonia, infection, pulmonary edema, atelectasis, intrapulmonary hemorrhage. Ventilate with positive end expiratory pressure if SpO_2 <90%.

Mannitol for cerebral edema. Mortality in grade 1–2 hepatic coma is 34% and with grade 4 is 80–90% without transplant.

Autoimmune Hepatitis

Ascites

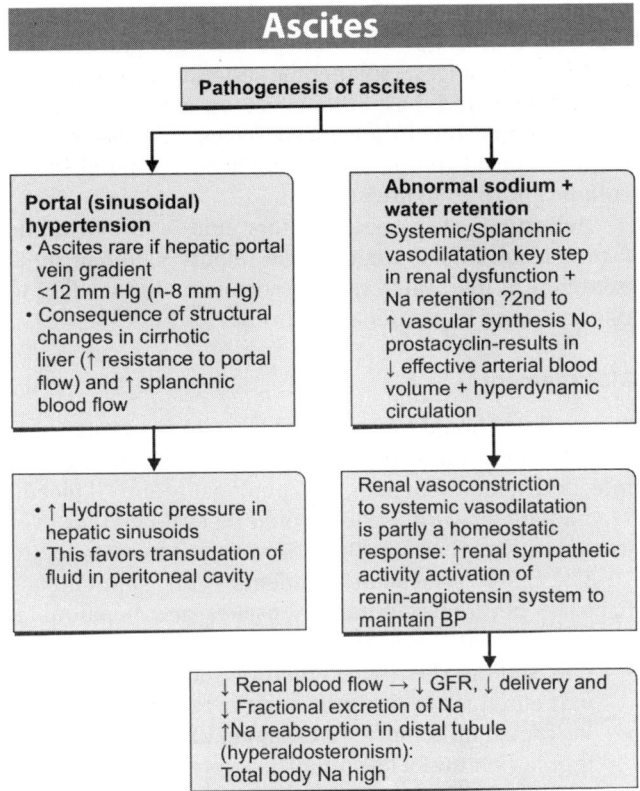

Ascites is the most common complication of cirrhosis and associated with poor quality of life, increased risk of infections and renal failure. Normal fluid content in peritoneal cavity is 25 mL.

Differential diagnosis of ascites	
Serum ascites albumin gradient (SAAG)	
>1.1 g/dL	<1.1 g/dL
Cirrhosis, CCF, hepatic failure, alcoholic hepatitis, liver metastasis, myxedema, Budd-Chiari syndrome	Peritoneal carcinomatosis, peritoneal TB pancreatitis, nephrotic syndrome connective tissue diseases

As portal hypertension (due to cirrhosis) develops, local production of vasodilators (nitric oxide) increases leading to splanchnic arterial vasodilatation causing increased intestinal capillary pressure and permeability and ascites.

In early stages, splanchnic arterial vasodilatation is moderate and has little effect on effective arterial blood volume but in advanced stages vasodilatation is so pronounced that it decreases effective arterial blood volume and arterial pressure.

Activation of vasoconstrictors and anti-natriuretic factors result in sodium and fluid retention, impair renal excretion of free water, renal vasoconstriction leading to dilutional and hepatorenal syndrome.

Management

Ascitic fluid should be examined to exclude spontaneous bacterial peritonitis, especially when there are signs of infection, abdominal pain, encephalopathy and GI bleed.

All patients with ascites should be evaluated for liver transplant (survival rate 30–40% at 5 yrs as compared to 70–80% after transplant). Patients with spontaneous bacterial peritonitis, refractory ascites and hepatorenal syndrome should be given priority.

- Low sodium diet (60–90 mEq or 1500–2000 mg/day) may eliminate or delay the onset of ascites.
- Restricted fluid intake (1 L/day) in dilutional hyponatremia (sodium <130 mmol/L in presence of ascites, edema or both).
- Diuretics either spironolactone (50–200 mg/day) or amiloride (5–10 mg/day) achieve the loss of fluids. Furosemide (20–40 mg) may be added for the first few days. Furosemide should be used with caution as excessive diuresis can lead to renal failure. Weight loss should be no more than 300–500 g/day.
- 24 hrs urinary sodium is helpful.
- Prophylaxis for all ascitic patients with norfloxacin for the duration of hospital stay or for life if previous episode of spontaneous bacterial peritonitis (SBP).
- *Spontaneous bacterial peritonitis (SBP)*: Spontaneous bacterial infection of ascitic fluid in the absence of intra-abdominal source of infection.

Its incidence is 10–30% and presence of 250 polymorphs/cubic millimeter of ascitic fluid is diagnostic. *E. coli* are most common organism and rarely grampositive organism.

It involves translocation of bacteria from intestinal lumen to the lymph nodes with subsequent bacteremia and infection of ascitic fluid.

Third generation cephalosporins are treatment of choice.

The most severe complication is hepatorenal syndrome which occurs up to 30% of patients.

Intravenous albumin 1.5 g/kg at diagnosis and 1.0 g/kg 48 hrs later helps to prevent hepatorenal syndrome.

Recurrence of bacterial peritonitis is 70% at one year which can be prevented by norfloxacin 400 mg/day. Quinoline resistant bacteria can be treated by trimethoprim + sulfamethoxazole.

Large Volume Ascites

Large volume ascites usually presents with abdominal discomfort which interferes regular daily activities. These patients usually have severe sodium retention (urinary Na <10 mmol/L).

There are two equal therapeutic strategies high dose diuretics and paracentesis.
Spironolactone (up to 400 mg/day and 160 mg of furosemide/day)

Paracentesis

Paracentesis can be performed with IV 20% albumin or plasma expanders (dextran 70 or polygeline) cover, 6 g/L fluid drained.

Correct pre-renal status before paracentesis and stop diuretics.

Close monitoring of renal function is required: hourly urine output and daily U and E.

Exclude spontaneous bacterial peritonitis.

Paracentesis contraindicated if platelet count <50,000 or INR >1.6 or prothrombin time (PT) more than 21 seconds.

Refractory Ascites

Ascites with lack of response to diuretics (Spironolactone 400 mg + furosemide 160 mg/day) and recurrent side effects (hepatic encephalopathy, hyponatremia, hyperkalemia or azotemia).

This usually is treated with repeated large volume paracentesis every 3–4 wks or with transjugular intrahepatic portosystemic shunts (TIPS).

Shunt decreases the activity of Na retaining mechanism and improves the renal response to diuretics.

Main disadvantage is shunt stenosis (75% in 6–12 months), high cost and lack of availability in some centers.

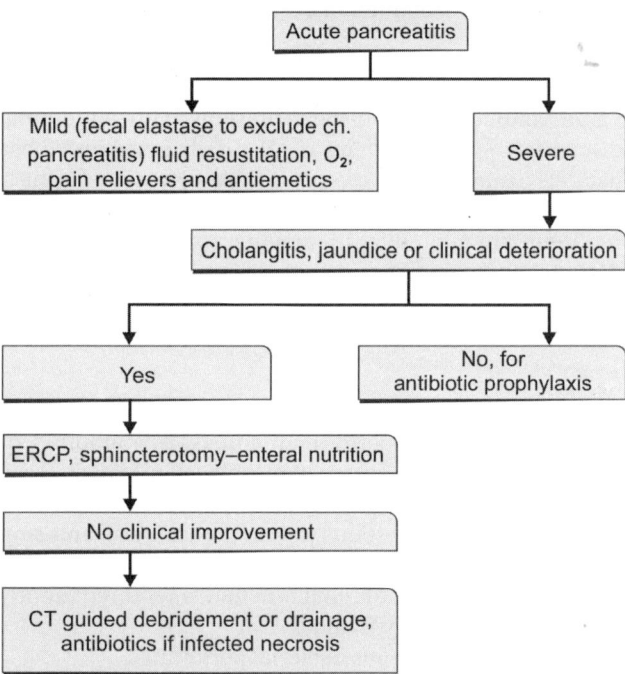

Presents as epigastric pain with hyperamylasemia (>amylase × 3).

Pain is usually continuous, occasionally colicky and is sometimes felt in the right or left upper quadrant with vomiting and fever due to septicemia (gram-negative 20–50%).

It radiates through to the back (50%). There is nausea and vomiting in 75% of patients. It can occasionally present as collapse. Hyperamylasemia usually regresses after 48 hrs and patients are often pyrexial.

Raised amylase 3 times the normal with abdominal pain is diagnostic of pancreatitis.

Level of serum amylase does not correlate with disease severity.

Overall mortality is 5–10% and half of deaths occur in first 14 days. There may be periumbilical bruising (Cullen sign) or flank bruising (Grey Turner's sign).

Investigations include X-ray abdomen, erect chest X-ray and ultrasound (US) of abdomen.

CT is diagnostic and excludes other diagnosis.

CT at >48 hrs—Necrosis predicts prolonged course. CRP is best predictive marker.

Risk Factors

Gall stones (raised ALT × 3, ALK × 3, bilirubin × 3 suggestive of gallstones), excessive alcohol intake, hypertriglyceridemia, bile duct obstruction, medications (thiazides, estrogen, azathioprine), hypercalcemia, obesity, some viral infections (mums, coxsackie B4), autoimmune disease, porphyria and trauma.

Pathogenesis

Inappropriate activation of trypsinogen to trypsin and lack of prompt elimination. Increased intracellular calcium activates intracellular proteases which causes cell necrosis.

Differential Diagnosis

- Perforated duodenal ulcer (DU)
- Acute cholecystitis.
- Biliary colic.
- Mesenteric infarction.
- Hypoxia is due to edema and toxic damage.
- Hypocalcemia is usually not treated.

Other Investigations

Consider ultrasound within 24 hrs or CT to confirm diagnosis, assess severity and development of any complications, and evaluate biliary tree for stones or dilatation.

Magnetic resonance cholangiopancreatography (MRCP) or endoscopy ultrasound (EUS) is helpful in common bile duct (CBD) stones. Consider dynamic CT in all severe cases between 3 and 10 days.

Treatment

The overall aim is to reduce pancreatic enzymes secretion (by decreasing stimulation) and complications, such as abscess and cholangitis.

Mild Pancreatitis

Intravenous fluids Hartmann solution (4-6 L/24 hrs), nil by mouth.

Analgesia with fentanyl patch or pethidine and antibiotics, imipenem or penicillin + ciprofloxacin + metronidazole or cefuroxime.

Endoscopic retrograde cholangiopancreatography (ERCP) as soon as possible after 48 hrs of antibiotics or immediately if patient not improving with antibiotics to clear the obstruction (gallstones) and decrease the high pressure in the CBD (normal 8-10 cm) usually >20 cm of H_2O.

For persistent vomiting a nasogastric tube is useful.

Moderate pancreatitis in which transient organ failure (renal creatinine >170 micromol/L, circulatory blood pressure < 90 mm Hg and respiratory) which resolves within 48 hrs or there is peripancreatic fluid collection with out organ failure.

Severe Disease

Modified Glasgow criteria during 1st 48 hrs are:
- Age >55.
- Albumin <32 g/L.
- Serum calcium <2.0 mmol/L.
- WBC >15000.
- AST >100 IU/L.
- LDH >600 IU/L.
- Blood glucose >10.0 mmol.
- Urea >16.0 mmol/L.
- PaO_2 <7.5 Kpa.

Patients with three or more of above criteria and all patients with hypotension, persistent oliguria after initial resuscitation, should be nursed in high dependency unit (HDU) or intensive care. Principles of management are the same as for mild disease.

They require intensive monitoring with CVP, hourly urine volumes,

Intravenous cefuroxime or imipenem 500 mg for TDS 14 days prophylactically if pancreatic necrosis on 48 hrs CT.

Consider ERCP with sphincterotomy in 1st 48–72 hrs in gall stone pancreatitis if bilirubin >70 mmol/L, high alanine amino transferase (ALT), not settling at 48 hrs and dilatation of ducts or cholangitis.

Endoscopic retrograde cholangiopancreatography (ERCP) is indicated at any time for deepening jaundice or cholangitis or clinical deterioration without explanation.

Necrotizing pancreatitis is suspected when there are persistent signs of systemic inflammation (temperature >38°C, heart rate >90/min, respiratory rate >20/min and WBC >12000) for more than 7–10 days after the onset of pancreatitis. Intervention in the 1st 2 wks of severe acute pancreatitis should be avoided until walled of necrosis has developed.

Early cholecystectomy in 6 wks after discharge before the risk of recurrent cholecystitis and pancreatitis.

Complications: Pseudocysts occur in about 50% of patients with severe pancreatitis, with half resolving spontaneously. Guided percutaneous/surgical/endoscopic drainage should be undertaken if infection or clinical deterioration present.

On discharge inform the patient of avoidance of alcohol for 6–12 months. After acute severe pancreatitis exocrine pancreatic functions should be tested by fecal elatase and pancreatic enzymes should be supplemented for at least 6 months and exocrine pancreatic functions should be tested again to ensure the recovery of functions.

Chronic Pancreatitis

Chronic pancreatitis is due to progressive inflammation resulting in destruction of secretory parenchyma and replacement by fibrous tissue leading to malnutrition and diabetes.

Pancreatitis begins as pancreastasis and prevention of acinar apical exocytosis triggered by reactive oxygen species (ROS).

Causes

About 95% alcohol or idiopathic (autoimmune disease with dense plasmocytic infiltrate, raised IgG4, antinuclear antibody (ANA) positive, rheumatoid factor positive).

It is related to gallstones (30%), smoking and drugs (thiazides, estrogen, valproate and azathioprine).

With alcohol, pancreatic juice is thick and viscid and blocks the small ducts.

Clinical

Presents with chronic epigastric pain radiating to left hypochondrium or dorsal spine relieved by sitting up or leaning forward or drinking alcohol.

Sometimes patients get postprandial pain with high fat and protein in the food, thus patients avoids food and loses weight. Nausea, malabsorption, diabetes mellitus (DM) and steatorrhea are other symptoms.

Fecal elastase is increased >200 µg/gm, serum amylase normal.

Pain is due to large duct obstruction or degranulation of mast cells or hydrogen sulfide.

There is calcification on plain abdominal X-ray.

Ultrasound abdomen, dynamic CT, MRCP, secretin enhanced MRCP, endoscopic ultrasound (EUS) help in diagnosis.

Check B_{12} and folic acid levels.

Treatment

- *Analgesics*: Paracetamol, tramadol, amitriptyline.
- Micronutrient therapy with vitamin C + methionine + selenium + vitamin E (Antox 2 tab tds).
- Anti-oxidant rich food.
- *Steatorrhea*: Pancreatin (nonenteric coated), low fat diet, H_2RA (H_2 receptor antagonist), i.e. Ranitidine or proton pump inhibitor (PPI), i.e. Omeprazole.
- Steroids for autoimmune pancreatitis (noncalcifying, raised IgG4) Prednisolone 30–40 mg/day tapered over 3/12 monitoring IgG levels. Long-term 5–7.5 mg/day.
- Surgery for pain, obstruction of the duct or pseudocyst.

Acute Diarrhea

- Frequent passage of small stools is due to proctitis, frequent passage of large volume stools is usually from small intestine and bloody diarrhea usually colonic.
- NSAID frequently cause bloody diarrhea.
- Pain and bloody diarrhea in an arteriopath may be due to ischemic colitis.
- Diarrhea can be watery or mixed with blood.

Causes

- *Infections*: Most common.
- *Drugs*: NSAID, metformin, antibiotics.
- *Colitis*: Ischemic, inflammatory bowel disease (IBD), radiation.
- History should be sought of foreign travel, antibiotic use, food history, occupation and other family members affected.

	Acute watery diarrhea	Dysentry (Diarrhea with blood)	Persistent diarrhea lasting more than 2 days
Rota virus	+	–	–
Enterotoxic *E. coli*	+	–	–
Enteroinvasive *E. coli*	+	+	+
Shigella	+	+	+
Salmonella (egg/chicken)	+	+	+
Campylobacter (milk/chicken)	+	+	+
TB	–	+	+
Giardia	+	–	+
Clostridium difficile	+	+	+
Entameba histolytica	+	+	+

- Tenesmus and urgency suggests proctitis.
- Acute diarrhea of less than 7–10 days is suggestive of an infective etiology.
- Ascertain any recent foreign travel (giardiasis, amebic dysentery), similar history among friends and family, any recent antibiotics or NSAID (in 2 wks).

- Also exclude malabsorption, thyrotoxicosis, laxative abuse, alcohol.
- Overflow and drugs, e.g. PPI, NSAID and bile acid malabsorption (BAM) by blood test for 7 alpha4 (OH) cholestene 3 one.
- Bloody diarrhea (colonic) is common feature of *Shigella, Salmonella, Campylobacter* enteritis, inflammatory bowel disease (IBD) and rarely (5%) in *Cl. difficle* infection.

Noninfectious Causes of Bloody Diarrhea

- Crohn's ulcerative colitis (UC), ischemic colitis, radiation colitis, Behçet's syndrome, colorectal carcinoma, and diverticular disease.
- 10% of flare up of UC have proven infection.
- Examine for tenderness, distension, volume depletion (pulse, temperature, postural hypotension, BP sitting and lying and mental state), arthritis, iritis, erythema nodosum, sepsis and toxic mega colon (marked abdominal distension and tenderness) and peripheral vascular disease (likelihood of ischemic colitis).

Investigations

- Full blood count (FBC), U and E, glucose, albumin, CRP, LFT.
- Stool microscopy and culture (hot stools for ameba), test for *Clostridium difficile* toxin in stool, blood culture if febrile.
- Sigmoidoscopy if bloody diarrhea, abdominal tenderness and erect abdominal X-ray and chest X-ray show marked distension.

CLOSTRIDIUM DIFFICILE COLITIS

- Colonization in the community 5%, surgical wards 20% and care home 30%.
- It is the most common cause of diarrhea acquired in the hospital.
- Acute diarrhea is due to toxin A (enterotoxin) and B (cytotoxin) produced by *Clostridium difficile*. Toxin assay sensitivity 63–99%.
- It is acute colitis, a complication of antibiotic therapy (Ampicillin, amoxicillin, cephalosporin and clindamycin).

- Diarrhea usually begins within 4–10 days of antibiotic treatment but sometime may not appear for 4–6 wks and elderly are more susceptible.
- Presentation range from mild self-limiting watery diarrhea to toxic mega colon.
- Diagnosed by detection of *C. difficile* toxins A and B in the stool and sigmoidoscopy may show adherent yellow plaques.

Risk Factors

Irritable bowel syndrome (IBS), use of PPI, immune suppression, recent surgery (in 30 days).

Treatment

- If hypervirulent strain 027—treat as severe as it produces × 23 time's toxins.
- Severity defined by raised temp >38.5, rise in creatinine >50% of base line, WBC >15000 and evidence of colitis.
- Supportive measures and isolation of the patient.
- Stop antibiotics if possible.
- *Mild*: Stools <3 (Bristol chart 5–7)/day, normal WBC—oral metronidazole 7–10 days.
- *Moderate*: Stools 3–5 (Bristol 5–7)/day, raised WBC <15,000—oral metronidazole.
- *Severe*: Stools 3–5 (5–7)/day, WBC >15,000, temperature >38.5 and X-ray signs—oral vancomycin.
- *X-ray signs*: Thickening of colonic wall, or loss of haustration, toxic dilatation or perforation and CT accordion sign alternate edema haustral folds and transverse mucosal ridges.
- Once WBC >49.000 and lactate >5 mortality with surgery is 63% and with medical treatment is 95%.

COMPLICATED *CLOSTRIDIUM DIFFICILE* COLITIS

- Hypotension, partial ileus or severe disease on X-ray or CT—oral vancomycin and IV metronidazole.
- In ileus give IV metronidazole + vancomycin by retention enema.
- Leukocytosis, shock and immune suppression are predictors of mortality.
- Surgery if age >65 yrs, WBC >20,000 and lactate >2.2.

- Life-threatening—complicating ileus or toxic mega colon—oral vancomycin and IV metronidazole plus consider subtotal colectomy.
- Around 20% will relapse due to germination of residual spores within the colon or reinfection or further antibiotic treatment. Give further course of metronidazole or vancomycin 125 mg 6 hrly for 7–10 days.
- Severely ill patients use vancomycin 500 mg 6 hrly otherwise 250 mg 6 hrly 14 days and then tapering three times daily for 7 days, reducing to twice daily for 7 days and then daily for 7 days.
- In severely ill patient vancomycin better than metronidazole.
- If unable to take orally then medication can be given IV metronidazole 500 mg 8 hrly for 7–10 days or IV vancomycin given through NG tube.

First Relapse

About 7–10 days course of metronidazole or vancomycin. Monitoring response to treatment by stool count, WBC, lactate and CRP.

Second Relapse

Metronidazole 400 mg tds for 7 days as for 1st relapse + probiotics.

Third Relapse

Vancomycin 125 mg 6 hrly if metronidazole used before or metronidazole if vancomycin used before, along with probiotics and monitoring as before. If at the end of 10 days, still not complete remission then pulse therapy or immunotherapy IgG 400 mg/kg or monoclonal antibody against toxin A and B.

Vancomycin 125 mg 6 hrly for on day 1, 3, 5, 7, 9, 11, 13, 15, 17, 19 and 21.

Further Relapse

Vancomycin as above plus colestyramine 4 gm bd or vancomycin 125 mg 6 hrly and rifampicin 600 mg bd for 7 days or IV immunoglobulin.

If previous *C. difficile* and patient is to go on antibiotics for any reason then add metronidazole 400 mg tds and for 3 days after stopping antibiotics.

CAMPYLOBACTER ENTERITIS

- Associated with fever, abdominal pain, and diarrhea; incubation period 2–6 days.
- Diarrhea initially watery later may contain blood and mucus.
- Usually self-limiting lasting 2–5 days but may be followed after 1–3 wks by Guillain-Barré syndrome.
- Diagnosed by culture of *Campylobacter jejuni* from stool.

Treatment

Ciprofloxacin 500 mg 12 hrly orally for 5 days or erythromycin 500 mg 12 hrly orally for 5 days.

NONTYPHOID SALMONELLAS

- Incubation period 1–3 days, associated with fever, vomiting, abdominal pain and diarrhea, may become bloody if colon is involved.
- Usually self-limiting.
- Diagnosed by culture of *Salmonella* species from stool.

Treatment

Ciprofloxacin 500–750 mg 12 hrly oral for 5 days or trimethoprim 200 mg 12 hrly for 5 days.

Known Inflammatory Bowel Disease or Sigmoidoscopy Suggests Ulcerative Colitis

Inflammatory bowel disease (IBD) is common in 3rd to 4th decade and M = F.

In ulcerative colitis (UC) there is diffuse superficial inflammation while in Crohn's disease (CD) is deeper transmural inflammation.

Appendectomy is protective in Crohn's disease and smoking may prevent ulcerative colitis (UC).

In rectosigmoid disease (limited disease) there is rectal irritation, tenesmus (sensation of incomplete emptying), small volume diarrhea and rectal bleeding predominates while in extensive colitis there is profuse bloody diarrhea, abdominal cramps, weight loss, fever and tachycardia.

If diarrhea is nocturnal then irritable bowel syndrome (IBS) is unlikely.

Crypt architecture is distorted in IBD while it is preserved in infectious diarrhea.

Exclude infection such as *Campylobacter, Shigella, Salmonella, Clostridium difficile* and amoebiasis.

Inflammatory bowel disease (IBD) is caused by IL23 (inter leukin), IL12b, IL10, genetics and immune response to unknown environment stimulus.

Fecal calprotectin test is surrogate marker for inflammatory bowel disease (IBD) and should be done to differentiate it from irritable bowel syndrome (IBS).

Other organs affected by UC by immune mediated inflammation,

Liver 5% (primary sclerosing cholangitis, autoimmune liver disease), joints 20% (seronegative arthritis of large joints, sacroiliitis, ankylosing spondylitis), eye 5% (scleritis, episcleritis, anterior uveitis) and skin 5% (erythema nodosum, pyoderma gangrenosum).

Mild Colitis

Apyrexial, pulse <90/min, Hb >120 g/L, ESR <10 and small amount of blood in stool.

Diarrhea stools <4/day in mild UC, >4 in moderate and >6 stools/day in severe UC.

Ultrasound is helpful in diagnosing ileal Crohn's (sensitivity 73–96% and specificity 90–100%).

Patients with Crohn's have impaired ability to clear bacteria from the gut and also have impaired blood flow.

Treatment

- 5-aminosalicylic acid (5-ASA) (Asacol or mezavant once a day) oral and local or local alone for proctitis or left sided disease. Mesalazine 2 gm/day if no response in 2 wks then switch to oral steroids or steroid enema if no infection.
- If diagnosis uncertain await stool culture and histology and consider barium enema or colonoscopy.

- Thiopurines/MTX (Methotrexate) used early in Crohn's disease (CD) as there is lack of efficacy of 5-ASA in CD and undesirability of steroids.
- Crohn's disease—Diagnosis → steroids—remission 55%, failure→AZA/MTX–remission 35%, failure 65% → Infliximab or adalimumab at wk 0, 2, 6 + AZA (Azathioprine).
- Budesonide 9 mg/day in Crohn's disease of terminal ileum.
- Tacrolimus has same effect as cyclosporine but beneficial in perineal Crohn's disease.
- If ASA started recently then stop.

ACUTE SEVERE COLITIS

Truelove and Witt's Criteria

Mild	Severe
Stools <5	>5 bloody stools/day
Temperature <37.5	Febrile >37.5°C
Pulse <90	Pulse >90/min
Hb >105	Hb <105 g/L
ESR <30	ESR >30
Small blood in stool	large volume blood in stools CRP >45 mg/dL and albumin<30 g/L.

Do not initiate 5-ASA drugs but if already on it then continue. Inform GI team, do abdominal X-ray (AXR) and stool culture × 3 including *C. difficile* toxin, FBC, U and E, LFT.

Treatment

- Intravenous hydrocortisone 100 mg 6 hrly for 5 days and then oral prednisolone 50 mg/day. Consider cyclosporine 2 mg/kg IV day 3–5 if not responding or infliximab 5 mg/kg if not in remission with steroids and azathioprine on discharge.
  All patients going on for azathioprine are tested for thiopurine methyltransferase (TPMT). This allows identification of 1/300 that develops bone marrow suppression due to deficiency of TPMT, or rectal steroid + oral prednisolone 50 mg/d + ASA (Mezavant XL 2.4 gm/day + local mesalazine).
- Prophylactic clexane to prevent thromboembolism 6.2% (atypical presentation of portal vein, mesenteric vein, cerebral sinus thrombosis).

- Correct fluid and electrolytes.
- Metronidazole
In severe UC infliximab + cyclosporin avoids colectomy.
On day 3 steroids if 8 + stools or CRP >45–85% get colectomy.
Transfuse if Hb <100 g/L.

Maintenance of Remission

Mezavant 2.4 g/day + salofalk (mesalazine) topical suppository 0.5 gm tds are corner stone, azathioprine for steroid dependent or frequent relapses.

Surgery

Perforation or massive hemorrhage, toxic mega colon, unresponsive acute stage or failed medical therapy.

Microscopic Colitis

Incidence 1–5/100,000, usually over 65 yrs, F:M 7:1,

Caused by celiac disease, NSAID, lansoprazole, aspirin, ranitidine, sertraline and sometimes luminal bacteria.

Presents as acute or chronic watery diarrhea, nocturnal diarrhea, fecal incontinence and abdominal cramps.

Differential diagnosis: Celiac disease, giardiasis, small bowel Crohn's, bile salt diarrhea, bacterial overgrowth of small bowel, lactose intolerance, irritable bowel syndrome (IBS), neuroendocrine tumors and postcholecystectomy syndrome.

Treatment

- Withdrawal of offending drug and use of antidiarrhea drugs.
- Treatment of celiac disease or with bile acid binding (Colestyramine).
- If persistent symptoms budesonide reducing course is effective.
- Other treatment options are metronidazole, 5 ASA (mesalazine).

Toxic Megacolon

- Toxic megacolon (TM) is colonic dilatation >6 cm + systemic toxicity (fever, tachycardia).
- Patient presents with diarrhea, abdominal pain and signs of systemic toxicity and abdominal tenderness. X-ray shows dilated colon >6 cm.
- Exclude low potassium (K), Low Mg, opiates and anticholinergic or antidiarrheal drugs as they can make dilatation worse.
- CT to diagnose perforation if localized pain or suspicion of perforation.
- Flexible sigmoidoscopy without preparation to confirm colitis and exclude cytomegalovirus.
- *Differential diagnosis*: Ulcerative colitis, Crohn's, *Clostridium difficile*, *Campylobacter* and ischemic colitis.

Pathology

Nitrous oxide (NO) inhibits muscle tone. Mucosa inflammation becomes transmural with neurogenic loss of muscle tone leading to dilatation of colon.

Treatment

Hydrocortisone 100 mg 6 hrly IV + oral vancomycin 125 mg 6 hrly + azithromycin 500 mg 6 hrly + fluids and correction of electrolytes. 50% of UC respond.

Next day abdominal X-ray, if dilation <6 cm continue medical management, if >6 cm or the same with toxicity then surgery.

Crohn's Disease

Cause

Chronic inflammatory disease of unknown etiology and can affect anywhere from mouth to anus but terminal ileum 35%, ileocecal valve 40% and colon 20%, 20–60 yrs of age and more common in women.

- There are skip lesions and affected bowel is thickened as a result of edema and fibrosis and there may be aphthous ulcers and transmural inflammation.

- Neutrophils are less marked in acute disease as compared to UC.
- Concordance in monozygotic twins is 37%.
- CARD15 (caspase recruitment domains gene) associated with ileal disease and chromosomes 6 HLA region associated with colonic involvement and presence of extraintestinal involvement.
- Smoking increases the risk 3 times.

Clinical Features

- Presents as diarrhea (70–90%), abdominal pain (45–66%), anal lesion (50–80%), rectal bleeding (45%), weight loss, (65–75%), fever (30–40%) and fistula (18%).
- Ileac disease often presents with malaise, weight loss, and abdominal discomfort and obstructive symptoms while colonic disease presents with rectal bleeding, perianal disease and extraintestinal manifestations.
- Rectum may be the only site involved in elderly patients and proctitis often accompanies ileal disease.
- Rarely mouth, stomach and duodenum are affected.

Complications

- Obstruction (ileal strictures are common), fistula formation (ileoilial, ileobladder or vagina) and perianal disease (fissures, fistula, abscess and fleshy skin tags violaceous hue in color). Strictures are more common.
- Recurrent UTI with pneumaturia indicates bladder fistula.
- Carcinoma in long standing crohns disease after 10 yrs is less than 5%.

EXTRA INTESTINAL MANIFESTATION OF CROHN'S DISEASE

- Iron, folate and B_{12} deficiencies are common.
- Raised ESR and C reactive protein are useful for monitoring disease activity.
- Fecal calprotectin (protein derived from neutrophils) can be used as an indicator of mucosal inflammation in IBD.

- Aphthous ulcers (20%), erythema nodosum (5-10%), pyoderma gangrenosum (0.5%), acute arthritis in large joints is transient and nondestructive (6-12%), conjunctivitis, uveitis and episcleritis (3-10%), sacroiliitis (18%), ankylosing spondylitis HLAB27 + (1-2%), gall stones, fatty change in liver (6%), amyloidosis and granulomata.
- Sigmoidoscopy and biopsy should be performed in all the patients as 33% of patients with small bowel involvement will have rectal Crohn's.

Investigations

- Small bowel enema (enteroclysis) barium directly introduced into small bowel by nasoduodenal tube and air-contrast barium enemas are for imaging intestine with barium.
- Technetium-99-HMPAO-labeled leukocyte scans demonstrate extent of inflammation if small bowel barium X-rays are equivocal.
- CT and MRI enteroclysis is helpful in determining small intestine strictures.
- Colonoscopy is useful to determine the extent of colonic involvement and obtaining ileal biopsy specimens.

Differential diagnosis: Acute terminal ileitis is usually due to *Yersinia* and these cases do not develop Crohn's. Major differential diagnosis of small bowel disease is TB.

Stool culture and antibody titer is not helpful. Trial of anti-TB therapy should be considered if there is a doubt.

Lymphoma, carcinoid, alpha chain disease, amyloidosis, Behçet's disease and carcinoma colon should also be considered.

For colonic disease, ulcerative colitis, ischemia, TB and lymphoma should be considered.

Full blood count, ESR, CRP and plasma protein electrophoresis will help whether further investigations are required.

Treatment

Previous management of Crohn's disease was combination of 5-ASA, intermittent steroids before moving on to immunomodulators (Azathioprine, methotrexate) and biologics.

Clinical features	Ulcerative colitis	Crohn's disease
Bloody diarrhea	Common	Less common
Abdominal mass	Rare	Common
Perianal disease	Less common	Common
Signs of malabsorption	None	Common (small bowel disease)
Rectal involvement	Invariable	Uncommon
Distribution	Continuous, mucosal	Segmental, transmural
Mucosa	Friable fine ulcers	Irregular deep ulcers, cobble stone appearance
Cellular infiltrate	Neutrophils, and eosinophils	Lymphocytes, plasma cells, macrophages
Glands	Gland destruction, mucin and crypt abscess	Gland preservation
Special features	None	Aphthous ulcers, granuloma, fissures

With this approach there is inevitable progression to stricture and fistula formation. With top down approach, using biologics and/or immunomodulators at or soon after diagnosis prevents these complications.

Diet: High fiber diet normally.
- Low residue diet if stricture, lactose free if hypolactasia and low fat if steatorrhea.
- Elemental diets (containing amino acids and glucose) and polymeric diets are as effective as steroids in active disease. But patients find them unpalatable and relapse rate is higher after remission by elemental diet. Parenteral nutrition is useful adjunct to medical therapy in malnourished patients.
- Folate, B_{12}, iron, vitamin D and other B complex vitamins are supplemented, if oral iron not tolerated then total intravenous dose of iron is given.

Steroids

Budesonide 9 mg (high rate 1st pass metabolism in liver, only 10% systematically available). Severe disease needs IV hydrocortisone 100 mg 6 hrly as in UC.

Prolonged steroids therapy is avoided.

Sulfasalazine 1 gm bd may be helpful in active colonic disease. Mesalazine may be helpful in active and long-term maintenance.

Azathioprine after thiopurine methyl transferase (TPMT) is the main enzyme for inactivating toxic products of azathioprine) test for continually relapsing or steroid dependent patients. This testing avoids bone marrow failure. The dose for azathioprine is 2–2.5 mg/kg/day. These drugs act slowly and effect may not been seen for several wks. Acute pancreatitis is uncommon complication of therapy. Treatment is effective for 5 yrs.

Methotrexate 25 mg/weekly in steroid resistant patients.

Metronidazole if associated sepsis (fistula or perianal disease) or bacterial over growth.

Infliximab 5 mg/kg IV, 0, 2, 6 wks for steroid resistant or perianal disease. Hydrocortisone 200 mg given 2 hrs before will avoid reactions.

Aloe vera and probiotics have also some beneficial effect.

Surgery for strictures, failure to respond to medical therapy, fistula and perianal disease. Resection should be minimal, covered by steroids and bypass procedures are avoided.

11
Blood

Sickle Cell Crisis

Sickle cell disease is autosomal recessive condition caused by mutation in B globulin gene of hemoglobin which changes glutamic acid to valine.

Sickle cell disease (HbSS) produces symptoms while HbAS (sickle trait) is asymptomatic.

Sickle hemoglobin (HbS) is insoluble when deoxygenated forms a long polymer with a rigid sickle shape cell with tendency to cause vaso-occlusion (infarction), hemolysis, vasculopathy, oxidative stress, hypercoagulability and inflammation.

It is common in Nigeria, democratic republic of Congo, African Americans, India, American-Africans and eastern Mediterranean.

HAND-FOOT SYNDROME

Sickle cell disease (HbSS) presents at the 6th months of life (when HbF has fallen to the adult level) as dactylitis as painful swelling of hands and feet as a result of vaso-occlusion. It is treated with analgesics and is rare after 2 yrs of age. Penicillin prophylaxis is given up to IST 5 yrs of life to prevent most frequent pneumococcal infections in childhood.

ACUTE PAIN IN LIMBS AND BACK

Acute pain is due to vaso-occlusion causing ischemic tissue damage, inflammation and pain in 10–30 yrs of age. On assessment look for infection, sepsis and dehydration. Initial treatment includes keeping warm, drinking plenty of fluids and analgesics.

Following are indications for hospital admission:
- Severe pain not responding to simple analgesics and weak opioids.
- Dehydration caused by vomiting or diarrhea for IV fluids.
- Severe sepsis temp >38°C or hypotension.
- Symptoms or signs of acute fall in hemoglobin.
- New neurological symptoms or signs. HbSS is the most common reason for stroke in children and presents as hemiparesis, speech problem, seizures and altered level of consciousness and are managed with blood transfusion to lower the HbSS levels. Urgently admit any patient with headache or any neurological impairment.
- Acute enlargement of liver or spleen or increase in jaundice.
- Hematuria or fulminant priapism recurrent episodes or lasting >2 hrs.

ACUTE CHEST SYNDROME

Chest pain, cough, tachypnea, oxygen saturation 5% below the steady state and signs of lung consolidation.

This is due to combination of infection, vaso-occlusion and endothelial dysfunction. The infectious agents are chlamydia, mycoplasma, respiratory syncytial virus and less often strep pneumonia due penicillin prophylaxis and vaccination.

Treatment is bronchodilators, broad-spectrum antibiotics, ventilator support and blood transfusion in severe cases. Patients with coexisting asthma are particularly vulnerable.

ANEMIA

In HbSS hemoglobin 70–80 g/L is common and well tolerated. Two common causes of acute fall in Hb >20% are splenic sequestration in which spleen rapidly enlarges and traps blood cells due to sepsis or parvovirus B19 causing slap cheek syndrome and reticulocytopenia. Urgent blood transfusion is lifesaving. Splenectomy is advised if two or more episodes of infection with splenic sequestration.

There is increased risk of osteomyelitis due to salmonella and acute chest syndrome in HbSS.

PREVENTION OF COMPLICATIONS IN HBSS AND HBS/BETA THALASSEMIA

- Penicillin prophylaxis at least up to age 5 yrs or throughout life.
- Routine childhood vaccination including protection against *Haemophilus influenzae* type B and *Streptococcus pneumoniae* and immunization against *Meningococcus*, influenza and hepatitis B.
- Dress adequately to prevent cold, windy weather and rainy season as precipitant of acute pain.
- Ensure adequate hydration.
- Avoid skiing because of exposure to cold provokes vaso-occlusion.
- Prolonged exercise in cold weather prohibited.
- Hydroxy urea usually started if more than two episodes of acute pain or after the severe episode acute chest syndrome. Hydroxy urea should be stopped 3 months before pregnancy. Regular blood transfusions are used in pregnancy with severe clinical course such as episodes of pain or acute chest syndrome.
- Progestin only or combined hormonal contraception was safe in women with sickle cell disease.
- Children with severe HbSS or HbS/Beta thalassemia should be offered stroke prevention with annual transcranial Doppler scan and blood transfusion.
- Chronic pain is related to tissue damage such as leg ulcers, avascular necrosis of head of femur or humerus or chronic osteomyelitis. Patients are monitored yearly for micro albuminuria (common in childhood) and treated with hydroxyurea and angiotensin converting enzyme (ACE) inhibitor when proteinuria approaches nephrotic range. Pulmonary complications include restrictive lung disease and pulmonary hypertension which are treated with blood transfusion, hydroxyurea and prostaglandins.

Chronic Myeloid Leukemia

Cause

Common in males 35–50 yrs, acquired chromosomes defect Philadelphia chromosome (PH), translocation of ABL gene from 9 PH to 22 PH) and translation of this oncogene (BCR-ABL) has increased tyrosine kinase which drives the overproduction of myeloid cells. Benzene and ionizing radiation are rare risk factors.

In chronic myeloid leukemia (CML) normal hematopoiesis is replaced by clone of cells with PH which affect the stem cell, so PH is present in red cells, granulocytes, platelets and lymphocytes.

Clinical Presentation

Patient presents with hypermetabolic symptoms such as weight loss, anorexia, lassitude, sweating, splenomegaly often >10 cm, hepatomegaly, anemia and gout.

Stable chronic phase usually lasts 3–5 yrs, accelerated phase with increasing white blood cell (WBC) and splenomegaly, myelofibrosis may develop and terminal blast crisis lasting 2–4 months.

Investigation

Anemia, raised WBC often 250×10^9 (250,000 per micro liter or per cubic mm), thrombocytosis. Neutrophil alkaline phosphatase low or absent differentiates it from leukemoid reaction. Blood film shows neutrophilia with several myelocytes and basophils.

Treatment

Tyrosine kinase inhibitor imatinib blocks BCR-ABL and produce very durable remissions (>10 yrs), along with allopurinol. Allogenic bone marrow transplant is curative but is dangerous over 50.

Chronic Lymphatic Leukemia (CLL)

There is excessive production of clone of abnormal lymphocytes involving blood, bone marrow and lymphoid tissue. These normal looking B lymphocytes functionally are useless, weakly expressing surface immunoglobulin.

Gene defect–trisomy 12, rarely under 40.

Clinical

Many asymptomatic patients are diagnosed on routine full blood count (FBC) and the disease progresses slowly, while others present with malaise, bone marrow failure, immune deficiency, hepatosplenomegaly, high lymphocyte count, lymphadenopathy and bone marrow invasion.

Recurrent opportunistic infections (pneumonia, aggressive herpes zoster with scarring and pain) are common. Autoimmune hemolytic anemia (5–10%) or autoimmune thrombocytopenia (1–2%) sometimes may be presenting feature

Lymphocytes $7–50 \times 10^{*}9$ (7500 per micro liter or per cubic mm) B cells with expression of marker CD5.

The 60% have hypogammaglobulinemia with low IgG and IgA.

Treatment

- Asymptomatic patients require no active therapy. Bacterial or herpetic infections are rapidly treated, if severe hypogammaglobulinemia, monthly IV immunoglobulin is given.
- If mass effect from lymphadenopathy then chlorambucil or fludarabine is given to reduce symptoms. Steroids are used if hemolytic anemia or thrombocytopenia is present.

Polycythemia Rubra Vera (PRV)

Cause

It is acquired mutation which activates genes for tyrosine kinase which regulates cell proliferation in the bone marrow. In PRV there is overproduction of red cells.

If there is overproduction of platelets resulting in essential thrombocythemia (ET) or overproduction of bone marrow matrix with disturbed functions resulting in idiopathic myelofibrosis.

Hematocrit (Hct) is raised >0.52 in men and >0.48 in women. Hemoglobin (Hb) is raised >18 gm in males and <16 gm in females, increased red cell mass, and platelet and WBC count may also be high.

Diagnosis

In secondary polycythemia erythropoietin is raised and red cell mass is normal. While in PRV erythropoietin is normal and red cell mass is raised. Blood is positive for Janus associated kinases (JAK2) V617F.

Clinical Features

About 50% present with arterial or venous thrombosis (CVA, MI, digital ischemia, DVT, thrombosis of portal, splenic or hepatic vein). Sometimes it can occur before the rise in HCT, so unprovoked arterial or venous thrombosis should prompt JAK2 testing.

Plethoric appearance with splenomegaly, loss of concentration, memory impairment, headache and dizziness are other symptoms. 10% suffer with gout and 15% have noticeable pruritus after hot bath or shower. Excessive bruising or bleeding from trauma or peptic ulcer is due to abnormal platelet functions. Massive splenomegaly suggests myelofibrosis.

Secondary polycythemia has raised erythropoietin. It is associated with high altitude, cyanotic congenital heart disease, pulmonary disease, hypoventilation, obesity, heavy smoking, renal disease (hypernephroma, cysts), hepatoma, cerebellar hemangioma and uterine fibroma.

Investigation

Full blood count (FBC) and film, JAK2V617F screen, ferritin levels and basic biochemistry. For diagnosis Hct (hematocrit) is >0.52 in men and 0.48 in women. O_2 saturation is always >92% (below 92% suggests secondary polycythemia).

Abdominal ultrasound and CT to exclude underlying renal pathology

Management

- Venesection (400 mL every 2–4 weeks) target Hct <0.45 and aspirin as antiplatelet.
- Cytoreduction if patient >60 yrs or unable to tolerate venesection or there is thrombocytosis, systemic symptoms or symptomatic splenomegaly.
- First line therapy is interferon <40 yrs old and hydroxycarbamide for >40 yrs.

ANEMIA

Iron-deficiency anemia (IDA) microcytic hypochromic—hemoglobin (Hb) <12.5 g% in males and <11.5 g% in females, ferritin <15 ng/L and MCV <76; if ESR raised then ferritin <50 and total iron binding capacity (TIBC) raised.

Screen for celiac disease, upper gastrointestinal (GI) blood loss by OGD and lower GI by colonoscopy.

Anemia of Chronic Disease (ACD), Normocytic Normochromic Anemia

Causes: Chronic inflammation, autoimmune diseases, cancer, chronic renal failure and chronic heart failure, causes raised hepcidin from liver.

Mechanism: Hepcidin binds ferroportin and blocks iron export from macrophages and hepatocytes and down regulates iron absorption from duodenum. RBC survival is decreased in ACD and normal response of increased erythropoietin to low Hb is also blunted. Serum iron levels are low. Ferritin is normal or high and total iron binding capacity (TIBC) low or normal. Serum iron levels and transferrin saturation are low but if ferritin is <100 ng/mL in ACD, it indicates coexistent IDA and will respond to iron supplementation oral/IV.

	IDA	ACD	Sideroblastic anemia	Thalassemia
Ferritin	Low	Normal/high	Increased	Normal
Serum iron level	Decreased	Decreased	Increased	Normal
Iron binding capacity	Increased	Decreased	Normal	Increased
Hepcidin	Low	Raised	Low	Low
Inflammatory markers	Low	Raised		
Transferrin saturation	Low	Low	Normal	Normal
Soluble transferrin receptor (sTfR)	High	Low		

Other causes of normocytic normochromic anemia (ACD) should be excluded, i.e. hemolysis, hypothyroidism, hypogonadism, myelodysplastic syndrome (MDS) and nutritional deficiencies.

Raised hepcidin is associated with vitamin D deficiency.

Strongyloides stercoralis: Diagnosed by stool test or serology test for IgG to filariform larval antigen. Treatment is with ivermectin 200 µg/kg two doses 2 wks apart or albendazole 400 mg twice daily for 7 days.

Blood Transfusion

Nonbleeding patients with hemoglobin <80 g/L can be transfused one unit of red cells at a time and reassessed.

Stop NSAID two weeks before orthopedic surgery, stop clopidogrel 3–5 days before surgery but aspirin can continue except neurosurgery or ocular surgery.

Emergency reversal of anticoagulation with warfarin is prothrombin complex 25–50 µg/kg and vitamin K 5 mg intravenous and for dabigatran or rivaroxaban is intravenous prothrombin complex.

12
Pulmonary

- Breathless patient with normal chest X-ray CXR
- Low PaO_2 [asthma, chronic obstructive pulmonary disease (COPD), pulmonary embolism (PE), pneumocystis, smoke inhalation, foreign body].
- Normal or high PaO_2 [metabolic causes like diabetic ketoacidosis (DKA), hyperventilation, anemia].

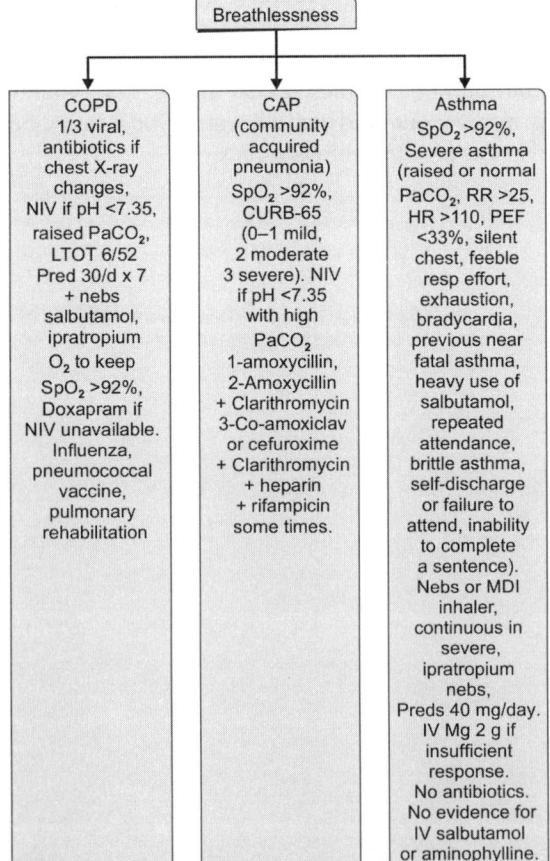

Breathlessness

COPD
1/3 viral, antibiotics if chest X-ray changes, NIV if pH <7.35, raised $PaCO_2$, LTOT 6/52 Pred 30/d x 7 + nebs salbutamol, ipratropium O_2 to keep SpO_2 >92%, Doxapram if NIV unavailable. Influenza, pneumococcal vaccine, pulmonary rehabilitation

CAP (community acquired pneumonia)
SpO_2 >92%, CURB-65 (0–1 mild, 2 moderate 3 severe). NIV if pH <7.35 with high $PaCO_2$
1-amoxycillin,
2-Amoxycillin + Clarithromycin
3-Co-amoxiclav or cefuroxime + Clarithromycin + heparin + rifampicin some times.

Asthma
SpO_2 >92%, Severe asthma (raised or normal $PaCO_2$, RR >25, HR >110, PEF <33%, silent chest, feeble resp effort, exhaustion, bradycardia, previous near fatal asthma, heavy use of salbutamol, repeated attendance, brittle asthma, self-discharge or failure to attend, inability to complete a sentence). Nebs or MDI inhaler, continuous in severe, ipratropium nebs, Preds 40 mg/day. IV Mg 2 g if insufficient response. No antibiotics. No evidence for IV salbutamol or aminophylline.

RESPIRATORY FAILURE

- Type 1 (Oxygenation failure)—normal $PaCO_2$ and low PaO_2 <8 kpa.
  Causes: Acute respiratory distress syndrome (ARDS), pneumonia, LVF, PE, pneumothorax, asthma and interstitial lung disease (ILD).
- Type 2 (ventilation failure) raised $PaCO_2$ and PaO_2 can be normal.
  Causes: Opiates, COPD, head injury, Myasthenia gravis (MG), Guillain-Barré syndrome (GBS), polio, cervical spine injury and motor neuron disease (MND).

Assessment

- RR usually >30, using accessory muscles, speaking sentences, tachycardia, decreased peripheral perfusion, altered level of consciousness (LOC), SpO_2 <92%, ABG.
- Noninvasive ventilation (NIV)/CPAP
- *COPD*: pH <7.35, $PaCO_2$ >6 KPa, RR >24

Contraindication to Noninvasive Ventilation

Facial trauma or burns, vomiting, confused or agitation, impaired conscious level, copious respiratory secretions, hemodynamic instability, focal consolidation on chest X-ray, pneumothorax, bowel obstruction, severe co morbidity, edentulous.

Lung volume reduction surgery in predominant upper lobe emphysema has significant benefit.

Acute Asthma

- Airway hyper-responsiveness, airway inflammation and airway remodelling (smooth muscle proliferation) are the main features of asthma.
- Most cases begin in childhood associated with atopy.
- Adult onset (often misdiagnosed because of similar characteristics to COPD) is usually nonallergenic.
- Smoking contributes to severity of asthma by enhancing steroid resistance.
- Usual presentation is breathlessness and difficulty in speaking, wheezy, chest tightness and cough with previous history of asthma.

- Symptoms are usually worse on rising or during night (3-6 am) and provoked by number of triggers. Onset may be rapid (hours) or gradual (days).

Mild Persistent

- Symptoms are more than once/wk but less than once/day, nocturnal symptoms once in 2 wks and normal lung functions between episodes.
- Treated with low dose inhaled corticosteroids 100–200 µg/day.
- Inadequate control on low dose corticosteroids 200–800 µg/day.

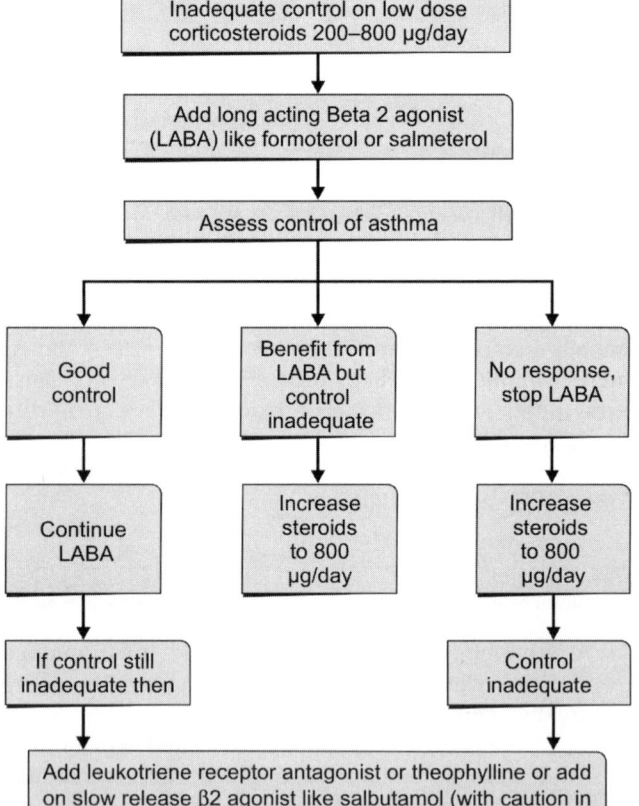

Moderate Acute or Persistent

- Daily symptoms, nocturnal symptoms at least 1/wk, exacerbations may affect sleep and activity.

- Peak expiratory flow (PEF) rate 50–75% of predicted or previous best. No features of acute severe asthma.
- Treated with inhaled corticosteroids budesonide up to 800 µg/day + long acting beta 2 agonist formoterol.

Severe Persistent

Symptoms daily, frequent exacerbations, frequent nocturnal symptoms and FEV1 <60% predicted, or

Acute severe asthma: Peak expiratory flow rate (PEFR) 33–50% of best, cannot speak a sentence in one breath, RR >25/min and pulse >110.

Life-threatening asthma: PEFR <33%, SpO_2 <92%, PaO_2 <8, $PaCO_2$ normal (4.6-6.0), silent chest, cyanosis, feeble respiratory effort, bradycardia, hypotension, exhaustion and confusion.

Near fatal asthma: Raised $PaCO_2$, needs ventilator.

Brittle asthma: PEFR variability >40% for 50% of the time or sudden severe attack in spite of good control. Oral steroids >50% of year or require inhaled steroids >1.2 mg/day.

Biomarkers

- Sputum cell count and fraction of nitric oxide (NO) <15 ppb in exhaled breath.
- Eosinophilic bronchitis is steroid responsive keeping eosinophil count <3%, while noneosinophilic bronchitis is usually not.

Controlled symptoms	Sputum eosinophil's	Symptoms not controlled
↓ Steroids ↓ Bronchodilators	<1%	↓ Steroids ↑ Bronchodilators
No change ↓ Bronchodilators	1–3%	No change ↑ Bronchodilators
↑ Steroids ↓ Bronchodilators	>3%	↑ Steroids ↑ Bronchodilators

Are All Symptoms due to Asthma? Differential Diagnosis

Consider rhinitis, bronchiectasis, COPD, pulmonary hypertension, cardiomyopathy, cystic fibrosis, gastroesophageal reflux disease (GERD), smoking, obesity, allergy to pets (cat, dog) at home and aspirin, paradoxical movements of vocal cords, dirty occupation (dusty environment), chronic infections and psychosocial morbidity.

Exacerbation-prone Asthma

It is the hall mark of severe asthma and poor outcome, low FEV1, African race, early onset, exacerbation in response to aspirin or NSAID or menses, depression and anxiety.

Asthma Defined by Age at Onset

Early onset asthma <12 yrs have greater likelihood of allergic sensitization (house dust mite, furred animals, season pollen and atopy), more likely have eczema or family history of asthma.

Allergic Asthma

Common in childhood asthma but also present in adults.

Occupational Asthma

- Accounts for 15% of adult onset asthma and immunologically mediated.
- Airway inflammation is similar to allergic asthma except in this there is fibrosis of bronchial wall, epithelial denudation and fibrohemorrhagic exudates in submucosa without eosinophil's.
- Asthma recedes if exposure promptly discontinued but once the process is established, symptoms continue even in the absence of exposure.

Precipitating Factors

- In severe asthma in 60% of patient's perennial allergens derived from house dust mite, cockroaches and fungi (*Aspergillus*, alternaria) contribute to on-going disease.
- Bronchopulmonary aspergillosis is rare but important as it leads to bronchiectasis.
- Air pollutants and infections have greater importance.
- Late onset asthma should raise awareness of occupational asthma (igE dependent) diagnosed by peak expiratory flow rate (PEFR) monitoring in and out of work pace. Smoking also causes deterioration and frequent exacerbations of asthma.

Adverse Drug Effects

- Asthma airways need constant B2 receptor stimulation, so beta-blockers are contraindicated.
- Angiotensin receptor blocker (ARB), adenosine, NSAIDs and aspirin intolerance are associated with deterioration of asthma. Obstructive sleep apnea and vocal cord dysfunction are also associated with severe asthma.
- Asthma is 2–3 times more common in women.
- There is strong association with menstruation and obesity.
- Relapses with thyrotoxicosis and improves in 2nd and 3rd trimester of pregnancy.
- Coexistence of nasal polyposis, chronic rhinitis and sinusitis also contributes to severity of asthma.
- In mild to moderate asthma mainly allergic pathway with inflammation are sensitive to steroids while severe asthma involves remodelling with Th2 (T helper cells), cytokines (TNF alpha, IL13), leading to submucosal fibrosis and changes in smooth muscle becoming more superficial and increased mucus production.
- Factors maintaining activation of epithelial-mesenchymal trophic unit (EMTU) are house dust mite, repeated viral infections and air pollutant including smoking.

Measurement of Airflow Obstruction

Reversible airflow obstruction is indicative of asthma:
- >20% diurnal variation in PEF (at least 60 mL) for >3 days a week for 2 consecutive weeks.
- >15% improvement in FEV1 (at least 200 mL) after 400 μg salbutamol via MDI and spacer or 2.5 mg nebulized salbutamol.
- >15% improvement in FEV1 (at least 200 mL) after a trial of steroids (30 mg/day for 14 days).
- Objective evidence of eosinophilic airway inflammation, sputum eosinophilia and blood eosinophilia.

Clinical Severity Markers

- Pulse >110/min, respiratory rate >25/min and too breathless to complete a sentence.
- PEF <50% of predicted normal or best known, predicts acute severe asthma and <33% as life-threatening.

- SpO_2 <92% and PaO_2 <8 kPa.
- $PaCO_2$ >6 kPa is ominous while normal $PaCO_2$ (4.6–6.0 kPa) implies life-threatening episode.
- Use of accessory muscles.
- Respiratory acidosis H+ >45 mmol/L or pH <7.35.
- If one or more of these signs are present inform ICU and anesthetist.
- Normal RR is consistent with patient being near to death if they are exhausted.
- Always check carefully for signs of pneumothorax.

Management

- Give O_2 40–60%,
- Salbutamol 5 mg nebulized driven by O_2 6 L/min if available and hydrocortisone 100 mg IV and/or prednisolone 40 mg orally.
- ABG if any feature of life-threatening attack or SpO_2 <92%.
- Intravenous access.
- Chest X-ray (CXR) to exclude pneumothorax and pneumonia.
- Repeat salbutamol nebulizer every 15–30 minutes if necessary.
- Add ipratropium bromide 500 µg to nebulized salbutamol if asthma severe or not improving.
    If no response to repeated nebulized bronchodilator and IV hydrocortisone then exclude upper airway obstruction (stridor, laryngeal edema) before considering IV magnesium sulfate.
- IV magnesium sulfate (1.2–2 g IV infusion over 20 minutes) if not improving after salbutamol and steroids. Repeated doses of magnesium sulfate can give rise to hypermagnesemia, muscle weakness and respiratory failure.
- Aminophylline infusion in acute asthma is not likely to result in any additional bronchodilation hence should be avoided.
    Methotrexate, cyclosporine, subcutaneous terbutaline and omalizumab (anti-IGE) are used as prednisolone sparing agents. Anti-TNF also increases airway response. Some patients with acute asthma require rehydration and correction of electrolyte imbalance. Hypokalemia can be caused or exacerbated by salbutamol or steroids and must be corrected.

Omalizumab is recommended for patients with severe persistent allergic IgE mediated asthma confirmed by history and allergy skin testing. If in previous year had >2 severe exacerbations requiring hospital admission or >3 severe exacerbations and one requiring hospital admission then consider omalizumab.

Assessment of Response

- Less distressed, able to talk sentences, decreased HR and RR.
- Louder breath sounds on auscultation.
- ABG should be repeated in 30 minutes if there is no or poor response to treatment.
- SpO_2 should be used to monitor if initial $PaCO_2$ was not high and patient is improving.
- PEF should be repeated after 30 minutes.
- Monitor HR and SpO_2 continuously.

Admit intensive unit (ITU)—if
- Exhaustion
- Confusion, drowsiness, coma
- Normal or high $PaCO_2$
- ABG worsening
- Deteriorating
- Worsening respiratory acidosis.

Antibiotics

Only minorities of asthma attacks are provoked by bacterial infection and antibiotics are not routinely prescribed. Antibiotics are prescribed if there is focal shadow on chest X-ray indicating pneumonia or fever or purulent sputum.

On discharge from hospital or A and E, oral prednisolone 40 mg/day for 7 days and then stop (taper if brittle or recent courses), inhaled steroid, salbutamol and correct inhaler for them.

Allergic Bronchopulmonary Aspergillosis

About 1–2% of asthmatics affected with colonization of lungs with *Aspergillus fumigatus*.

Clinical Features

Asthma, proximal bronchiectasis and pulmonary infiltrate on chest X-ray, positive skin prick test to aspergillus, IgE >400 kU, eosinophilia, mucus plugs containing aspergillus or polymerase chain reaction (PCR) on bronchial alveolar lavage (BAL) or respiratory fluid.

Suspect aspergillosis if unresolving pneumonia on antibiotics or unresolving wheeze despite being on steroids or cavitation on CXR/CT, new nodules on CT or poorly controlled asthma.

Risk Factors

Neutropenia, on steroids, low CD4, COPD, cirrhosis, bilateral infiltrates. Multi cavity is the hall mark of cavitating pulmonary aspergillosis.

Treatment

Voriconazole 4 mg/kg bid or itraconazole 400 mg/day in addition to the treatment already on helps.

Community-acquired Pneumonia (CAP)

Symptoms

Suspect pneumonia if there are acute respiratory symptoms cough, purulent sputum, breathlessness, pleuritic chest pain, rigors, fever, malaise and myalgia.

Nonrespiratory symptoms include confusion, upper abdominal pain and diarrhea.

Consider contact with birds (Psittacosis); travel abroad or hotel stay (*Legionella*), contact with farm animals or cats (*Coxiella burnetii*).

Majority are due to *Streptococcus pneumoniae*, *Mycoplasma* (11%), *Legionella* (common in September–October) 50% related to travel.

Signs

Abnormal chest signs (dullness, crackles, bronchial breathing, and pleural rub at the site) present in 80% of patients. Other signs are tachypnea (RR >20), tachycardia, cyanosis, sputum (mucopurulent, rusty or blood stained) and herpes labialis.

Prognostic Factors

- CURB-65 ccore
- C (confusion) AMT <8/10
- U (urea >7 mmol/L)
- R (respiratory rate 30 or >30)
- B (blood pressure systolic <90 mm Hg or diastolic 60 or <60 mm Hg)
- Age 65 or >65.

Additional Features

- Presence of co-existing disease
- Hypoxia SaO_2 <92%, PaO_2 <8 kPa
- Bilateral or multi lobular involvement.

CURB 65 score 0–1: Mortality low 1.5% and are suitable for home treatment.

CURB 65 score 2: Mortality intermediate 9.2%, consider hospital supervised treatment short stay in patient or outpatient.

CURB 65 score 3 or more: Managed in the hospital as severe pneumonia and ICU if score 4 or 5.

Intensive Treatment Unit (ITU)

If hemodynamically compromised:
- PaO_2 <8 kPa (type 1 respiratory failure) despite adequate supplemental O_2
- Progressive hypercapnia PCO_2 >6.5 (type 2 respiratory failure)
- Severe acidosis pH <7.26
- RR >30–35, SpO_2 <92%.

Noninvasive Ventilation (NIV)

If pH <7.35, $PaCo_2$ >6, RR >30.

Noninvasive ventilation (NIV) contraindicated if facial trauma, vomiting, impaired consciousness, confusion or agitation, copious respiratory secretions, edentulous and pneumonia on X-ray.

NIV: EPAP 5–8 cm, IPAP 12–15 cm, rate 15, regular assessment 1–2 hrly along with ABG.

If Neutropenic

If temperature >38°C for 4–6 hrs or patient is toxic, assume septicemia and start broad-spectrum antibiotics after blood culture, piperacillin and netilmicin + vancomycin? Continue antibiotics until a febrile for 5 days. If fever persist consider CMV, pneumocystis (Co-trimoxazole 60 mg IV 12 hrly 14 days) or fungal (*Candida*, *Aspergillus*) Fluconazole 50–200 mg/day.

Investigations

- Chest X-ray.
- Full blood count, U and E.
- Urine analysis and urine for pneumococcal and *Legionella* antigen testing (greater sensitivity rates then blood or sputum cultures and are less effected by previous antibiotic use).
- ABG if SpO_2 <92% (record FiO_2 concentration).
- Blood culture (can be omitted in patients with non-severe CAP and no comorbid illness).
- Sputum culture.
- C-reactive protein (CRP) if less than 50 then consider other diagnosis but level does not correlate with prognosis. Serial CRP is useful, if CRP level does not fall by 50% within 4 days then consider failure of treatment or development of complications.
- Serology for titers (*Legionella*, *Mycoplasma*).
- Differential diagnosis of pneumonia
  - Pulmonary embolism
  - Pulmonary edema
  - Bronchial carcinoma
  - Pulmonary vasculitis
  - Pulmonary hemorrhage
  - Acute extrinsic allergic alveolitis
  - Subdiaphragmatic abscess.

Empirical Antibiotic Choices in an ill Patient

CURB65 1–2 moderately sick: Amoxycillin or amoxicillin + clarithromycin.

CURB65 3 or more: Co-amoxicav or cefuroxime + clarithromycin.

If preceding influenza and cavitation on chest X-ray consider Staph and add flucloxacillin and treat for 3 wks.

Co-amoxiclav covers everything that cefuroxime does and upper GI anerobes, orally active.

Gentamicin	Gram-negative sepsis
Ceftriaxone	Neurological features
Soft tissue infection	Benzyl penicillin and flucloxacillin
Metronidazole	Lower GI tract.

COMMUNITY-ACQUIRED (CA) METHICILLIN-RESISTANT *STAPHYLOCOCCUS AUREUS* (MRSA)

Treated with ciprofloxacin or cotrimoxazole or clindamycin.

METHICILLIN-RESISTANT *STAPHYLOCOCCUS AUREUS* (MRSA) PANTON–VALENTINE LEUKOCIDIN (PVL)

If recurrent skin/soft tissue infection, narcotizing pneumonia/narcotizing fasciitis/purpura fulminans, severally ill (RR >30, HR >140), young, multilobar pneumonia, hemoptysis, leukopenia and evidence of influenza infection before consider community acquired MRSA. Gram's stain and culture of sputum or bronchial lavage/brush is helpful. Treat with linezolid 600 mg bd + clindamycin 1.2 gm qds as these will switch of PVL (Panton valentine leukocidin) Staph. If not improving then IV + IgG + rifampicin.

HOSPITAL-ACQUIRED (HA) METHICILLIN-RESISTANT *STAPHYLOCOCCUS AUREUS* (MRSA)

Vancomycin intravenous 1 gm bd.

Initial Treatment of CAP

- O_2 (high concentration) to correct hypoxemia and to keep SpO_2 >92% or PaO_2 >8 kPa. Monitor $PaCO_2$ in COPD patients.
- Intravenous fluids (3 L/day) to correct hypovolemia and prevent renal dysfunction.
- Bronchodilator therapy with nebulized salbutamol and ipratropium should be given to patient's if previous history of COPD or asthma.
  Exceptions to standard therapy
  - *Alcoholics*: Increased risk of aspiration and legionella, cover with metronidazole + macrolide.

- *Nursing homes*: Gram -ve and anerobes, lower threshold for metronidazole.
- *Bronchiectasis*: Most will be colonized with pseudomonas and will require tazocin or ceftazidime and aminoglycosides.

Consider PCP (*Pneumocystis jiroveci* pneumonia) even if chest X-ray normal if IV drug user or suspected immune compromised. Treat with high dose co-trimoxazole

- Nonsevere CAP without comorbidity in the community
  Amoxicillin 0.5–1.0 g 8 hrly or IV ampicillin 0.5–1.0 g 6 hrly.
  Clarithromycin 500 mg 12 hrly in patients allergic to penicillin.
- Nonsevere with comorbidity (COPD, CCF, immune suppression, renal failure, liver disease and diabetes)
  Amoxicillin 500 mg–1.0 g 8 hrly PO or IV plus Clarithromycin 500 mg 12 hrly.
  Alternatively levofloxacin 500 mg bid po or moxifloxacin 400 mg od po.

Consider adding rifampicin 600 mg bid IV in *Legionella* infections.

If the patient already had antibiotics from GP, find out what and for how long and modify the treatment accordingly.

If atypical pneumonia is suspected add clarithromycin 500 mg bd.

In pneumococcal pneumonia—treat until a febrile for 3 days.

In *Mycoplasma, Legionella, Chlamydia,* staphylococcal, pneumonia treat for at least 2 wks.

Rough Guide

Severe pneumonia: Aminoglycosides or ciprofloxacin + pipercillin/tazobactam or ceftazidine/imipenem.

If MRSA then teicoplanin/vancomycin.

Nonresponding Patient

- *Incorrect diagnosis*: Consider PE/bronchial carcinoma/ eosinophilic pneumonia, foreign body, unexpected pathogen and pneumococcal resistance.
- *Local/distant complication*: Parapneumonic effusion/ empyema
- *Simple parapneumonic effusion*: Clear fluid, pH >7.2, gram stain and culture negative.
- *Complicated parapneumonic effusion*: Clear/cloudy or turbid, pH <7.2, LDH >1000.

Empyema

Frank pus: Pleural fluid to be sent for pH (in ABG syringe), culture including AFB in blood culture bottles, for protein, LDH, glucose and cytology.

Treatment

Intercostal drain, IV cefuroxime or tazocin + metronidazole for 21 days.

Early involvement of cardiothoracic surgeon if it fails to resolve. No role for intrapleural streptokinase.

Postoperative Patient with Pneumonia or PE

Acute dyspnea and fever are features of both. Pneumonia is favored by initial fever > 39°C, WBC >15000 and purulent sputum. If you remain uncertain, treat for both conditions until VQ or CT pulmonary angiography (CTPA) scan is done.

Aspiration Pneumonia

Suspect aspiration if pneumonia develops in patients with disordered swallowing or after a period of reduced conscious, cardiopulmonary resuscitation, stroke, poisoning with alcohol, psychotropic drugs and ketoacidosis. Antibiotics cover should be broad range (before culture results) Amoxicillin/clavulanate or ciprofloxacin plus clindamycin or metronidazole.

Discuss with a chest physician whether bronchoscopy should be done to remove the particulate matter from the airways.

INDICATIONS FOR BRONCHOSCOPY

- Suspected foreign body inhalation
- No organism identified from blood or sputum and patient not responding to antibiotics (especially in immune compromised patient or if TB is suspected).
- Cavitating pneumonia with negative sputum microscopy and culture.
- Lobar or segmental collapse with significant hypoxia.
- Persistent (>1 wk) segmental or lobar collapse.

- Slow resolution of symptoms and signs (CXR shadowing may take up to 6 wks to clear completely)
- Recurrent pneumonia at same sight.

Pleural Effusion and Empyema

Patient presents with breathlessness and chest pain (implies pleural inflammation and suggestive of exudative process, e.g. malignancy, pleural infection or infarction).

Massive effusions are commonly malignant. Mesothelioma is increasingly common cause of effusion and history of asbestos exposure should be elicited from occupational history, i.e. work in construction, insulation, ship building industry, electrical repair, carpentry or plumbing.

Investigations

Chest X-ray

- Pleural effusion is visible on CXR at volumes of 200 mL and clinically at 500 mL.
- *Pleural fluid analysis*: Aspiration of pleural fluid (except LVF) is an important investigation for appearance, protein, LDH, pH, culture and sensitivity, cytology and additional tests (glucose, amylase and triglycerides).
- Simple effusion pH >7.2, complicated effusion pH <7.2.
- Transudate (pleural fluid protein <30 g/L) and exudates (pleural fluid protein >30 g/L).
- Transudate is the result of increased hydrostatic pressure or decreased osmotic pressure in the microvascular circulation while exudate is due to increased capillary permeability and or impaired lymphatic drainage.
- When pleural fluid protein is 25–35 g/L then Light's criteria is used to distinguish transudate and exudates.

Light's Criteria

Pleural effusion is exudate if it meets one or more of the following criteria:
- Pleural fluid protein to serum protein ratio >0.5
- Pleural fluid LDH to serum LDH >0.6
- Pleural fluid LDH more than 2/3 the upper limit of normal LDH.

Causes

Transudate	Exudate
LVF	Parapneumonic effusion and empyema
Cirrhotic liver disease	Malignancy
PE (10–20% are transudates)	PE
Nephrotic syndrome	Mesothelioma
Hypothyroidism	TB, RA, SLE and other connective tissue diseases
Malignancies 5% are transudate	Esophageal rupture, pancreatitis
Atelectasis	Chylothorax and drug induced

Drug-induced pleural effusion: Amiodarone, nitrofurantoin, phenytoin, methotrexate, carbamazepine, procainamide, propylthiouracil, penicillamine, granulocyte colony stimulating factor (GCSF), cyclophosphamide, bromocripitine.

Low pH Effusions

A very low pH <7.3 may follow bacterial or tumor cell metabolism and often is accompanied by low pleural fluid glucose (<3.3 or pleural fluid glucose/serum glucose <0.5).

This type of effusion is common in para pneumonia effusion or empyema, malignant effusion, RA, TB, esophageal rupture and lupus pleuritis.

Pleural fluid amylase is raised in esophageal rupture, pancreatitis and pleural malignancy.

Disruption to thoracic duct (by trauma, lymphoma) results in chylothorax with milky appearance of pleural fluid and high TG >110 mg/dL.

Computed Tomography Chest

Pleural Biopsy

Computed tomography or ultrasound or thoracoscopy guided for exudative effusions. Thoracoscopy biopsy has 80–95% sensitivity for malignancy and pleurodesis can be done at the same time. Bronchoscopy is unhelpful and blind (Abram's) biopsy is insensitive in TB.

Treatment

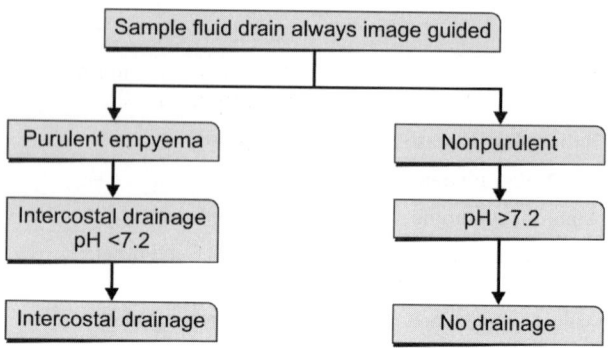

If community-acquired: Cefuroxime + metronidazole or coamoxiclav or vancomycin + ciprofloxacin + metronidazole.

If hospital acquired: Vancomycin + meropenem.

Contrast-enhanced CT if Still Substantial Effusion

Fluid can be removed for symptomatic relief by aspiration 1–1.5 L or intercostal chest drain. With the drain there is significant morbidity and mortality and always use ultrasound guided technique.

Parapneumonic Effusion

It complicates half of all pneumonias, common in young people usually sterile and resolves with antibiotics for pneumonia, but in few becomes infected (empyema) and requires drainage procedure.

The pH of the fluid <7.3 and LDH >1000 is highly suggestive of infection (empyema) and has a mortality of 20%.

	Empyema score	
R–renal –urea >7	0–2	Mortality 2–3% drainage + antibiotics
A–age >65	3	Mortality 25% Earlier referral and aggressive treatment
P–protein <25	4–5	Mortality 68%
I–in patient empyema		
D–diastolic BP <70 mm Hg		

Malignancy

This is the most common cause of exudative infusion over 60 yrs.

Most cases represent metastatic disease, the primary sites being lung, breast, lymphoma, genitourinary tract and gastrointestinal tract but in 10% primary site remains unknown.

Pleural fluid cytology is sensitive 60% for the diagnosis of malignancy.

Pleural thickening on CT is highly suggestive of malignancy and image guided or thoracoscopic pleural biopsy is required in cytology negative cases.

Malignant pleural disease generally has poor prognosis with a survival of 3-12 months from the diagnosis.

Mesothelioma

It is a malignant tumor of pleura and peritoneum resulting from asbestos exposure with lag time of 20-40 yrs between exposure and disease.

Pleural fluid cytology is relatively insensitive for mesothelioma but confirms alternative diagnosis. Mesothelioma has tendency to invade needle and biopsy tracks in the chest wall so minimal definitive investigations (image guided CT or thoracoscopic biopsy) should be done. All pleural aspiration or biopsy sites are marked with ink tattoo for prophylactic radiotherapy which is effective in preventing chest wall invasion.

Treatment is supportive including pleurodesis for symptomatic effusion. There is no benefit from surgery or chemotherapy at present and median survival 8-14 months.

Acute Exacerbation of Chronic Obstructive Pulmonary Disease (COPD), Long-term Oxygen Therapy (LTOT) and Noninvasive Ventilation (NIV)

DEFINITION

Chronic slowly progressive disorder characterized by airway obstruction with FEV1/FVC <70%, abnormal response to gases (cigarettes) and raised CD4, CD8 involved in pathogenesis of COPD and this immune mechanism of inflammation persists even after stopping smoking.

- *Mild*: FEV1 80% or less.
- *Moderate*: FEV1 >50 % or <80%.
- *Severe*: FEV1 >30% or <50%.
- *Very severe*: FEV1 <30%.

Usual smoking history is of 20 pack years (20/day/yr = 1 pack year) or more.

Most of the lung functions impairment is fixed with some reversibility with bronchodilators.

Exclude (AAT) alpha1 antitrypsin deficiency if COPD in less than 45 yrs.

Alpha 1 antitrypsin is a protein secreted in liver, neutralizes neutrophil elastase which digest the wall of alveoli.

These patients with family history of COPD and with irreversible lung function tests, if present are treated with stopping smoking, yearly pneumococcal and influenza vaccine, intensive COPD therapy and ultimately bilateral lung transplant if needed.

Asthma is excluded by its characteristics such as larger day to day variation, earlier onset, coexistence of other atopic diseases and marked nocturnal symptoms.

In unclear cases the response to 14 days of systemic steroids 30 mg/day or 6–8 wks of inhaled corticosteroids with increase in FEV1 (300–400 mL) confirms asthma.

Type 1 Respiratory Failure

It is characterized by hypoxia, low or normal $PaCO_2$, impaired gaseous exchange across alveolar membrane.

Causes

Pneumonia, pulmonary edema, pulmonary fibrosis, pulmonary embolus (PE), pneumothorax, pulmonary artery hypertension and acute respiratory distress syndrome (ARDS).

Type 2 Respiratory Failure

High $PaCO_2$ with hypoxia.

Causes

Alveolar hypoventilation, COPD, myasthenia gravis, polyneuropathies and CNS diseases.

Symptoms

- Increased breathlessness (more than usual and recent change).
- Increased wheeze (more than usual and recent change).
- Chest tightness.
- Increased cough and sputum volume (more than usual volume/purulence recent change)
- Effort tolerance usual (ability to cope with daily activities, distance walked on the flat, number of stairs climbed without stopping) and recent change.
- New or increased ankle edema.
- Requirement for home nebulized bronchodilator and O_2 therapy.
- Social circumstances and quality of life, whether living alone or alone with support or whether house bound.
- Number of previous admission to hospital, ICU and whether previously ventilated.
- Smoking history.

Signs

- Confusion and decrease conscious level
- Cyanosis
- Tachypnea (RR >20)
- Wheeze, use of accessory muscles with increased work of breathing
- Pyrexia and/or purulent sputum
- *Signs of cor pulmonale*: Raised JVP, right ventricular heave, right ventricular gallop, loud P_2, congested liver, ascites, and peripheral edema.

Investigations

- Full blood count, U and E, PEFR, theophylline plasma levels for patients on theophylline
- Chest X-ray
- Arterial blood gases (ABG), record inspired O_2 concentration.
- Normal pH = 7.38–7.42, PaO_2 = 13.3 (100 mm Hg), $PaCO_2$ = 5.3, base excess –2 to +2,
- ECG
- Sputum culture and blood culture (if febrile or focal shadowing on chest X-ray).

Causes

- Usually 50% viral and 50% bacterial and 25% both.
- *Bacteria*: Haemophilus influenzae, Streptococcus pneumoniae, Haemophilus parainfluenzae, Moraxella catarrhalis, Pseudomonas aeruginosa.
- *Viruses*: Rhino, influenza, parainfluenza, respiratory syncytial and corona virus.
- *Pollutants*: Ozone, sulfur and N_2 dioxide.

Treatment

Smoking cessation with combination therapy (Salmetrol, Fluticasone and Teotropium) reduces inflammation and is helpful in prevention and treatment of exacerbations. In severe air flow limitation (FEV_1 <50% predicted normal) or two or more exacerbations a year add on therapy of inhaled corticosteroids to long acting bronchodilators is suggested as a long-term.

- *Oxygen*: Give O_2 28% via venturi mask 4 L/min or 2 L/min via nasal prongs to maintain SaO_2 >90%, and salbutamol 5 mg plus ipratropium 500 µg nebulized while making rapid clinical assessment.

  If $PaCo_2$ is normal then aim for SaO_2 is 94–98%, if $PaCO_2$ is raised then the aim is 88–92%. Nebs are driven by air and not O_2 if $PaCO_2$ is raised or pH <7.4.
  - O_2 nasal prongs 1 L (venturi 2–4 L/min) = 24%, O_2 range in normal 96–98%
  - 2 L (venturi 4–6 L/min) = 28%, O_2 range in COPD 88–92%
  - 4 L (venturi 8–10 L/min) = 35%, O_2 target in COPD >92%
  - Venturi 10–12 L/min = 40%
  - Venturi 12–15 L/min = 60%

  Face masks up to 50%, venturi system up to 50%, and reservoir bag up to 80%.

- ABG should be done with in 60 minutes of starting O_2 or changing inspired O_2

  Aim to keep PaO_2 >6.6 kPa and H^+ <55, if the PaO_2 is responding and the effect on H^+ is modest then increase the inspired O_2 to achieve PaO_2 >7.5 kPa.
  - If pH <7.35 or H >45 nmol/L and $PaCO_2$ >6.0 consider NIV.
  - If pH > 7.35 or H <45 nmol/L and $PaCO_2$ >6.0 kPa keep SpO_2 88–92% and nebs driven by air and not O_2
  - If $PaCO_2$ <6.0 keep SpO_2 94–98%.

- SpO$_2$ is indirect measurement of oxygen content of blood by oximetry.
- PaO$_2$ or PaCO$_2$ is direct measurement by ABG (arterial blood gases sampling).
- *Bronchodilator*: Nebulized salbutamol and ipratropium bromide can be repeated 4–6 hrly. For distressed patient, salbutamol can be repeated more often. For patients with hypercapnia, use compressed air for nebulizer and deliver O$_2$ via nasal prongs.
- Aminophylline IV 250 mg (5 mg/kg) infusion over 20 minutes, only if patient is not improving after repeated salbutamol nebulizer and is not on oral theophylline's. Follow this with an infusion of aminophylline 750–1500 mg over 24 hrs.
- Prednisolone 40 mg/daily should be given to all patients for 7–14 days unless contraindicated. Give 200 mg hydrocortisone IV if patient cannot take orally. No need to taper off if steroids given for <3 wks.
- *Antibiotics*: Give antibiotics if signs of infections, Amoxicillin (Erythromycin in penicillin allergic patient) nonsevere without comorbidity, coamoxiclav (nonsevere with comorbidity) or ceftriaxone or coamoxiclav + clarithromycin (severe with comorbidity).
- Diuretics indicated if there is raised JVP with peripheral edema.
- Long-term O$_2$ therapy (LTOT) when PaO$_2$ <7.3 on 2 occasions 3 wks apart and patient stable. PaO$_2$ 7.30–7.38 if polycythemia, pulmonary hypertension, nocturnal hypoxemia or peripheral edema.
  - *Benefits of LTOT*: Increased survival, prevention of deterioration of pulmonary hypertension, reduction of secondary polycythemia, improved sleep quality, reduction in cardiac arrhythmia, reduction in exacerbation and hospitalization and neuropsychological improvement.
- If active and desaturates on 6 meters walk test SpO$_2$ <90 prescribe O$_2$ LTOT, if low activity then cylinder short burst for relief of breathlessness.
- In air flight if SpO$_2$ >95%—O$_2$ not needed
  - SpO$_2$ 92–95%—O$_2$ not needed
  - SpO$_2$ 92–95% with risk factors Ca lung, weak respiratory muscles, FEV1 <50%—O$_2$ needed 2–4 L/min.
  - SpO$_2$ <92%—O$_2$ needed.

AF if present should be rate controlled with digoxin. LMWH used for thromboprophylaxis in all patients. Attention should be given to hydration and nutrition.

Relative Contraindication to Early Assisted Hospital Discharge

Acute onset, confusion, worsening peripheral edema, new chest X-ray abnormality, poor performance status, concomitant unstable disorders, adverse social condition, acidosis or marked hypercapnia or hypoxia.

- NIV (noninvasive positive pressure ventilation via face mask) BIPAP should be 1st line of management after 1 hr of medical treatment if patient is still acidotic pH <7.35 with respiratory rate >23. If pH between 7.3–7.35 and patient reluctant to NIV then continue medical therapy. However if pH <7.3 or <7.25 NIV strongly advised.
- NIV provides positive inspiratory pressure (14/7 cm of H_2O, starting with 10 and max 20), reduces work of breathing and off loads tiring respiratory muscles and positive expiratory pressures (5 cm of H_2O, max 10) splints open the airways, reduces the atelectasis and the work of breathing.
  - Continuous positive air pressure (CPAP) for type 1 respiratory failure, e.g. pulmonary edema, pneumonia and obstructive sleep apnea and bilevel positive air pressure (BiPAP) for type 2 respiratory failure, e.g. COPD.
  - BiPAP can also be used in pulmonary edema along with buccal or IV nitrate. It is indicated in acute exacerbation of COPD.
  - Cardiogenic pulmonary edema.
  - Hypoventilation syndrome due to obstructive sleep apnea syndrome (OSA), obesity and hypoventilation syndrome. Hypoxic respiratory failure in immune suppressed.
- Check ABG after 1 hr starting NIV and improvement in pH, $PaCO_2$ or reduction in RR are good prognostic signs. If no improvement check patient is wearing the mask, it is comfortable with out leaks and ventilator is in synchrony with the patients' effort. Check ABG in 4 hrs.

Indication of NIV

- Patients with respiratory failure SpO_2 <88–90%, PaO_2 <7.5 kPa, $PaCO_2$ >6 kPa, pH <7.35 or H+ 45–55 nmol/L and rising $PaCO_2$, RR >25/min, use of accessory muscles, awake and strong cough.
- Failure to respond to optimal conventional treatment.
- Respiratory distress with use of accessory muscles should be considered for NIV and respiratory team should be involved.

  Patient with impending respiratory arrest (feeble respiratory effort, deteriorating conscious level) should be considered for endotracheal intubation and mechanical ventilation.

  Benefit from doxapram infusion is the same as from NIV and only considered if NIV not available.
  - H^+ after maximum standard therapy >55 nmol/L then ventilate if H^+ 45–55 then either NIV or doxapram infusion.

Factors to Encourage NIV

- Demonstrable, remedial reason for current declines.
- First episode of respiratory failure.
- Acceptable quality of life before admission, avoids intubation, decreased need for sedation, able to eat and drink, improve ability to communicate.

Following do not Benefit

Altered conscious state, pH <7.25, noncompliance, confusion, agitation, uncontrolled vomiting, GI bleeding, facial/cranial trauma, copious respiratory secretions, pneumonia on chest X-ray, pneumothorax, asthma, hemodynamically unstable.

Factors to Discourage NIV

- Previously diagnosed severe COPD, fully assessed and unresponsive to therapy.
- Poor quality of life (e.g. house bound) despite maximal therapy.
- Severe comorbidity, decreased ability to cough, facial skin necrosis, increased aspiration risk.
- Copious respiratory secretions.

How to Apply

- Explain and choose correct interfaces and size (total face mask (covers mouth nose and eyes), nasal mask, mouth piece and helmet.
- Set pressures, start low (pressure support 8 cm of water and peep 4–5 cm of water.
- Place interface gently over the face and start ventilation.
- When patient tolerant tighten the straps to avoid leaks but not too tight.
- Set FiO_2 on ventilator aiming SpO_2 >90%.
- Consider use of mild sedation.
- Humidification if application >6 hrs.

Doxapram infusion 1 mL/min (5% 500 mL dextrose containing 2 mg/mL) may be considered if mechanical ventilation is not appropriate and NIV is not available.

ABG should be checked after 1 hr and if PaO_2 <6.5 kPa and pH <7.25 or H+ >55, increase the infusion rate to maximum of 2 mL/min.

Patient not Improving Despite Treatment

Wrong diagnosis: Consider pneumonia, PE, pulmonary edema, pneumothorax and other causes of respiratory failure.

Inadequately treated infection: Consider changing to cefuroxime or cefotaxime IV and adding erythromycin.

Inadequate bronchodilator therapy: Check that nebulizers are being run at the correct flow rate. Nebulized salbutamol and ipratropium can be given 2 hrly.

Check plasma K as salbutamol and steroids may result in significant hypokalemia.

Treat multifocal atrial tachycardia with verapamil if HR >110/min.

On discharge long acting beta 2 agonist and tiotropium (moderate COPD with FEV1 > 50% and <80%) and corticosteroid inhalers (if severe COPD with FEV1 >30% and <50% and repeated exacerbations) reduce exacerbation.

Lung Volume Reduction Surgery

It is helpful in patients with primary upper lobe emphysema and low exercise capacity with FEV1 >20%. No effect on mortality but improves exercise capacity.

PNEUMOTHORAX

Consider pneumothorax in any patient with sudden breathlessness or chest pain, particularly in young fit adults or after invasive procedures, e.g. subclavian vein puncture, lung biopsy, chest aspiration, acute exacerbation of COPD or asthma.

Clinical signs are reduction in lung expansion, a hyper resonant percussion note and diminished breath sounds on the affected side. Presence of hypotension and tachycardia may indicate tension pneumothorax.

Consider computed tomography (CT) chest if loculated pneumothoraces, to distinguish pneumothorax from large bullae and radiologically guided drain insertion.

It can be classified as primary and secondary.

SECONDARY PNEUMOTHORAX

This is caused by lung disease or trauma and requires admission in the hospital for at least 24 hrs and also requires more active management.

A rim of air <2 cm on inspiratory chest X-ray (CXR) film is regarded as small pneumothorax and a rim >2 cm is large pneumothorax and implies >50% of hemithorax is filled with air.

Pneumothorax is large when >2 cm measurement from lung margin to chest wall at the level of hilum.

PRIMARY PNEUMOTHORAX

There is increased porosity in the visceral pleura.

Pneumothorax on inspiration on chest X-ray (CXR) <2 cm rim (small) and >2 cm rim (large).

Risk Factors

Smoking, tall, thin, male, 15–34 yrs. Marfan syndrome., thoracic endometriosis (pneumothorax associated with menses).

Height is thought to be a risk factor as pressure gradient increases from base to the apex of the lung. So apical alveoli are subjected to far greater distending pressure in taller patients, which may precipitate subpleural cyst formation.

All patients admitted for observation should receive high flow O_2 (10 L/min by mask) unless COPD. Air reabsorption is 2%/day and increases to 8%/day with O_2 as O_2 displaces nitrogen in the pleural spaces.

Needle Aspiration

Identify 3rd–4th intercostal space in mid axillary line. Infiltrate with lidocaine down to pleura over the pneumothorax. This should follow explaining the procedure and thorough cleansing of the skin.

Connect a 21G (green needle) to a three-way tap and 60 mL syringe.

With the patient semirecumbent (45 degrees) needle into the pleural space withdraw air and expel it via the three-way tap. Obtain chest X-ray to confirm resolution of pneumothorax.

Stop Aspiration

- If more than 2.5 L aspirated
- Resistance is felt
- Excessive coughing.

Chest drains (10–14 F catheter) are required in the following:
- Tension pneumothorax
- Failed aspiration of primary pneumothorax (unsatisfactory resolution or breathlessness).
- All patients with secondary pneumothorax except asymptomatic patient with small pneumothorax <50 yrs old and these can be aspirated.
- History of chest trauma (CPR related pneumothorax and CVP line).
- Ventilated patient.

Surgical Advice Should be Sought

- If there are bilateral pneumothoraces
- Lungs fail to re-expand after intercostal tube drainage in 3–5 days.
- History of previous one or more pneumothoraces on the same side as the current episode.
- History of pneumothorax on the other side.
- A persistent air leak or hemothorax.
- Divers, pilots and others with an occupational risk.

TENSION PNEUMOTHORAX

Tension pneumothorax is a clinical diagnosis, not radiological.

Signs

- Patient looks as though they are about to die.

Pulmonary

- Gasping respiratory effort.
- Asymmetrical chest being prominent on side of tension.
- Cyanosis, low SpO_2 and low PaO_2.
- Hypotension with raised JVP.
- Raised airway pressures if ventilated.
- Tracheal deviation away from the side of clinical signs.
- Reduced air entry, reduced expansion and hyper-resonance to percussion, vocal resonance and vocal fremitus on side of pneumothorax.

Management

- 100% O_2.
- 10–14 G cannula inserted perpendicular to the skin. Aspirate mid-axillary line above the level of nipple on the affected side.
- This can be converted to a temporary underwater seal drain with a blood giving set and a container of water until formal chest drainage is achieved.
- Give analgesia.
- Formal intercostal drain insertion.

Chest X-ray (CXR) to check position and re-expansion.

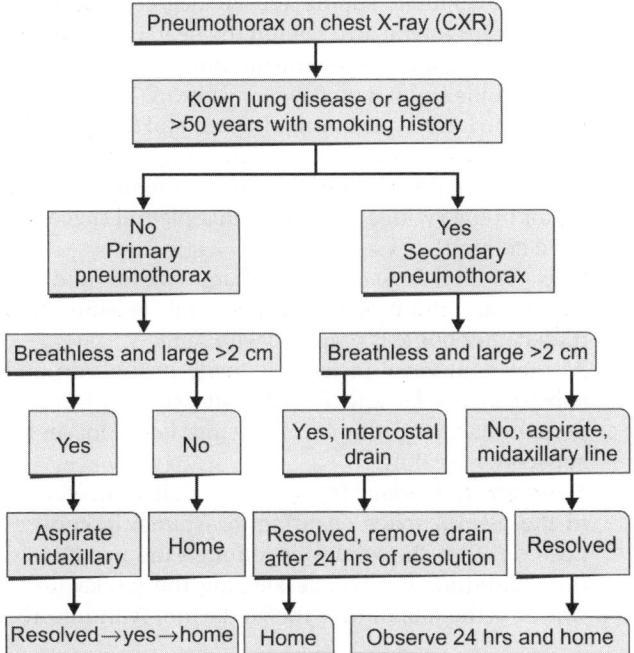

Aspirate midaxillary line above the level of nipple on the affected side.

Fit to fly after six weeks but should avoid flying for 1 yr as increased risk of recurrence.

No diving permanently.

Consider suction (-10 cm H_2O) after 48 hrs and after thoracic surgical opinion. In professionals (divers or pilots) thoracic surgical opinion should be sought in the beginning.

Intercostal Drainage Tube Insertion

- Explain the procedure to the patient.
- O_2 and IV access.
- Flumazenil and atropine should be available as profound bradycardia can occur during pleural manipulation.
- Premedicate anxious patient with midazolam 1–2.5 mg IV. Analgesia including morphine may be required.
- Look at the chest X-ray and mark the site (4th or 5th inter costal space in midaxillary line) with pen on the patient chest (line of nipple).
- Place the patient supine (20–30 degrees) with the patient's ipsilateral arm behind the head (note patient 45 degree supine in needle aspiration).
- Wash hands and put on gown and gloves.
- Clean the lateral chest wall, drape it and infiltrate the skin with 1% lidocaine 10–20 mL using initially blue needle later green aspirating intermittently (looking for air in the syringe to confirm that pleural space has been entered).
- Select 10–14 F chest drain tube (large size for fluid).
- Check all drain connections and ensure that underwater bottle is prepared with fluid.
- A small transverse incision is made in the skin and subcutaneous fat and two 2/0 silk sutures inserted perpendicular to the incision and leave loose for subsequent sealing.
- *Seldinger technique*: Insert the supplied needle in to the pleural space ensuring to aspirate to confirm position. Pass the guidewire through the needle and then withdraw the needle keeping the guidewire *in situ*. Pass the dilator over the guidewire. Withdraw the

dilator and pass the chest drain over the guidewire in the pleural space and withdraw the guidewire.
- Connect drain to underwater seal bottle, release clamp (look for bubbling and swinging of water column confirming position in the pleural space) and secure drain with 2/0 suture (one loop through skin and 4 ties on tube).
- Apply dressing (swab and elastoplast), and secure with plaster.
- For check chest X-ray (CXR).
- Instruct patient to keep water bottle below waist level and prescribe adequate analgesia.
- Tube should not normally be clamped under any circumstance.
- Suction should not be applied for 48 hrs.
- Chemical pleurodesis with talc or tetracycline derivative (minocycline) only should be considered if on going air leak and not fit for surgery.

13
Bronchiectasis

Patient may be under weight, clubbed, breathless, frequent productive cough, sputum pot nearby (copious sputum), inspiratory crackles heard with unaided ear over the zone or with stethoscope and wide spread rhonchi.

Differential diagnosis: Carcinoma lung (heavy nicotine staining, lymph nodes), fibrosing alveolitis (no copious sputum), lung abscess and cystic fibrosis. In this usually there is lack of smoking history, young age and recurrent exacerbations of chronic obstructive pulmonary disease (COPD) like symptoms.

There is permanent dilatation of bronchi and bronchioles with impaired mucociliary clearance leading to bacterial colonization with *Pseudomonas aeruginosa* of normally sterile airways and excessive bronchial inflammation.

Investigations

Sputum culture, protein electrophoresis, *Aspergillus* IgE, high resolution computed tomography (HRCT) and bronchoscopy.

Assessment of Severity

Sputum color and volume: In severe disease sputum is purulent and volume >25 mL/day.

Lung functions: Obstructive usually but may be restrictive.

Causes

Respiratory infections in childhood (whooping cough, measles, TB), cystic fibrosis (<40 yrs, *Staphylococcus* in sputum, primary male infertility, upper lobe disease and diagnosed by sweat chloride).

Hypogammaglobulinemia, yellow nail syndrome (curled yellow nails, bulbous finger tips, lymph edema), bronchial atresia and Kartagener's syndrome (ciliary immotility, dextrocardia, situs inversus, dysplasia of frontal sinuses, sinusitis, otitis media).

Treatment

- Chest physiotherapy, postural drainage (twice daily) or active cycle breathing.
- Bronchodilators before physiotherapy or nebulizer with hypertonic saline (7%).
- Lung functions tests for reversibility before long-term bronchodilators with long acting agents and anticholinergics.

Antibiotics

Long-term (6/12) antibiotics erythromycin or azithromycin may be considered who have >3 exacerbations /year.

Try to get the sputum sample. If organism are *Streptococcus pneumoniae* or *Haemophilus influenzae* then amoxycillin 500 mg tds or 1 g bd or 3 g bd (severe cases) as 1st line and clarithromycin 500 mg bd 2nd line.

Haemophilus influenzae (B Lactamase+) or *Moraxella catarrhalis* then co-amoxiclav 625 mg tds 1st line and doxycycline 100 mg bd or clarithromycin 500 mg bd or ciprofloxacin 500 mg bd or ceftriaxone 1–2 g daily IV as 2nd line.

Staphylococcus aureus: Flucloxacillin 500 qds as 1st line and clarithromycin 500 mg bd.

Methicillin-resistant *Staphylococcus aureus* (MRSA)

Oral therapy: Rifampicin 600 mg OD + trimethoprim 200 mg bd as 1st line and rifampicin + doxycycline 200 mg OD. Rifampicin dose reduced if weight <50 kg to 450 mg daily.

Vancomycin or teicoplanin IV as 1st line and linezolid oral or IV as 2nd line.

Coliform (*Klebsiella, Enterobacter*): Ciprofloxacin 500 mg bid as 1st line and ceftriaxone 1–2 gm daily IV.

Pseudomonas: Tazocin 4.5 gm tds IV or ciprofloxacin 500 mg bd or 750 mg bd (severe infection) as 1st line and ceftazidime 2 gm tds IV or meropenem 1 gm tds IV or aztreonam 2 gm tds IV or each of the above can be combined with gentamicin or tobramycin or colomycin as 2nd line.

If no previous sputum samples or mixed flora then amoxicillin 500 mg tds or clarithromycin 500 mg bd.

Bronchodilators and mucolytics (Carbocystein).

No role of steroids.

Surgery: Localized disease not responsive to medical therapy or severe hemoptysis.

Transplantation if <60 yrs, FEV1 <30%, respiratory failure, pulmonary hypertension and rapid deterioration.

PNEUMOCYSTIS PNEUMONIA

Caused by *Pneumocystis jirovecii*.

Suspect in immune suppressed patients on steroids 20 mg/day for 4/52, on immunosuppressant's methotrexate (MTX), cyclophosphamide, TNF alpha inhibitors, cancer patients on cytotoxic drugs, ALL patients on antileukemic therapy, HIV not on HAART, CD4 <400, Hodgkin's and non-Hodgkin's lymphoma.

Symptoms

New onset of dyspnea, cough, fever, indolent pneumonia on chest X-ray (CXR), oral candidiasis, Seborrheic dermatitis and Kaposi sarcoma.

Assessment

PaO_2 <8 severe, PaO_2 -8-11 moderate and PaO_2 >11 mild. Adjuvant steroids if PaO_2 <9.3.

Treatment

Cotrimoxazole 120 mg/kg/day for 3 days in divided doses, then 90 mg/kg/day IV for moderate to severe disease and oral for mild for 17 days in non-HIV. 4–7 days of treatment is needed before improvement occurs in temperature, hypoxia and symptoms.
- IV pentamidine
- Clindamycin + primaquine
- Dapsone + trimethoprim
- Atovaquone
- Caspofungin.

Causes of Treatment Failure

- Fluid overload, pneumothorax, intercurrent infection, methemoglobinemia and postbronchoscopy deterioration.
- Start highly active antiretroviral therapy (HAART) as soon as improvement is evident on chest X-ray and clinically (after 2/52 of cotrimoxazole).

14
Carcinoma of Bronchus

Clubbing of fingers, nicotine staining, loss of weight, persistent cough and lymph node in the neck are highly suggestive.

On examination sinus rhythm (SR), jugular venous pressure (JVP) normal, trachea central, percussion note (PN) decreased (stony dullness), vocal fremitus, vocal resonance and breath sounds decreased over R/L base indicating Ca bronchus causing pleural effusion.

Lymph nodes in axilla, wasting of small muscles of hand and sensory signs including loss of pain over T1 and Horner's syndrome (ptosis, miosis, enophthalmos, ipsilateral anhidrosis), may further suggest the possibility of carcinoma of bronchus.

The R/L thoracotomy scar, trachea deviated R/L, expansion diminished, PN more resonant and breath sounds harsher. Patient has lobectomy in the past to remove the tumor.

Diagnosis is carcinoma of lung and Pancoast tumor in the latter case. Bronchoscopy is usually diagnostic.

Complications:
- SVC obstruction
- Edema of face and upper limbs, nonpulsatile engorged neck veins and dilated superficial veins, stridor and hepatomegaly (metastasis).

Nonmetastatic complications: Hypertrophic pulmonary osteoarthropathy, neuropathy, cerebellar degeneration, encephalopathy, proximal myopathy, polymyositis, reversed myasthenia or Eaton-Lambert syndrome, SIADH, ectopic ACTH, ectopic PTH, gynecomastia, DVT or thrombophlebitis migrans, nonbacterial thrombotic endocarditis, anemia, acanthosis nigricans and herpes zoster.

Pneumonectomy or Lobectomy

There is deformity of the chest with flattening on R/L with thoracotomy scar. The trachea is deviated to the R/L side and apex beat is displaced in the same direction. Expansion is reduced and percussion note is dull and breath sounds are diminished. There may be bronchial breathing in the R/L upper zone (over deviated trachea).

After lobectomy signs are more localized, there is deformity of the chest, thoracotomy scar, lower ribs pulled in, tracheal central or displaced to the side, percussion note dull and breath sounds diminished and usually no bronchial breathing (unlike in pneumonectomy).

Surgery has little role in small cell carcinoma. About 25% nonsmall cell Ca undergo surgical resection after CT chest, abdomen, bone scan and LFT. Surgical resection of solitary pulmonary nodule is considered some times for bronchiectasis (recurrent hemoptysis when other treatments have failed).

Idiopathic Pulmonary Fibrosis (IPF) or Usual Interstitial Pneumonia (UIP)

Short of breath on exertion, cough, clubbing, cyanosis and fine mid or late inspiratory velcro like crackles or crepitation's.

Causes to excluded—Chronic obstructive pulmonary disease (COPD), asthma and connective tissue disease like rheumatoid arthritis (rheumatoid hands, rheumatoid nodules), systemic sclerosis (mask like faces, telangiectasia, sclerodactyly), SLE (typical rash), Sjögren's syndrome (dry eyes, dry mouth), polymyositis (proximal muscle weakness and tenderness), dermatomyositis (heliotrope rash over eyes, back of hands, around knuckles, nail fold telangiectasia, subcutaneous edema around eyes and polymyositis), ulcerative colitis, chronic active hepatitis (CAH) and drugs (Amiodarone, nitrofurantoin, bleomycin and busulfan).

Diagnosis: Age >50 yrs, bibasal inspiratory velcro like crackles.
- Unexplained gradual onset of breathlessness >3/12.
- Bibasal reticular abnormality on high resolution CT (HRCT).
- Abnormal pulmonary functions restrictive (low VC) and diffusion abnormality low PaO_2 and DLCO.

Treatment: Pirfenidone when forced vital capacity (FVC) 50-80% of predicted in mild to moderate disease. If there is drop in FVC by 10% in 1 yr then stop pirfenidone.

15
Obstructive Sleep Apnea Syndrome

Obstructive sleep apnea syndrome (OSAS) diagnosis requires repetitive apnea/hypopnea >5/hr and symptoms of sleep fragmentation and excessive day time sleepiness.

Mechanism

In sleep there is loss of pharyngeal dilator muscle tone resulting in narrowing of the airway and if combined with retro positioning of lower mandible or narrowing of lateral pharyngeal wall with fat pads.

Suspect in overweight, plethoric patient with excessive day time sleepiness, who snores loudly, has morning headaches, not refreshed by sleep and have nocturnal apnea.

They often have impaired concentration, mood disturbance and increased risk of road traffic accidents and cardiovascular mortality.

Investigation

Full polysomnography [Electroencephalogram (EEG), electromyogram (EMG), oximetry, oral/nasal flow, respiratory effort, snoring] for diagnosis.

Indications for sleep study:
- Symptoms of excessive sleepiness or Epworth sleepiness score >11.
- Recurrent witnessed apnea.
- Nocturnal choking, gasping or dyspnea.
- Headache in the morning.
- Unrefreshing sleep despite adequate sleep time.

- Near miss of events or incidents when driving caused by reduced vigilance.
- Unexplained pulmonary hypertension or polycythemia.

Treatment

- Lose weight and sometime bariatric surgery
- Alcohol reduction, smoking cessation
- Avoid sleeping on the back
- Stop sedatives.

Continuous Positive Air Pressure (CPAP)

In CPAP pressure inside the mask remains positive throughout the respiratory cycle splinting open the collapsible upper airway while the patient self ventilates.

Other causes of excessive day time sleepiness with fragmented night time sleep: Narcolepsy which is usually associated with cataplexy which is sudden loss of muscle tone and collapse, vivid dreams, hypnagogic hallucinations and sleep paralysis with positive family history in response to emotional stimulus.

Treatment: Narcolepsy (modafinil) and cataplexy (clomipramine).

Percutaneous Needle Stick Injury

Precautions, safer needle devices and proper disposal of sharps containers reduce the indices of viral transmission but do not eliminate.

The risk of transmission after a single percutaneous exposure from a positive source is Hep (hepatitis) B (one in 3), hepatitis C (one in 30) and HIV (one in 300).

Rapid HIV test: Usually results are available in a few hours if negative HIV infection not present, but positive test is presumptive evidence of HIV infection and confirmatory tests (enzyme immunoassay) should be performed since false-positive results do occur.

Transmission: Following exposure it takes 48–72 hrs before HIV can be detected in regional lymph nodes and up to 5 days before detection in the blood.

Postexposure prophylaxis (PEP) 28 days of regimen of triple combination therapy Truvada (fixed drug combination of tenofovir disoproxil and emtricitabine) and kaletra for 4 wks ASAP postexposure. Truvada can rarely cause reversible proximal tubulopathy, fanconi syndrome and kaletra causes GI side effects, so anti diarrhea and anti-vomiting drugs are given proactively. If Index case with consent or without when immediately of clinically benefit, is determined to be HIV negative then no treatment is required.

Presenting <72 hrs

A—Index patient HIV positive: First squeeze out and clean the wound with spirit and save serum for testing to exclude pre-existing HIV and in 3 months to detect occupation exposure.

High risk exposure characteristics: Deep injury, hollow bore needle, visible blood on the device, device used for insertion into artery or vein, death of patient within 2 months, high RNA viral count, low CD4 count or the bite resulting in punctured wound or bleeding.

Give PEP triple combination ideally with in 1 hr.

Suture needles or intact skin in contact with contaminated blood; have been much less implicated as source of infection.

If index case has seborrheic dermatitis, symmetrical persistent (>3 months) generalized lymph adenopathy, oral candidiasis, Kaposi sarcoma, needle marks, tattoo, evidence of weight loss, CMV retinitis, genital herpes, molluscum contagiosum on face and multidermatome herpes zoster, consider high risk exposure.

Risk of Infection Transmission

Receptive anal intercourse (3%), receptive vaginal intercourse (0.1%), insertive vaginal or anal intercourse (0.1%), needle stick injury (0.3%), sharing injecting equipment (0.6%), mucous membrane exposure (<0.1%).

HIV sero-prevalence in the community: Homosexual men (10%), injecting drug users (1–2%), heterosexuals-UK (0.11%), Sub Saharan Africa (20–39%), SE Asia (1.8%), Caribbean (1.2–6.1%), Latin America (0.1–2.7%).

If Index patient HIV unknown: If index high risk of HIV infection, test the index case (after permission) for HIV and consider PEP till results available, if positive continue PEP or unable to test index case. If index case low risk do not prescribe PEP.

Presenting >72 hrs: PEP is generally not recommended when presenting >72 hrs.

Malaria

Sporozoites after injection by the bite of anopheles mosquito, develop in the liver for 7 days → merozoites emerge and infect RBC causing signs and symptoms of malaria.

P. vivax and *P. ovale* may cause persistent liver forms (hypnozoites).

Clinical

Severe malaria is common in children, pregnant mothers, and travelers.

Fever, prostration, headache, back pain (flu-like symptoms), vomiting, diarrhea, abdominal pain and cough.

In severe infection sometimes impaired consciousness (coma), respiratory distress, pulmonary edema (tachypnea), seizures, shock (SBP <90 after repletion), abnormal bleeding, anemia, leukopenia, thrombocytopenia, jaundice, acute renal failure and macroscopic hemoglobinuria is associated with severe complications and increased mortality.

Incubation period: 9–14 days.

Common in rural areas than big city.

On investigation they may have severe anemia, hypoglycemia, metabolic acidosis (bicarbonate <15 and pH <7.25), parasitemia >5% and raised ALT, bilirubin with disseminated intravascular coagulation (DIC).

Differential diagnosis: Typhoid, meningitis and gram-negative septicemia should be considered. Antimalarial prophylaxis does not rule out malaria. Prophylaxis is 70–90% effective.

Immediate thick and thin film for diagnosis, three films if 1st is negative.

Treatment

For severe malaria: If patient can swallow, then riamet (each tablet contains artemether 20 mg with lumefantrine 12 mg) 4 tabs twice daily for 3 days or quinine 600 mg tds for 7 days followed by single dose of 3 tabs of fansidar (Sulfadoxine/pyrimethamine) or doxycycline 100 mg daily for 7 days.

If patient cannot swallow, intravenous artesunate 2.4 mg/kg 12 hrly on day 1 and daily for another 2 days (total 4 doses) followed by 1 wk of doxycycline or intravenous quinine 20 mg/kg max 1400 mg over 4 hrs then 10 mg/kg over 4 hrs twice daily. When quinine is being given patient should be on cardiac monitor and BM monitored.

Clindamycin or atovaquone-proguanil or mefloquine are other alternative.

Blood cultures should be done to exclude other bacterial infections.

Atovaquone-proguanil or quinine (3 day course followed by 1 wk of doxycycline or clindamycin) or mefloquine are other options.

For P. vivax, P. ovale and P. malariae: Chloroquine 600 mg stat and after 6 hrs 300 mg and two further doses of 300 mg at 24 and 48 hrs. In *P. vivax* and *P. ovale* chloroquine should be followed by primaquine 15 mg/day/2 wks.

Prophylaxis

Essential for residents living abroad and going on holidays to the SE Asia and tropical areas. It is a major risk if prophylaxis not taken or taken irregularly.

A (awareness), B (bite avoidance), C (compliance with chemoprophylaxis) and D (prompt diagnosis).

Plasmodium falciparum common in sub-Saharan Africa, *P. vivax* in Indian subcontinent, Mexico, central America and China and both species common in SE Asia and south America.

A—peak time for mosquito bite is dust to dawn, during these times using repellents and covering with clothing with long sleeves and pants, full coverage foot wear with socks, impregnated with permethrin and sleeping under impregnated bed nets.

B—*Repellents*: Deet 20-50% gives 6-12 hrs protection, picardine 20%. Lemon eucalyptus oil is effective but needs frequent re-application.

Ineffective malaria preventive practices: Homeopathic, yeast, garlic, marmite vitamin B_1, electronic mosquito repellents, and oil of citronella (effective only for 30–60 minutes).

Prophylaxis Regime

A—Chloroquin resistant areas: Malarone (atovaquone 250 mg—proguanil 100 mg) once daily, can be used in children >11 kg, not used in pregnancy, started 2 days before and finish 7 days after the trip, contraindicated if GFR <30.

Mefloquine (Larium) 250 mg once weekly, can be used in children and pregnancy, started 2 wks before and finished 4 wks after the trip. Contraindicated if recent depression, psychosis, seizure disorder and A-V node conduction abnormality. Side effects include insomnia, night mares, vivid dreams, mood alteration, 1st degree A-V block and prolonged QT interval.

Doxycycline 100 mg once daily. Not used in children or pregnancy, started 2 days before and 4 wks after the trip. Taken after meal with full glass of liquid and remain in upright position for 1/2 hr. Yeast vaginitis is sometimes a side effect in women.

B—Chloroquine sensitive areas: Chloroquine 500 mg once weekly, can be used in children and pregnancy, started 1 wk before and finished 4 wks after the trip. Not to use if psoriasis or psychosis or prolonged QT interval present. Rarely causes retinopathy (>100 gm).

Primaquine 30 mg base once daily can be used in children but not in pregnancy, G6PD testing essential before the 1st dose, must be taken with meal.

C—3,4,5 for chloroquine resistant falciparum malaria.
- Chloroquine alone
- Chloroquine + proguanil
- Atovaquone + proguanil (malarone)
- Doxycycline
- Mefloquine.

Side effects: Headache sleep disorders (neuropsychiatric problems).

Continue taking prophylaxis for 4 wks after returning except atovaquin (1 wk).

Primaquine can be used 2 line after testing for G6PD (glucose-6-phosphate dehydrogenase) deficiency.

Standby prophylaxis: Where risk is low traveller carries antimalarial and takes at the 1st sign of fever.

Pregnant women should avoid travelling to endemic areas. Chloroquine and proguanil are safe, no theoretical risk in atovaquone + proguanil.

Mefloquin avoided in 1st trimester, safe in 2nd and 3rd trimester. Doxycycline avoided. Deet impregnated nets are useful in pregnancy.

Human Immunodeficiency Virus

Thirty million are HIV positive and 3 million have AIDS mostly in women and children in sub-Sahara Africa. Human immunodeficiency virus (HIV) is double stranded RNA retrovirus transmitted by sexual contact including oral, infected blood products, IV drug abuse and perinatally.

It is a retro virus 120 nm in diameter, 1/60th of RBC (single stranded two copies of RNA virus which upon entry to the cell converted to double strand DNA virus by reverse transcriptase and fuses with host cell DNA with integrase), which causes acquired immune deficiency syndrome (AIDS) in which immune system begins to fail and leads to serious life threatening opportunistic infections.

Human immunodeficiency virus (HIV) occurs by transfer of blood, semen, pre-ejaculate, breastmilk and birth process. Virus is present as free as well as in infected cells. Genital epithelium preferentially sequesters virus and spermatozoa carry CCR3 and CCR5 receptors and responsible for carrying virus.

Transmitted by unprotected sexual intercourse when sexual secretions of infected person come in contact with oral, genital or rectal mucus membrane.

Spermicides and diaphragm increase the risk, so not advised while circumcision decreases the risk.

Saliva, tears and urine contain low HIV virus and has not been reported to transmit, so negligible risk of HIV.

Also transmitted by contaminated or sharing needles, tattoos, breastmilk and transfer at pregnancy and birth or cesarean (25% if untreated and 1% if treated with antiretroviral drugs). Screening of blood products has eliminated risk of infection by blood transfusion in developed countries.

Risk of infection 1/10,000 exposures if not using condoms.

Blood transfusion—1/9000, child birth—1/2500, sharing needles—1/67, receptive anal intercourse—1/50, percutaneous needle stick—1/30, receptive penile-vaginal intercourse—1/10, insertive anal intercourse—1/6.5, insertive penile-vaginal intercourse—1/5, receptive fallaltio—1, insertive fallatio—0.5.

About 50-80% of individuals after 2-6 wks of post-exposure develop transient glandular fever like illness, malaise, myalgia, pharyngitis, maculopapular rash, oropharyngeal ulceration and rarely neurological symptoms (meningitis, neuropathy, encephalopathy and myelopathy).

If headache with CNS signs and symptoms of fever, then in the CSF look for following pathogens.

If CD4 count >200—standard pathogens and *Listeria*
- *CD4 count <100*: Toxoplasmosis
- *CD4 count <50*: Cryptococcus, CMV.

Ask them if on antiretroviral drugs (ARV) or taking prophylactic drugs.

Differential Diagnosis

Viral: EB virus, cytomegalovirus (CMV), primary herpes simplex virus, rubella/measles, adeno virus, hepatitis B/C,

Bacterial: Syphilis, streptococcal pharyngitis, brucellosis, disseminated gonococcal infection.

Protozoal: Toxoplasmosis.

Others: Lymphoma, drugs, sarcoidosis and autoimmune diseases.

It is pandemic and WHO thinks AIDS has killed 25 million people since December 1, 1981 and 1/3 in sub-Sahara Africa. HIV infects T helper cells (CD4), macrophages and dendritic cells. Macrophages and microglial cells are infected in CNS, adenoids and tonsils.

Low CD4 is due to direct killing by the virus, increased rate of apoptosis and killing by CD8 cytotoxic lymphocyte. Cell mediated immunity is lost or low when CD4 count is very low and individual is more susceptible to opportunistic infections and eventually develops AIDS. 9 out 10 persons with HIV develop AIDS in 10-15 yrs and die from opportunistic infections or malignancies.

Incubation: About 2—4 wks after exposure and asymptomatic.

Acute infection period lasts 28 days with fever, lymphadenitis, pharyngitis, rash, myalgia, malaise, mouth and esophagus sore, sometimes thrush, weight loss and nausea usually lasting a wk and not all patients get acute symptoms.

Latency usually lasts 2 wks to 20 yrs and patient is asymptomatic but infectious.

AIDS: Symptoms of opportunistic infections, weight loss, recurring respiratory infections, rashes, prostatitis, oral ulcers, *Candida*, shingles, herpes simplex, TB, Kaposi sarcoma, lymphoma, PCP (*Pneumocystis carinii* pneumonia), CMV and *Mycobacterium avium* infections.

HIV Test: HIV is tested by ELISA if positive then retested by ELISA if positive then confirmed by western blot or IFA, if positive is declared HIV positive.

Treatment: Started before the CD4 count fall below 380 and is highly active antiretroviral therapy (HAART) which contains 2 nucleoside reverse transcriptase inhibitor and 1 protease inhibitor). HAART stabilize the patient but it does not cure or alleviate the symptoms. New therapy with trecombinase and recombinase enzyme will cure the disease. Stem cells from patient are treated with these enzymes cured of virus and injected back when cells will seek out the infected cells.

16
Toxicology

Clues to identify cause of unconsciousness after overdose.

Small pin-point pupil, respiratory depression—Morphine overdose—give naloxone.

Dilated pupil with tachycardia—tricyclics overdose.

Deeply unconscious with normal pupils and respiratory depression—benzodiazepines overdose.

Calcium Channel Blockers Overdose

Calcium channel blockers (CCBs) cause severe cardiovascular toxicity with combination of peripheral vasodilatation, myocardial depression and arrhythmias.

Slow release (SR) preparations cause delayed and prolonged toxicity, like diltiazem 500 mg or verapamil 1000 mg.

Case history: A 44 year-old lady admitted 4 hrs after ingestion of 30 × 120 mg verapamil SR, on arrival asymptomatic, HR 88, BP 124/82 mm Hg, RR 12

Initial management—IV access, ECG, U and E, whole bowel irrigation and screen for coingestant. Two hours later she is confused, now her BP 80/40 mm Hg, HR 64, fluid challenge and catheterized. Ten milliliter 10% calcium gluconate intravenous (IV) and repeated over 20–30 min if BP remains low keeping serum calcium 2.8–3.0 mmol/L. Watch IV site to prevent extravasations.

Four hours later after 500 mL of crystalloid and 40 mL of 10% calcium gluconate IV, her BP 64/38 mm Hg, HR 60/min, blood glucose 14 mmol/L and urine output 10 mL/hr.

Myocardium relies on free fatty acid (FFA) for energy supply but during shock glucose is main substrate. CCB decrease insulin release, decrease myocardial glucose uptake, causes shock, decreases insulin release and increase insulin resistance.

Insulin loading dose 1.0 U/kg in 50% dextrose, give 25-50 mL and then 10% dextrose infusion with insulin 0.5 U/kg/hr. Keeps an eye on K checking 1-2 hrly and check blood glucose (BM) every 15 minutes for 1st hr and then every hour. If required insulin can be increased to 1-1.5 U/kg/hr.

Tricyclic Overdose

Present with sedation, coma, seizures, tachycardia, arrthymias, hypotension, dilated pupil, dry mouth and urinary retention.

The ECG shows QRS duration >100 msec, deep S wave in AVL and tall R-wave in AVR.

Treatment

Activated charcoal if <2 hrs.

If seizures treat with benzodiazepines and not with phenytoin.

Opioid (Heroin) Overdose

Symptoms

Drowsiness, coma, pin-point pupils, slowed respiration RR <12.

Treatment

- Check A (airway), B (breathing), C (circulation).
- Respiratory support
- Naloxone 5 mg IV/IM.

Cocaine

Causes euphoria, confidence, talkative, mentally alert, hyper active, restless, reduced appetite. Risk of coronary ischemia greatest in the 1st hr, but may be delayed 4-6 hrs.

Mode of Action

- Blocks reuptake of dopamine and noradrenaline causing euphoria, increases heart rate, constricts the blood vessels causing coronary vasospasm and raises the blood pressure.
- Blocks sodium channels causing numbness of nerves, weakens heart action and local anesthetic.
- Activates platelets causing platelet aggregation.

Crack (Free Base) Cocaine

Crystals (rocks) each 100–200 mg inhaled through pipe after vaporizing in a flame (187C). Produces intense euphoria with in 30 secs and effects lasts 30–60 minutes. There is danger of thermal injury/upper air ways burns.

Emergency Situations

- Myocardial ischemia/infarction (ACS) use troponin for diagnosis.
- Seizures, cerebrovascular accidents.
- Thermal injury from inhalation.
- Pneumothorax, rhabdomyolysis and renal failure.
- Premature labor (abruption).
- Agitated delirium.
- About 84% have abnormal ECG and use troponin for diagnosis of ACS.

Treatment

- Oxygen, diazepam, aspirin (for coronary), nitrates (GTN infusion to control hypertension)
- Do not use beta-blockers or thrombolysins (tPA).

Cocaine Induced Chest Pain

- Oxygen
- Diazepam 5–20 mg IV
- GTN buccal or IV
- Aspirin 300 mg orally
- Diamorphine as indicated
- Do not use beta blockers or thrombolysin (increased risk of intracranial bleeds)
- Second-line—Verapamil, phentolamine, coronary angiography, angioplasty or intracoronary GTN.

Electrocardiogram (ECG)

- *If normal*: Follow local chest pain guideline
- *Abnormal*: ST-T changes usually resolve within 12 hrs. If arrhythmias then treat as usual and avoid beta blockers.
- Infarction-treat as infarct. Thrombolysis contra-indicated <30.

Excited delirium: Shouting, paranoia, agitation, violence, hyperthermia, removing clothes, dilated pupil, unexpected strength then sudden tranquillity and death likely.

Cocaine Dependence

Unable to control doses used, high dose, episodic consumption, increased anxiety, depression, paranoid ideation and weight loss.

Ecstasy (MDMA)

Recently 7 patients died from 3, 4-methylenedioxymethamphetamine (MDMA) toxicity. All had been dancing at clubs, taken 2–5 tablets, presented as collapse or convulsions, hyperpyrexia (40–43°C), tachycardia, hypotension. One died from asystole, six developed DIC, four rhabdomyolysis and acute renal failure.

CLINICAL FEATURES

Mild over dose: Sweating, dry mouth, anxiety, dehydration. Some may have hyponatremia due to drinking water to excess.

Severe features: Hypertonia, hyper-reflexia, hallucinations, hypertension, supraventricular tachycardia (SVT), coma, convulsion, hemorrhagic stroke, hyperpyrexia, rhabdomyolysis, metabolic acidosis, acute renal failure, DIC and multiorgan failure.

Management

- Activated charcoal with iced water should be considered up to 1 hr postingestion.
- Benzodiazepine should be used for agitation, psychosis and it also lowers the BP.
- If BP still high then other antihypertensive should be considered (alpha-blockers, labetalol or vasodilators).

- Hyperpyrexia should be treated as a standard manner (cold sponges) and dantrolene if temperature >40°C
- Prolonged CPR if required due to cardiotoxicity, NaHCO$_3$ for hypotension.
- Hyponatremia should not be treated with fluids, use hypertonic saline or furosemide.
- MDMA: Long-term
- Psychosis, depression, panic attacks, visual changes, memory impairment and late development of depression.

Aspirin

- *Moderate toxicity*: 500–750 mg/L (blood salicylate levels)
- *Severe toxicity*: >750 mg/L.

CLINICAL FEATURES

- Tinnitus, deafness, sweating, pyrexia, hypoglycemia, vomiting, nausea, hematemesis, hyperventilation, hypokalemia, and dehydration.
- In severe cases coma, hyperpyrexia, pulmonary edema and metabolic acidosis.

Treatment

- Activated charcoal,
- Intravenous n saline
- Intravenous sodium bicarbonate 1.26% (keeping urine ph >7.5)
- Repeat ABG and salicylate levels every 2 hrs till salicylate levels are falling and metabolic acidosis improving.
- Supplement glucose if altered mental state. Vitamin K and glucose is used to correct hypoglycemia and hypoprothrombinemia.
- Alert renal team for hemodialysis if altered mental state, pulmonary edema, cerebral edema, clinical deterioration in spite of supportive care and blood level of salicylate >1000 mg/L.
- Levels >1000 mg/L hemodialysis.
- Levels <800 mg/L and ill patient forced alkaline diuresis NaHCO$_3$ 1.26% 500 mL over 2 hrs keeping urine ph >7.5.

Paracetamol

- Metabolism (step 1) paracetamol normally converted to benzoquinoneimine which is normally conjugated with glutathione. Toxicity is more with enzyme inducible drugs.
  Risk factors: Inducible pathway by barbiturates, phenytoin, carbamazepine, rifampicin, St John's wart and ethanol.
- Metabolism (step 2) glutathione dependent affected by starvation, cachexia, eating disorders, alcoholism and HIV.

Clinical features: Nausea and vomiting only 1st 24 hrs.

Treatment

Check FBC, LFT, U and E, INR and paracetamol levels.

- Administration of activated charcoal if patients present within one hour after drug ingestion of >150 mg/kg or 12 gm, will benefit from activated charcoal 50 gm (240 mL) which will bind in the stomach and prevent absorption.
- Before 4 hrs elapsed after ingestion blood levels not interpretable. If significant overdose 12–16 gm start to administer acetylcysteine while waiting for blood levels.
- Between 4 hrs and 8 hrs, depending on the blood levels treat with acetylcysteine IV 150 mg/kg in 200 mL of 5% dextrose over 60 minutes, then 50 mg/kg in 500 mL of 5% dextrose over 4 hrs and 100 mg/kg in 1000 mL of 5% dextrose over 16 hrs or oral methionine 2.5 gm stat and then 2.5 gm 4 hrly for 12 hrs (rarely used), both 100% effective.
- After 8 hrs blind treatment with acetylcysteine started if the patient has ingested paracetamol > 150 mg/kg or 12 gm. Acetylcysteine can be stopped if the level when available is below the threshold of treatment.
- Acetylcysteine is also used in paracetamol overdose irrespective of plasma paracetamol levels in circumstances where overdose is staggered or there is doubt over time of ingestion.
- Beyond 24 hrs acetylcysteine is most effective when given early in preventing liver damage. Effect of acetylcysteine declines after 12 hrs; it is given even after 24 hrs to treat liver failure and not as a paracetamol antidote.

Pseudoallergic reactions are common and should be treated with antihistamine (Chlorpheniramine).

History of previous reactions is not a reason to deny treatment with acetylcysteine.

A small number of patients develop renal damage so creatinine should be checked before discharge.

Prothrombin time (PT) and INR is sensitive indicator of liver damage and should be checked twice daily and acetylcysteine infusion should continue till INR is normal. Reduce conscious level >72 hrs, exclude hypoglycemia and consider hepatic encephalopathy and contact liver unit. All patients should be seen by psychiatrist before discharge.

Refer for liver transplant if INR >1.3, lactate >3.5, creatinine >300 micromol/L, prothrombin time (PT) >100 sec and pH <7.3.

Carbon Monoxide Poisoning

Carbon monoxide (CO) is odorless, colorless, tasteless, nonirritating.

Source: Poorly functioning heating system, improper vented fuel burning device, motor vehicle operating in poor ventilated area.

Symptoms

Confusion, drowsiness, chest pain, potentially fatal, under diagnosed.

Carbon monoxide 240 times potent in combining with Hb as compared to O_2.

SaO_2 normal as capillary probe cannot distinguish between carboxy hemoglobin and oxyhemoglobin.

Treatment

- ECG and pregnancy test should be done if applicable.
- Activated charcoal 1 gm/kg (max 50 gm) oral if presenting with in 4 hrs.

Consider hyperbaric oxygen if patient is:
- Unconscious, CO >25%, metabolic acidosis, ECG changes with chest pain.
- Pregnancy with CO >20%.
- Focal neurological signs.

Carbon monoxide half-life room air: 5 hrs
100% O_2: 1 hr
Hyperbaric O_2: 30 minutes.

Index

A

Abciximab 212
Abdomen, acute surgical 7
Abdominal mass 324
Abdominal pain 268
Acid-base balance 177
Acquired immune deficiency syndrome (AIDS) 376
Acute coronary syndrome 19, 20, 205, 235
    management of 204
Acute kidney injury 119, 240
    causes of 120, 121
Addison's disease 154, 156, 158, 296
Adenoma sebaceum 102
Adenoma, bleeding in 167
Adenosine 226
Adrenal crisis 157
Adrenal failure 154
Adrenal insufficiency, secondary 155
Adult basic life support 10
Adult polycystic kidney disease 124
    treatment 125
Advanced life support (ALS) 11
Advanced renal disease 132
Air pressure, positive 317, 356
Airflow obstruction, measurement of 339
AKI *See* Acute kidney injury
Alanine amino transferase 299
Albumin creatinine ratio 126
Alcohol chronic liver disease 293
Alcohol induced cirrhosis 301
Alcohol withdrawal syndrome 295
Alcoholic hepatitis 293
    signs of 293
    symptoms of 293
    treatment 294

Aldosterone
    high 240
    low 240
Allergic granulomatosis 198
Alport's syndrome 131
Alzheimer's disease 115, 116
Aminophylline 355
Amiodarone 168, 369
Ammonia 280
Amoxicillin 5, 346
    in children 74
Amyloid precursor protein 107, 116
Anaphylaxis, acute 3
Anemia 129, 327, 332
    causes 129
    microcytic 192
    normocytic normochromic 332
    of chronic disease 332
Angiofibroma 102
Animal bite 9
Ankle jerks 93
Anovulation 175
Antibiotics 5, 135, 365
Anticoagulation, reversal of 262
Antidiuretic hormone 50
Antithrombotics 220
Anti-thyroid drugs 165
Aortic dissection 206, 240
    acute 242
        management 243
Aortic regurgitation 250
    causes 250
Aortic stenosis 247
    causes of 248
Aortic valves 254
Aphasia 42
Aphthous ulcers 323
Apomorphine 113
Apraxic gait 107
    causes 107

Arrhythmic death syndrome 229
Arrhythmogenic right ventricular cardiomyopathy 231
  treatment 231
Arterial blood gases 177
Arthritis 181
  acute 181, 192
Ascites 305
Aspartate amino transferase 284
Aspergillus fumigatus 341
Aspirate synovial fluid 186
Aspiration pneumonia 347
Aspirin 32, 36, 211, 383
Asthma
  acute 335
    severe 337
  allergic 338
  by age 338
  exacerbation-prone 338
  life-threatening 337
  occupational 338
  symptoms to 337
Ataxia to MS 101
Ataxia to tabes dorsalis 101
Atlanto axial subluxation 192
Atrial fibrillation 218, 222
  ablation therapy 218
Atrial flutter 224
Atrial septal defect 245
Autoimmune hepatitis 299
Autoimmune thyroid disease 160
Autosomal dominant 171
AV node re-entry tachycardia 226
Axonal neuropathy 88

B

B cell targeted therapy 195
Back, acute pain in 326
Barter's syndrome 144
Basal pneumonia 268
Basilar artery thrombosis 38
Basilar migraine 69
Behçet's syndrome 41, 314
Benzbromarone 185

Benzodiazepine 82
Beriberi 255
Beta amyloid 116
Biliary sepsis 7
Bleomycin 369
Blood 326
  glucose 135, 138
  pH 135
  transfusion 333, 377
Bloody diarrhea 313, 324
  noninfectious causes of 314
Bradyarrhythmia 12
Bradycardia 233
Bradykinesia 109
  of foot 109
Brainstem 96
Brisk knee jerks 100
Bronchiectasis 364
Bronchodilator 355
Bronchopulmonary aspergillosis, allergic 341
Bronchus, carcinoma of 368
Brown-Sequard syndrome 75
Brugada syndrome 224, 231
  treatment 231
Budd-Chiari syndrome 280, 300
  causes 300
  treatment 300
Busulfan 369

C

Calcium channel blockers 35
  overdose 379
Calcium gluconate 123, 379
Calcium pyrophosphate 186
  dihydrate 185
Campylobacter 188, 318
Campylobacter enteritis 317
Campylobacter jejuni 317
CAP, treatment of 345
Carbamazepine 300
Carbon dioxide, pressure of 177
Carbon monoxide
  poisoning 385
  symptoms 385
  treatment 385

Cardiac arrest, prevention of 1
Cardiac arrhythmia 15
Cardiac defibrillator, implantable 237
Cardiac patient 266
Cardiac resynchronization therapy 205, 237
Cardiovascular system 50
Cardioverter defibrillator 213 therapy 205
Carotid arterectomy 35
Carotid arterial dissection 38
Carpal tunnel syndrome 88
Catechol-o-methyl transferase inhibitors 114
Cauda equina syndrome 94
Cefotaxime 275
Cefuroxime 5
Celiac disease 320
Cellular infiltrate 324
Cellulitis 8
Central nervous system 157
Cephotaxime 74
Cerebellar ataxia 105
   causes 105
Cerebellar stroke 18
Cerebellopontine angle syndrome 83
Cerebellum 96
Cerebral artery
   anterior 23
   posterior 23
Cerebral salt wasting syndrome 152
Cerebral vasoconstriction syndrome 59
Cerebrospinal fluid 41
Cervical cord 95
Cervical myelopathy 92
Charcot foot and osteomyelitis, distinguish between 141
Charcot's joints 100
Charcot-Marie-Tooth disease 87, 92
Chest pain 327
Chest syndrome, acute 327
   in HBSS 327
Chlamydia 188
   infections 27

Chlordiazepoxide 294
Chloroquine sensitive areas 375
Chloroquine resistant areas 375
Chlorpheniramine 385
Cholangitis, ascending 308
Cholestatic hepatitis 300
Cholesterol emboli 121
Chronic kidney disease 126
Churg-Strauss syndrome 90, 198
Ciprofloxacin 5, 6, 141
Cirrhosis, severity of 277
Cirrhotic liver disease 349
Clarithromycin 5
Clindamycin 141
Clopidogrel 211
Clostridium difficile 313, 318
   colitis 314, 315
CNS disease, acute 64
Co-amoxiclav 5
Cocaine 380, 381
   dependence 382
   induced chest pain 381
Cold 167
Colitis, acute severe 319
   treatment 319
Coma 43
Community-acquired pneumonia 342
Congestive cardiac failure 82
Coning and tentorial herniation 56
Coning causes 56
Coning management 56
Conus syndrome 77
Cord compression 98
Cortical basal degeneration (CBD) 111
Cough 327
Coxiella burnetii 342
C-reactive protein 344
Crohn's disease 100, 317, 321, 322
   cause 321
   complications 322
   management of 323
Crossed syndrome 22

Cullen sign 309
Cushing disease 173, 174
Cushing's syndrome 144, 173, 242
Cyclosporine 182, 183, 185
  or cyclophosphamide 191
Cytomegalovirus 75

D

de Quervain's disease 166
Deep vein thrombosis 257
Delirium 79
Delirium tremens 82, 295
Demyelinating neuropathy 88
Dextran 307
Dextrocardia 255
Diabetes mellitus
  noninsulin dependent 144
  type 2 150
    ketosis prone 135
    new drugs in 146
Diabetic amyotrophy 88
Diabetic control 216
  on oral hypoglycemic
    drugs or insulin 148
Diabetic foot 8, 141
Diabetic ketoacidosis 135, 268
Diabetic management 148
Diabetic neuropathic pain 142
Diabetic neuropathy 141
Dialysis 123
Diarrhea, acute 313
Diet pills 242
Digoxin toxicity 238
  treatment 238
Dilated cardiomyopathy 255
Discitis 8
Disseminated intravascular
  coagulation 3
Dix-hall pike test 17, 85
Dopamine 2
  agonist 113
  dysregulation 113
Doxycycline 5, 74, 375
DPP4 inhibitors 150
Dry eyes 191
Dry mouth 191
DVT prophylaxis 135
DVT, upper limb 263

Dysarthria 22
Dysdiadochokinesia 105
Dysphagia 22,

E

Ear, pain radiating to 167
Eaton-Lambert syndrome 179
Ecstasy 382
Electrophysiologist, referral
  to 224
Empyema 347, 350
Endocarditis 8
Endocrine hypertension 239
Endoscopy risk score 274
ENT and bronchoscopy 247
Entameba histolytica 313
  enteroinvasive 313
  enterotoxic 313
Enzyme immunoassay 371
Eosinophilic esophagitis 275
Epilepsy 62, 64
  causes 64
  drugs used in 67
Epileptic seizure, first 62
Episcleritis 191
EPO, side effects of 130
Epstein-Barr virus 75
Eptifibatide 212
Erythema nodosum 323
Essential tremor 110
Ethambutol 183
Extensor plantars 93

F

Faints 17
Falciparum 72
Fascicular tachycardia 229
Fatty liver 292
Fever 27
Fits 16
Flexor digitorum profundus 90
Flucloxacillin 5
Focal muscle damage 132
Foot drop 92, 106
  causes 106
Fresh frozen plasma 221
Friedreich's ataxia 94, 101, 105

Frontotemporal dementia 118
Full blood count 331
Fulminant hepatic failure 279, 301

G

Gait disturbances 105
Galactorrhea 172
Gamma glutamyl transpeptidase 281
Gastrointestinal bleeding 278
    acute upper 269
Gastrointestinal loss 144
GBS *See* Guillain-Barré syndrome 77
Genetic prothrombotic conditions 41
Gentamycin 5, 6
Giant-cell arteritis 71
Glasgow alcoholic hepatitis score 295
Glasgow coma score 48
Glomerular filtration rate 119
Glomerulonephritis 121
Glucocorticoid insufficiency 170
Glutamic acid decarboxylase 136
Glycoprotein IIB/IIIA receptor inhibitors 211
Goiter 165
Gout 181
    treatment of 183
Graves' disease 166
Guillain-Barré syndrome (GBS) 75, 87, 145, 179, 317, 335
    management of 77

H

Haemophilus influenzae 365
Hand-foot syndrome 326
Hartmann's solution 31
Hashimoto's disease 166
HBV infection, stages of 287
Headache 68
    analgesic 69
    cluster 70
    retro-orbital 172
    tension 70
        treatment 70
    thunderclap, causes of 71
Heart 192
Heart block
    first degree 233
    second degree 234
Heart failure 199
    mild 235
    moderate 235
Heart, embolism from 39
Helicobacter pylori 27
Hematoma
    extradural 27
    subdural 27
Hemianopia 39
Hemiparesis 42
Hemiplegic gait 106
Hemiplegic migraine 69
Hemochromatosis 297
Hemodialysis, complications of 131
Hemofiltration 123
Hemorrhage 280
Henoch-Schönlein purpura 121
Heparin 262
Hepatic encephalopathy 270, 279, 282
Hepatic failure, chronic 302
Hepatic vein obstruction 300
Hepatitis
Hyperventilation 43
Hepatocellular carcinoma 277
Hepatorenal syndrome 283, 306
    treatment 284
Hereditary spinocerebellar degeneration 101
Heyde's syndrome 274
Hirsutism 175
HIV sero-prevalence in community 372
HIV test 371
Horner's syndrome 83, 99, 104, 368
Human bite 9
Human immunodeficiency virus (HIV) 376

Hydrocephalus, acute 59
Hypercalcemia 158
    causes 158
    signs 159
    symptoms 159
    treatment 159
Hyperglycemic hyperosmolar syndrome 135
Hyperkalemia 1, 133
Hyperosmolar hyperglycemic syndrome (HHS) 140
Hyperphosphatemia 123
Hypertension with hypokalemia 144
Hypertensive emergencies 238
    causes 238
Hyperthyroidism 160
Hypertrophic cardiomyopathy 12, 15, 230, 256
    treatment 230
Hyperuricemia 182
Hypocalcemia 1, 157
    causes 157
    treatment 158
Hypoglycemia 46, 146
    etiology 146
    management 147
    mild 147
    symptoms 146
Hypokalemia 1, 144, 216
    alkalosis 144
    causes 144
    symptoms 145
    treatment 146
Hyponatremia 151
    management 151
    symptoms 151
Hypopituitarism 176
    causes of 176
Hypotension 1, 304
Hypothermia 47
    causes 47, 48
    complications 49
    investigations 48
    management 50
Hypothyroidism 169
    causes 169
Hypovolemia 1, 215
Hypoxemia 304
Hypoxia 1
Hypoxic respiratory failure 356

I

Infarction 172
Inflammatory bowel disease 41, 317
Inflammatory polyneuritis, acute 75
Insulin 135, 138, 380
    fixed dose 138
    varying dose 138
Interstitial nephritis, acute 121
Interstitial pneumonia 369
Intra-articular corticosteroid 187
Intracerebral hemorrhage 35
Intracranial hypertension
    benign 70
    idiopathic 19
Iron-deficiency 129
    anemia 332
Irritable bowel syndrome 268
Ischemic heart disease 26, 36
Ischemic stroke 32

J

Jugular venous pressure 247, 368

K

Kallmann syndrome 176
Ketones
    in blood 135
    in urine 135
Korsakoff's psychosis 304
Kyphoscoliosis 99

L

Lambert-Eaton myasthenic syndrome 78
Larium 375
Levetiracetam 67
Levofloxacin 5
Lewy body 107
    dementia 112

Lhermitte's phenomenon 98
Liddle's disease 144
Limbs, acute pain in 326
Liver disease
   acute 301
   chronic 301, 302
      signs of 280, 281
Liver failure
   acute 279
      cause of 282
   chronic 279
   complications in 304
Liver transplant 301, 302
Lobectomy 368
   signs of 369
Long QT syndrome 231
   causes 231
Lugol's iodine 165
Lumbar puncture 41
Lung carcinoma 364
Lung disease 359
Lung volume reduction surgery 358
Lymphatic leukemia, chronic 329

M

Malabsorption, signs of 324
Malaria 72, 373
   treatment 72
Mallory-Weiss tear 271
MAO-B inhibitors 114
Marfans syndrome 242, 359
Median medullary syndrome 105
Median nerve palsy 88
Mefloquine 375
Meniere's disease 85
Meningitis 7, 28, 51
Menopause 181
Menstrual disturbances 175
Mesothelioma 351
Metabolic acidosis 136
   causes of 179
Metabolic alkalosis, causes of 179
Metabolic disturbance 64
Metalloproteinases-3 188
Metatarsal phalangeal joint 181
Methotrexate, treatment with 194
Methylenedioxy-methamphetamine toxicity 382
Migraine 68
   prophylaxis 69
   treatment 69
Miller-Fisher syndrome 88
Mineral and bone disorder 130
Mitral regurgitation
   causes 251
   symptoms 251
Mitral stenosis 253
Mono sodium urate crystals 181, 182
Motor neuron disease 94, 98, 335
Motor response 45
Mucolytics 366
Mucopolysaccharides 170
Multiendocrine neoplasia 171
Multinodular goiter 165
Multisystem atrophy 111
Murmurs, intensity of 254
Muscle damage 132
Muscle specific kinase 77
Myasthenia gravis 77, 335
Mycobacterium avium 378
Myeloid leukemia, chronic 328, 329
Myocardial infarction 268
Myocardial perfusion scan 213
Myopathic waddling gait 106, 107
   causes 107
Myxedema 89

N

Nasal decongestants 242
Nausea 132
Necrotizing small vessel vasculitis 199
Needle aspiration 167, 360
Nephrotic syndrome 119, 125
   causes 125
Nephrotoxic drugs 119
Nervous system 199
Neuritic plaques 117

Neurofibromatosis type 1 102
Neuroleptic malignant like syndrome 115
Neurological deterioration or complications 61
Neurological emergencies 20
Neuropathic osteoarthropathy 141
Neuropathic pain 132
Neuropathy 142
Neutropenic sepsis 7
Niacin 183
Nitrofurantoin 369
Nonalcoholic fatty liver disease 291
Nonalcoholic steatohepatitis 291
Nonepileptic attack disorder 65
Noninvasive ventilation (NIV) 351
Nonischemic mitral regurgitation 252
Nonlocalized sepsis 7
Nonmetastatic complications 368
Nonsteroidal anti-inflammatory drugs 3, 77, 119
Non-thyroid illness 170
Non-tissue hypoxia 179
Nontoxic goiter 166
Nontyphoid salmonellas 317
treatment 317
Non-VTA, reversal of 221
Norepinephrine 2
Nutrition 165

O

Obesity and hypoventilation syndrome 356
Oliguria 119
Ophthalmoplegia nystagmus 282
Opioid (Heroin) overdose 380
Optic neuritis 95
Orbital cellulitis 9
Organ transplant 182
Orthostatic hypotension 15
Orthostatic syncope 16
Osmolality 135
Osteoarthritis 188
flare-up of 188
treatment 189
Oxygen saturation 327
Oxygen therapy, long-term 351
Oxygenation failure 335

P

Pacemaker 233
treatment 233
Paget's disease 158
Pancreatitis
acute 308
chronic 311
Pansystolic murmur of TR 252
Panton-valentine leukocidin 345
Paracetamol 384
Paraganglioma 171
Parapneumonic effusion 350
Parkinson's disease 15, 47, 107, 112, 114
drug induced 110
treatment for 112
Parkinsonian gait 106
Parkinsonism plus 111
Paroxysmal atrial fibrillation 218
Partial dysautonomic 16
Partial pressure of oxygen 178
Patent foramen ovale 28
Penicillin G 5
Penoxybenzamine 172
Perianal disease 324
Periarticular inflammation 181
Pericarditis 215
Peripheral neuropathy 86
Peritoneal dialysis 131
complications 131
Peritonitis 7
Peroneal nerve palsy 92
Petrosal sinus sampling 174
pH effusions, low 349
Phenytoin 66, 300
Pheochromocytoma 171, 240, 242

Philadelphia chromosome 328
Photophobia, neck stiffness 52
Pituitary apoplexy 172
Pituitary disease 173
Pituitary or thyroid releasing hormone 169
Plasmodium 72
    falciparum 72, 374
Pleural effusion
    and empyema 348
    drug induced 349
Pneumocystis carinii pneumonia 378
Pneumocystis jirovecii 366
Pneumocystis pneumonia 366
    symptoms 366
    treatment 366
Pneumonectomy 368
Pneumothorax 359
    secondary 359
Polyarteritis nodosa 199
Polycystic ovarian syndrome 175
    treatment 175
Polycythemia 27
    rubra vera 330
Polymyalgia rheumatic 196
Polyuria, causes of 177
Portal hypertension, management of 277
Postcardiac arrest, treatment 12
Postendoscopic management 274
Postpartum thyroiditis 160
Postural orthostatic tachycardia syndrome 15
Potassium 135
Pregnancy with stroke 36
Presenaline gene 116
Presyncope symptoms 13
Primary adrenal failure 154
    causes 155
    management 156
    signs of 155
    symptoms of 155
Primary biliary cirrhosis 282, 296, 301
    treatment 296
Priorities 60
Probenecid 184
Prostatitis 8
Prosthetic mitral 254
Prosthetic valve endocarditis 246
Pseudoallergic reactions 385
Pseudogout 185
    treatment of 186
Pseudomonas infections 2
Ptosis 84
Pulmonary artery pressure 264
Pulmonary disease 351
    chronic obstructive 6, 364, 369
Pulmonary edema 373
Pulmonary embolism 257
    in pregnancy 257
Pulmonary fibrosis, idiopathic 369
Pulmonary hypertension 15, 264
    idiopathic 264
Purines 181
Pyogenic meningitis 53
Pyrazinamide 183

R

Radial nerve palsy 91
Raynaud's disease 296
Reactive arthritis 188
    treatment 188
Rebleeding after endoscopy 273
Receptive anal intercourse 372
Rectosigmoid disease 318
Refractory ascites 307
Renal artery
    stenosis 242
        presentation 127
Renal disease 185
    itching 132
    pain 132
Renal failure 304
    acute 119, 199
    chronic 126
Renal hypo perfusion 119

Renal parenchyma disease 242
Renal transplant 131
Renal tubular acidosis 121
Renal unit, referral to 127
Renin
  high 240
  low 240
Renovascular disease 127, 238
Resistant hypertension 238, 241
Respiratory acidosis 179
Respiratory alkalosis, causes of 179
Respiratory depression 379
Respiratory distress 373
Respiratory failure 335
  type 1 352
  type 2 352
Respiratory infections in childhood 364
Respiratory rate 1, 46
Resuscitation 10
Rhabdomyolysis 132
Rheumatic heart disease 248, 251, 253
  symptoms 248
Rheumatoid arthritis 189, 296
  management of 192
Rheumatoid nodules 191
Rifampicin 300
Right ventricular failure 215
Right ventricular infarction 215
Rituximab 195
RNA flavivirus 289
Rota virus 313
RVOT tachycardia 229

S

Salmonella 188, 313
Scleritis 191
Scleromalacia 191
Sclerosis, multiple 95
Seldinger technique 362
Selenium deficiency 255
Sensory ataxia 106
  causes 106
Septic arthritis 8, 186
  in prosthetic joint 8
  treatment of 187
Septic shock 2
Shigella 188, 313, 318
Shock, cardiogenic 216
Short Synacthen test 156
Sick euthyroid syndrome 168
Sickle cell
  crisis 326
  disease 326
Sickle hemoglobin 326
Sinus thrombosis 41
Sjögren's syndrome 191, 198, 296, 369
Skin infection 187
Sleep apnea 175
  obstructive 242, 370
Small bowel enema 323
Small pin-point pupil 379
Solitary nodule 166
Spastic paraparesis 74
Spastic paraplegia 105
Spinal artery thrombosis
  anterior 43, 73
  treatment 74
Spinal cord
  compression 73
  hemisection of 75
Spinal injury, acute 76
Spinal stenosis 95
Spinocerebellar degeneration 94
Spontaneous bacterial peritonitis (SBP) 7, 294
Sporadic tumors 171
Spurious hypocalcemia 157
Stable angina 210
Staphylococcus 364
Staphylococcus aureus 187, 246
  community-acquired methicillin-resistant 345
  hospital-acquired methicillin-resistant 345
  Methicillin-resistant 345, 365
Status epilepticus 62, 64
Status migraines 69
Stem cells 378

Sterile pyuria 122
Streptococcus bovis 246
Streptococcus pneumoniae 54, 187, 328
Stress 68
   testing 212
Stroke 21, 28
   acute 20
      management of 31
      causes of 39
      mimics 27
Strongyloides stercoralis 333
Sub-acute combine degeneration 86, 100
Subarachnoid hemorrhage 28, 57, 60
Subdural hematoma 40
   chronic 39
   or tumor 27
Sudden cardiac death 229
Sulfinpyrazone 184
Superior vena cava syndrome 264
Supranuclear palsy 111
Supraventricular tachycardia 224, 382
Sympathetic neurones C8/T1 99
Syncope 14, 65
Syndrome of inappropriate antidiuretic hormone secretion (SIADH)
   causes 153
   chest disorders 153
   drugs 153
   malignant diseases 153
   neurological disorders 153
   treatment 154
Syringomyelia 91, 99, 100
Systemic diseases 41
Systemic inflammatory response syndrome 2
Systolic hypertension 127

T

T cell targeted therapy 195
T1 nerve roots, compression 99
Tabes dorsalis 106
Taboparesis 94, 101
Tachyarrhythmia 217
Tachycardia, broad complex 227
Tachypnea 327, 373
Tazobactam 141
Tazocin 5
Temporal arteritis 71, 196, 197
Temporal artery biopsy 71
Tension pneumothorax 360
   management 361
   signs 360
Thiazides 183
Thiopurine methyl transferase 319, 325
Third degree atrioventricular block 234
Thoracic endometriosis 359
Thoracotomy scar 369
Thrombocythemia 27
Thrombolysis 22, 33
Thrombolytic therapy 208
Thrombolytics 207
Thrombosis of cerebral veins and sinuses 40
Thymectomy 79
Thyroid 167
   acropachy 162
   adenoma 166
   disease 296
   functions in pregnancy 168
   hormone 168
Thyroiditis 167
Thyrotoxic crisis 164
Thyrotoxicosis 160
   crisis treatment 164
   signs of 164
Thyroxin abuse 167
Tirofiban 212
Tissue hypoxia 179
Tissue inhibitor of metalloproteinases 188
Tissue plasminogen activator (TPA) 33, 207
Torsades-de-pointes tachycardia 232
   causes 232
   management 232

Toxic adenoma 167
Toxic megacolon 321
  treatment 321
Toxic multinodular goiter 165
Toxicology 379
Toxins 4
Transient ischemic attack 35
Transvenous temporary pacing 234
Tricyclic overdose 380
Trimethoprim 6
Troponins 203
Tuberous sclerosis 102
Tumor necrosis factor 120
Tyrosine kinase inhibitor 329

U

Ulcerative colitis 317
Ulnar nerve palsy 90
Unfractioned heparin 211
Unstable angina 210
Upper motor neuron signs 111
Urate nephropathy, chronic 183
Uric acid stones 185
Uricemia 183
Uricosuric drugs 184, 185
Urinary catheterization 32
Urinary retention 73
Urinary tract infection 6

V

Vancomycin 5, 246, 316
Variceal bleeding 275
Vascular dementia 117
Vascular disorders 82
Vascular parkinsonism 110
Vasculitis 198
  causes of 198
Vasovagal syncope 15
Vena caval filter, placement of 263
Venous thromboembolism 32
Ventilation, noninvasive 335
Ventricular hypertrophy 230
Vertigo 17, 84
  benign paroxysmal positional 17, 85
Vestibular failure, bilateral 18
Vestibular neuronitis 18, 85
Vestibular ocular reflex 17
Viral encephalitis 55
  treatment 56
Viral hepatitis 284
  A 284
    virus 284
  B 281, 285, 371
    infection 287
    virus, testing for 285
  C virus 281, 289, 290
  chronic active 282
  E 284
Viral thyroiditis 166
Vitamin
  B deficiency 87
  B_1 375
  B_{12} 87
Vivax 72
von Recklinghausen's disease 102
von Willebrand disease 274

W

Wallenberg's syndrome 104
Warfarin 36
Wernicke's encephalopathy 115, 304
Wilson's disease 297
Wolff-Parkinson-White Syndrome 219

Y

Yersinia 188